Here There be Soul-Eaters
Sacred Journeys of Nurse Healers

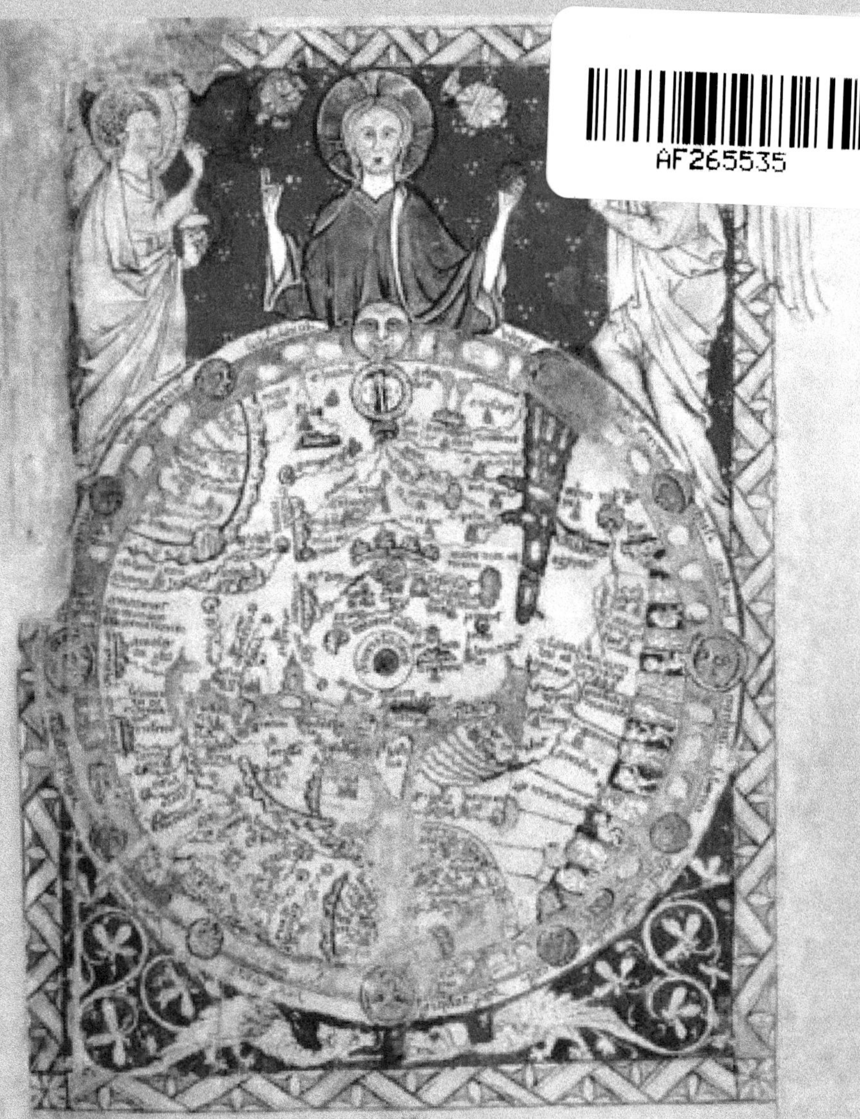

Dr Martin Hemsley, PhD

Here There be Soul-Eaters
Sacred Journeys of Nurse Healers

Dr Martin Hemsley, PhD

Dr Hemsley presents the stories of eleven nurse healers, on their journeys of inner and outer transformation. Achingly honest, always challenging and often heart-breaking, these accounts chart the healer's path beyond the edge of ordinary reality and back. Often associated with shamanism, these stories, viewed through the lens of Process Work, offer new vistas on the path of heart and healing. This is a book not only for nurses and therapists, but for all of us seeking to live and work more consciously and with deep integrity.

Eldership Academy Press is a platform for elders of any age from all walks of life. Elders in our view are lifestyle artists for personal aliveness, relationships and community building. Eldership Academy Press strives to provide our culture with guides for living meaningful, compassionate lives, in our publications, research and creative media.

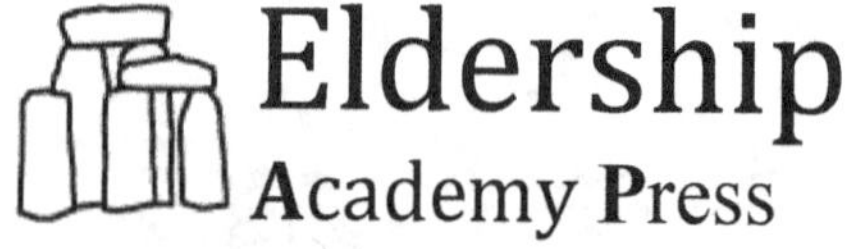

Eldership
Academy Press

Eldership Academy Press

ISBN-13: 978-0-6486824- 0-0

Designed in San Francisco, California
Printed in Australia

Table of Contents

Section One—Beginnings 1

Section Two—Stories of Nurse Healers 30

Section Three—Transmutation   223

Contents

Figures and Illustrations

Contents

Disclaimer All reasonable efforts have been made to source, acknowledge and compensate the original creators of images in this book for permission to reproduce.

Contents

Dedication

To Emerald, who arrived in the nick of time

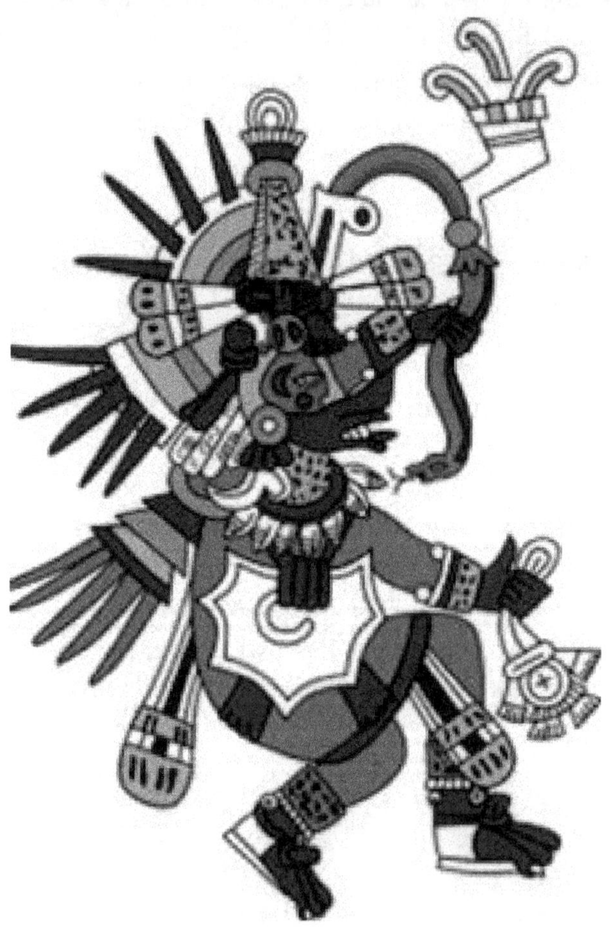

Acknowledgements

First of all, I must acknowledge the eleven nurse healers who co-created this work with me. Meeting these eleven nurse healers and entering so deeply into their worlds was an immense privilege, and this has replayed for me throughout the writing of this book. To them, for the generosity of their stories, I am always indebted.

Thanks to my supervisor, Doctor Gerald Maclaurin, for encouraging the writing of this as my thesis towards the Diploma of Process Oriented Psychology. He prompted me to be more myself in this writing, and has imparted the dreaming of his Jungian soul and love of the poetic. This book owes much to his friendliness, his love and wisdom. In the background of the writing of this have been the other members of my study committee in the Australian and New Zealand Process Oriented Psychology faculty, Dr. Jane Martin and Andrew Lindsay, along with my training therapist, Dr. Susan Hatch, cheering me on and sending me their love. It was Andrew who first suggested I turn my PhD thesis into a book as the thesis for my studies towards the Diploma.

Thanks also must go to Professor Nel Glass, who at the beginning of this millennium supervised the PhD upon which this book is based. Her love and deep engagement with me and the work was of incredible value.

To my editor, Shelley Kenigsberg, many thanks are owed for the sensitive and inquisitive way she has edited the transcripts of my interviews with the nurse healers who participated in the original research, so that they can be read as autobiographical stories. I have very much enjoyed and prospered from how she has walked the paths of this book with me.

Big thank you to Edan Chapman for his elegant and insightful artwork throughout.

To my wife Susan, many thanks also for your forbearance and love, and for being a great support in the times I struggled in writing this. And, of course, thanks to my lovely children Rebecca and Sebastian, a big part of whose childhoods were spent with a Dad so preoccupied with this work.

Preface

This, Jim, is what I see as the unknown terrain that psychotherapy must either explore or become meaningless. This is the white space on the map, Jim, where the ancient navigators wrote, "Here There Be Soul-Eaters" [1]

Around 1994, I underwent a time of great inner turmoil and upheaval which culminated in a period of wild and intense spiritual experiences. During this foment, I found myself to be, for a time, a healer. My life was completely changed in ways I could not have imagined or even wished for. Out of this period came a desire to explore this kind of experience, and the experiences of nurse healers especially, as I was, and still am, a nurse. Hence, in the early 2000s, I embarked on the exploration of the mysterious inner and outer lives of healers, specifically nurse healers. I wanted to contribute to my profession by increasing the knowledge understanding of nurse healers.

In this research, prompted by my own journey, I was particularly interested in the experience of coming to be a healer, and living as a healer. What transformations in a person's inner and outer worlds would lead to being a healer? How does the journey to become a healer change one's inner and outer lives? I wanted to know what is distinctive about the terrain these people traverse, know about their extraordinary experiences? It is evident that being a healer is not something we all identify in ourselves. Is this a talent, something learned or is something else going on in these people? This research — my PhD — forms the basis of this book you are now reading.

Early on in this research there were strong indications that what I was investigating was intimately related to shamanism, the ancient spirituality of the natural world and the spirits, that has dwelt within cultures all over the world. I had a lot of thoughts about this myself, as I had gone through shattering personal experiences leading to being able to channel healing for others in certain ways, being cast into the awesome, thrilling and bewildering world of what might be called shamanic experience. Thus, it was of deep personal interest to learn more about this, about other people who had these kinds of experiences, and to share it with others. I was also very drawn to make connection with other nurse healers.

The research I conducted on this was presented in a thesis, *Walking Two Worlds,* through the Nursing School at Southern Cross University in 2003 for my PhD.[2] It explores the extraordinary and transformational journeys of nurse healers. I also published two papers from the thesis.[3,4]

Unlike the thesis, written at an earlier time in my life, this book is directed towards Process Oriented Psychology (POP, or Process Work). This book stands as my thesis, part of my studies towards the Diploma in Process Work, through the Australia and New Zealand Process Oriented Psychology (ANZPOP) school. Accordingly, I have in the following pages highlighted Process Work's relevance to this area of practice and study, how in turn this research can fruitfully inform Process Work and psychotherapy. Thus, beyond being a conversion of my PhD thesis into a book, this work reflects how I am now influenced by Process Work, and also seeks to speak to Process Work and how it relates to the fundamental experience of being a healer and shaman.

I found Process Work towards the end of writing the PhD thesis; seeing a Process Worker for therapy helped me get through it. Becoming a Process Worker myself has been largely about bringing the shamanic part of myself into relationship with the everyday part, to find some friendliness between these wild and gnarly branches of my life myth.[5] I sense the writing of this book is in some ways a completion of this personally, as well as the completion of my studies for the Process Work Diploma.

From his early writings, Arny Mindell, the founder of Process Work, has been influenced by shamanism, and there are many indications that he functions as a shaman. He certainly writes with great respect of his experiences with Australian Aboriginal and African shamans, whose perspectives on the world have come to influence how Process Work is practiced, and how the world is viewed through the process-oriented lens.

Carlos Castaneda's accounts of his training with the shamanic "Man of knowledge" Don Juan also significantly inform the thinking and practices of Process Workers. Arny wrote his mesmerising book *The Shaman's Body* from his PhD studies which investigated and integrated Castaneda's insights into psychotherapy and personal development.[6]

The wonderful capacity of Process Workers to work therapeutically with others experiencing powerful altered and extreme states of consciousness is, in no small part, due to the integration of skills and "metaskills" based in Castaneda's revelations.

As a research report, *Walking Two Worlds* was preoccupied with locating the research within nursing's theoretical and research scholarship traditions. In writing this book, however, I wanted to showcase the stories of the nurse healers who participated in this research, and thus promote their insights to the broader world of healing, therapy, shamanising and personal development. My desire is to give the reader the full benefit of these resonant and beguiling accounts of a little-illuminated area of human experience. Here in this work, I am not focused on academic concerns unique to nursing, nor detailing of methodology or method. Anyone interested in these can easily find my doctoral thesis online.[2]

With the encouragement of my supervisor, Gerald Maclaurin, I have brought myself quite prominently into this work, which is another significant departure from the PhD thesis upon which it is based. In this, I hope the personal account makes the work more accessible to the reader.

In the following chapters, I have kept the original understandings that the co-creators of that work applied to their experiences. My interpretations are mostly unchanged from the original work although, of necessity, have shifted as I have evolved over the years. Yet, I feel that these phenomenologically rich stories emerging from the human spiritual adventure of healing and shamanism are still fresh and vital.

One of the nurse healers who participated with me in this research (pseudonym, Chris[7]) lamented — in her uniquely left-field way — that nursing texts are not sacred texts. In some ways this book may be one of those, not in the sense of being divinely inspired but in that it gives voice to those nurses — those who work from the very core of their beings to bring the sacred to their practice, describing their joys, struggles, fears, insights and moments of empowerment and healing along the way.

This book is about nurse healers but I believe it also has a lot to say about, and to, healers, shamans, therapists and spiritual adventurers from all walks of life. I hope you agree that accounts in this book have some fresh things to say to Process Workers and nurses, and others curious about the lesser-known and numinous corners of human experience.

Section One

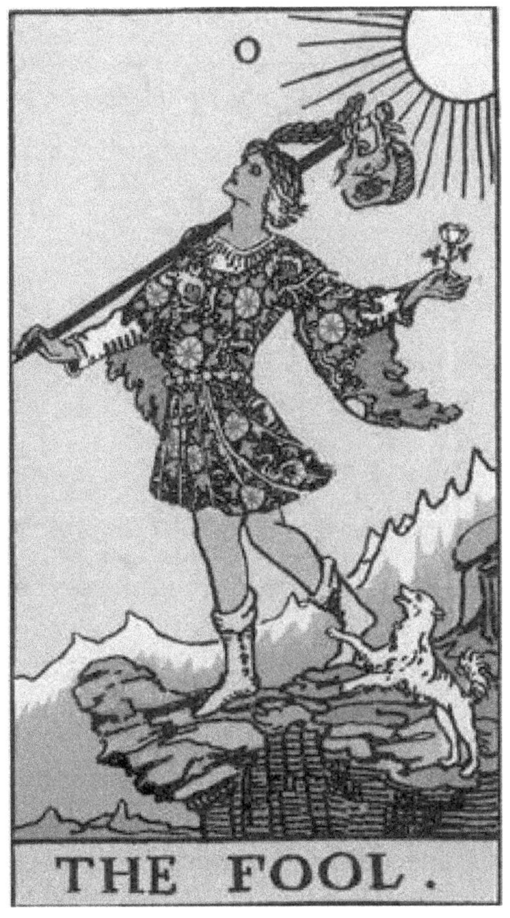

Beginnings

Chapter One

OPENING

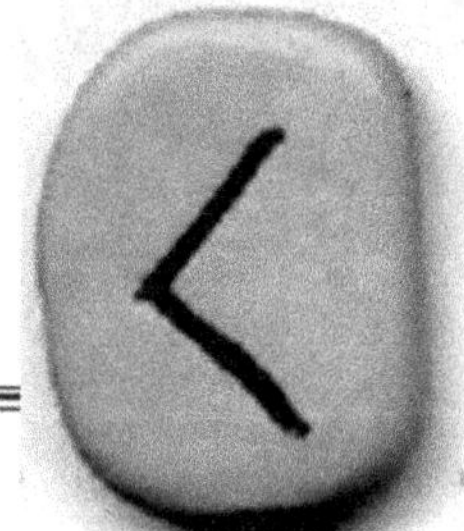

KANO — An opening

When you are in the darkness, an opening with light is the best and most gracious thing to have bestowed upon you. This is a great time for putting energies into new opportunities. [8]

A shaman of the Tavgy people of Siberia recounted his initiatory passage through the underworld to the Russian anthropologist Andrei Popov:[9]

The Great Underground Master told me that I would have to travel the path of every illness. He gave me a stoat and a mouse as my guides and together with them I continued my journey further into the underworld. My companions led me to a high place where there stood seven tents. "The people inside these tents are cannibals," the mouse and stoat warned me. Nevertheless I went into the middle tent, and went crazy on the spot.

These were the Smallpox People. They cut out my heart and threw it into a cauldron to boil. Inside the tent I found the Master of my Madness, in another tent I saw the Master of Confusion, in another the Master of Stupidity. I went round all these tents and became acquainted with the paths of various human diseases.

Then I went through an opening in another rock. A naked man was sitting there fanning the fire with bellows. Above the fire hung an enormous cauldron as big as half the earth. When he saw me the naked man brought out a pair of tongs the size of a tent and took hold of me. He took my head and cut it off, then sliced my body into little pieces and put them in the cauldron. There he boiled my body for three years. Then he placed me on an anvil and struck my head with a hammer and dipped it into ice cold water to temper it.

He took the big cauldron off the fire and poured its contents into another container. Now all my muscles had been separated from the bones. Here I am now, I'm talking to you in an ordinary state of mind. And I can't say how many pieces there are in my body. But we shamans have several extra bones and muscles. I turned out to have three such parts, two muscles and one bone. When all my bones had been separated from my flesh, the blacksmith said to me, "Your marrow has turned into a river," and inside the hut I really did see a river with my bones floating on it. "Look, there are your bones floating away!" said the blacksmith and started to pull them out of the water with his tongs.

When all my bones had been pulled out onto the shore the blacksmith put them together, they became covered with flesh and my body took on its previous appearance. The only thing that was left unattached was my head. It just looked like a bare skull. The blacksmith covered my skull with flesh and joined it onto my torso. I took on my previous human form.

Before he let me go the blacksmith pulled out my eyes and put in new ones. He pierced my ears with his iron finger and told me, "You will be able to hear and understand the speech of plants". After this I found myself on the summit of the mountain and soon afterwards woke up in my own tent. Near me sat my worried father and mother.

The above account, wild and outrageous as it is, aptly sets the stage for this work. There is no doubt that the inner and outer worlds of healers and shamans are populated by deep and confounding events and figures. Each has to negotiate and learn from these, to be obedient to extraordinary forces in order to not only bring healing to others, but maintain their own health and sanity. Such experiences may occur very early in life, or at some point during adulthood, but few who are called to heal others are granted straightforward passage through life.

The title of this chapter, 'Opening' describes, pretty well, the beginning of this work. At a certain time in my life I went through a series of experiences which could be described as an opening, and through that opening I came to inhabit a quite different terrain. This led to an experience of living which was at the same time thrilling and confounding, and presented to me a set of challenges in living within this new ground of experience.

At a point in this period, I understood myself to be undergoing a transformation to be a healer. Later, in this understanding, I conceived my Honours and PhD research. More recently, I understand this shift in life path in the frame of shamanism; it looks and feels like the kind of shift that shamans throughout the world have been reporting for at least centuries and probably millennia. The opening I refer to was preceded by incredibly difficult months of disruption of my identity and usual operating in the world, where I was filled with anxieties and haunted by spectres of madness and dysfunction. Nonetheless, I knew that I was undergoing an important transitional experience and this knowledge funded the courage I needed to undergo this ordeal.

Astonishingly, at the point I was considering psychiatric treatment, a wild shaman healer came to my home, saw what I was going through, and undertook a healing journey with me where I became both her apprentice and her healer. My personal account of this is Chapter Fourteen, 'My story'.

A few years into this change, in I embarked on research into the lived experience of nurse healers in the nursing profession.[10] One of the essential themes identified in that research, my Honours thesis — 'Evolving' — concerned how the nurse healers I interviewed described their personal experiences of evolution and transformation as healers.

One of the participants (Brigit) articulates the intriguing glimpse into an almost unknown world that was offered to me at that time:[11]

> *Initially, as I went through my own journey of discovery about what I was meant to do on the planet, my sensitivities rose to such a level that I was extremely impacted by the patients that I cared for, impacted by the unjustness of these children having cancer and having to fight for life, impacted by their struggle, impacted by their disease — sometimes I would come home with the symptoms of their stuff.*
>
> *We all know now that is about "taking on stuff", but at the time I had no idea. I had no idea why I understood what unconscious children required. So it was a very confusing time, in that I hadn't any real guidelines, hadn't established myself as having any clairvoyance, any telepathic control, power or anything — I just had all these feelings. It was a real struggle. It was a struggle how to maintain a professional image... [With] some children I literally would go near, and I would have to leave, because I was so impacted I would be in the toilet vomiting from their "stuff". And I had no support from within the nursing profession. Nobody could understand this sensitivity.*

Clearly, what Brigit experienced was not only vitally significant to her personally and as a nurse healer, but was one kind of experience which others exploring healing in nursing (such as myself) might also encounter. The following from another participant in my earlier study (Freyr)[12] spoke to the necessity for nurse healers to undergo extraordinary and challenging experiences, such as those Brigit mentioned:

> *The biggest challenge, I think, for nurse healers is that once you embrace the concepts of holism, and health, it can't become separate to... it can't be just what you do. It becomes who you are. It's like, it's not just a philosophy any more, or a nursing theory. It's a way of life. It becomes part of you. Once you go down that road, there is no turning back. You will never not be a healer. You can't just turn it off. Once you make that choice, you call in challenges that you have to face. It is much easier to be the unemotional, the non-recognising of spirit, the great technician. And pay your mortgage. That is an easier road, there is no doubt.*

These words might suggest that many of the unknown numbers of nurses, Process Workers, therapists, social workers, doctors and other helpers who know themselves as healers will be undergoing powerful and confusing experiences with little understanding or support from their professions. Further, such experiences are not, as far as I can determine, addressed comprehensively in the ordinary professional discourses, nor even in the published writings of holistic practitioners.

Such thoughts fuelled my curiosity and my passion to deeply explore these kinds of experiences, this book is wrought from the deep and unusual experiences of eleven nurse healers I spoke with.[13] Although they worked in various areas of nursing, all eleven of these strongly identified as healers. There are interesting and valid questions around whether everyone or no one is a healer, whether healers are shamans, and whether shamans are healers. But for me, it was enough that these people identified and lived as healers, and were at least recognised as such by peers and colleagues. Some were also known as academics and teachers of healing, and some were well known simply for the healing they brought to others. It was a great pleasure and privilege to have these conversations with people who disclosed their inner worlds so generously, and I will always treasure the time I spent with them, as well as the gifts of their life experiences and insights.

It is with joy that I share these with you, the reader, in the following pages, in the hope of bringing more knowledge and understanding to areas of experience which are so tender, so hard-come-by, and which hold much that is esoteric or sacred, and often hidden or held secret from a world that can be harshly disbelieving, judgmental and tending to pathologise. And let's not forget that witches used to be burned.

The descriptions of experience in the following chapters depict or assume certain understandings of reality which are not mainstream, and many may call them misguided, erroneous or heretical or right-out delusional. And indeed not all of the participants hold the exact same interpretations of their experiences of the wider terrain they traverse. This refers particularly to spirituality and an individual's understandings of the subtle experiences perceived in meditative states or in healing sessions, or even just the ways of interacting with the world.

As I write, I am reminded that there is a big part of me that can be harshly disbelieving, judgmental and tending to pathologise. This is a big part of my personal journey — how I often do look askance at my wilder, odd, madcap experiences; how it often seems safer and more sensible to deny what transpires in my other ways of being, in non-ordinary states of consciousness, and see them as bizarre and of no consequence, maybe even a sign of mental derangement. And on the other side, in the experiences of these non-ordinary realms, the shaman in me can be unkind to the ordinary me, not accommodating to the need to appear composed and in control, and to give clear and reassuring messages to the everyday world. This dynamic, as I understand it, is my "life myth", a deep interplay of characteristics and circumstances that has structuredmy experiences throughout this life; and several times over the years I have had recollections and insights that tell me that this dynamic has been present through many lifetimes.

And so, as you read this book, you will be not alone if you find some of the things you encounter herein hard to accept, and you question the reality or validity of what you find in these pages. I have been there, in that situation, regarding my own experiences, and you will read how many of the healers I spoke with have also struggled along the way, been confronted by their experiences, and questioned their reality at times. It is part of the journey into the unknown realms where be dragons, where there be soul-eaters (as the early cartographers imagined).

To address the challenging nature of the experiences described in the following pages, the next chapter, 'Initiation', offers a conceptual milieu for the experiences of the nurse healers who shared their sacred journeys with me. I aspire in this to give a frame and context to their experiences as they have reported them. Thus, I aim to show that although much of what they say is beyond the normal, particularly in terms of mainstream Western culture's dominant paradigm, there are accounts from other writers and other spiritual adventurers which talk about these kinds of experiences. The experiences of my collaborators are in many ways extraordinary, but not unique in the overall human experience.

In the following chapter I also give a brief description of Process Work (PW), especially as it speaks directly to this topic. In my own personal journey of healing, PW has played a crucial role, and has supported me to self-transform beyond some very murky and bewildering places. As I have found Process Work to be commensurate with my world view, and that of nurse healers generally, I have been inspired to study it, over the past decade and more. Thus, I have aspired to grow myself and to support others in their journeys of healing and transformation.

Beyond the chapter on framework, the following chapters are the personal accounts of the nurse healers I interviewed back in 2000. They are crafted from the transcripts of my conversations with each of them, edited so they are focused conversational autobiographies. I've removed my side of each conversation, so the accounts are more coherent and flow more smoothly. Some passages have also been deleted where, usually due to my clumsy questioning, they perseverate or are off topic. To preserve anonymity, the accounts have been changed to remove identifying details.

These conversations were structured by the following questions to each participant, which were flagged in invitation correspondence I sent:

- ***Please describe your emotional and spiritual experiences associated with your coming to be a nurse healer?***

- ***What experiences unique to your journey as a healer have you encountered? Can you talk about the challenging aspects of these?***

- ***How did you meet these challenges?***

- ***How has the process of coming to be a healer, and living as a healer changed you?***

- ***What stories do you have that would illustrate what you have told me?***

There is something about storied accounts which speaks so directly to another's experience. In the personal descriptions of profound experience, as is held in these biographies, is the potential to be both deeply resonant and also initiatory of such experience in the readers.

The nurse healer Margi Martin spoke powerfully to this when she wrote: "One person who speaks in a certain way can literally open up the universe for others".[14]

Furthermore, storied accounts, as form the core of this book can, I believe, bring to life for the reader these mysterious and little-understood aspects of human experience, beyond the explanatory power of more measured analytical writing. Full understanding of these usually- hidden phenomena involves a kind of knowledge that is difficult to conceptually hold and rationally substantiate, inhering mysteriously in the stories of those who tread that path.

Cognitive psychologists such as Abelson & Schank[15] have pointed out how humans are "hardwired" for story, and consequently storied knowledge is more meaningful, understandable and memorable than information presented in more rationalised and structured forms.

And there are deeper, more mysterious aspects to our storied nature. The following passage drawn from the story of one of the collaborators of this work, Chris, illustrates how story is intrinsic to our makeup, and she uses it to address the forgotten wholeness of those she helped:[16]

> *I'm learning better now how to use the talk to knit a whole... If the person's come to you, and they're kind of broken; if their heart's broken, their soul's broken, and their body's broken, then no amount of touching or quietness is going to fix that. Really, in the amount of time. If we've got an hour, I might knit them up with story. And in that, I'm using my hands, and my voice becomes kind of like patches and I know precisely what I'm saying, and how I'm saying it. So, I have now lots of stories. Big stories, little stories.*
>
> *And sometimes they're a long way away. You know, the meat and bones are here, but they are like, away up in the trees a long way away. They may not even know where they are. And so, I'm always talking to their soul. Wherever their soul is. And I don't go looking for their soul... And that's a real key thing, because what happens is, they might not have seen their soul for a long time. And so, I have — it just happens — a sense of speaking with the essence of them.*

Following the stories are the chapters on the themes which I have gleaned from them. Drawing out themes makes it possible to discuss the commonalities in these experiences, and to gain a sense of what is be essential and fundamental on this topic. Max van Manen wrote that themes:

> *...are like knots in the webs of our experiences, around which certain lived experiences are spun and thus experienced as lived wholes. Themes are the stars that make up the universes of meaning we live through. It is by the light of these themes that we can navigate and explore such universes.[17]*

Hence, Chapters Fifteen to Twenty set out these themes, illustrated by excerpts from the stories, as well as the literature of healers, shamans and others. In the spirit of Van Manen, I hope these themes help you navigate and explore the universes of these eleven nurse healers who collaborated with me in this project, as they have disclosed their sacred journeys.

Chapter Two

INITIATION

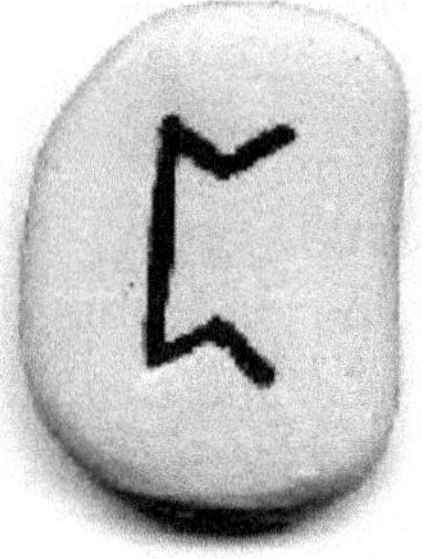

PERTH — Things unexplainable (Initiation)

A hieratic or mystery Rune pointing to that which is beyond our frail manipulative powers. This Rune is on the side of Heaven, the Unknowable, and has associations with the phoenix... Its ways are secret and hidden.[18]

The realities of the healer

The practice of healing throws the individual into experience of realms of experience which in everyday consciousness (or in Consensus Reality) are not perceptible. These non-ordinary realms of experience can be astounding and beautiful, as well as frightening and confusing. There are a few possible explanations why many healers encounter this.

For example, as attested by nurse healers such as Janet Quinn[19] and Dolores Krieger,[20] it can be said that the healer must work within and through levels of consciousness more expanded than ordinary states of mind. Some healers report having conscious contact with these non-ordinary realms of experience throughout their lives.

Also affecting the experiences of the nurse healers I spoke with is a pervasive critical attitude within the profession, and Western health systems in general, concerning healing and spirituality. Nurse healers are nearly always working within highly bureaucratised, hierarchical and scientifically founded systems. These systems, which significantly background their evolvement as healers, are ever vigilant to stamp out what they denote deviant ideas and practices. Therefore, it is relevant to look at the experiences of nurse healers within these systems, as another way to give context to the accounts in the following chapters. Below, I discuss this in reviewing some of the literature around Therapeutic Touch.

Nurse healer as mystic and the dilemma of secularism

Therapeutic Touch (TT) is a healing modality developed by nurses and taught and practised in nursing settings. There is a considerable body of research and other writing on it. While by no means are all nurse healers practitioners of Therapeutic Touch, the experiences of those who have practised and written about TT may serve as exemplars of the understanding of healing evolving both within nursing and throughout the contemporary Western healing experience.

Therapeutic Touch practitioners

From the early days of teaching and practicing Therapeutic Touch within nursing, practitioners have presented and conceptualised it as a secular modality, which may be practised by people of any or no religious faith.

This has been important in its propagation — nurses are given a tool whereby they may offer comfort, relaxation and healing to their patients, without imposing religious beliefs which may not be shared by their patients. The secular nature of TT was reinforced by a growing body of research supporting its value and efficacy, and by its systematic association with recognised scientific nursing theory (Rogers' Unitary Science).

Notwithstanding TT's projecting of a secular image within nursing and the other health care professions, the accounts of practitioners and recipients have often been anything but mundane or prosaic, and described, in a number of instances, as significant spiritual experiences for both practitioners and recipients. I focus on the experiences of the nurses offering the healing.

The two nurses most prominent in the propagation and research of TT in the USA over the last three decades of the twentieth century, Dolores Krieger and Janet Quinn, described their experiences as TT practitioners as significant for their personal spiritual evolution. Krieger, in the early days of TT, published research on the measurable physiological benefits of receiving TT.[21] In her 1987 book, by contrast, Krieger framed the experience of practicing TT in terms of her understanding of Hindu esoteric spiritual philosophy.[22] Thus, the Indian notions of prana (subtle energy) and chakras (centres of energy in the human esoteric bodies) came to help Krieger conceptualise the energetic occurrences at the core of TT practice.

In Krieger's 1987 book, *Living the Therapeutic Touch*, she presented the committed and ongoing practice of TT as a kind of yoga, or path of spiritual evolution and development, much the same, I imagine, as one might undertake as an initiate to a monastic order, or in an ashram, at the feet of a spiritual master. Thus, for Krieger, the practice of healing is a spiritual or mystic practice, and the experience of being a healer is an introduction to the spiritual realms, and to the ensuing inner transformation. Krieger's book is essentially a treatise on how healing, as a spiritual practice, could bring powerful change into the life of the healer.

Janet Quinn extensively researched and theorised TT after learning the modality from Krieger in 1974.[23] For Quinn, TT was a secular practice, which she quite early theorised in terms of Martha Rogers' "Unitary" theory of nursing.[24] (Rogers was influenced by writers on mysticism such as Teilhard de Chardin, but presented her theory as scientific, employing particularly the ideas of systems theorists such as Ludwig von Bertalanffy[25] and James Miller[26]). In a 1996 interview, Quinn disclosed how years of practising TT had led her to profound and life-changing spiritual experiences, despite the painstaking secularism she brought to the practice over decades.[27]

> *I was raised a Catholic, but promptly left the church at age eighteen. Meanwhile, I learned Therapeutic Touch, and since 1974 I have been asking to be used as an instrument of healing. Therapeutic Touch, at its core, is the offering of unconditional love and compassion, and so I asked over and over again for years to be an instrument for unconditional love and compassion. This, of course, was a spiritual practice, but I did not realise it. Then, quite suddenly, … I had an ongoing series of spiritual experiences that, at the time, were terrifying to me. I thought it was happening out of the blue, out of nowhere. But my sense of it now is that it was the natural product of years of spiritual practice by another name. All our careful language, our conceptual frameworks, the way we describe things, cannot constrain the Divine.*

The challenge to secular views of reality

It is clear that the experiences of healers points to a reality which, in terms of conventional scientific ontology, is completely extraordinary and lacking rational or empirical substantiation – even bizarre. Accounting for healing in secular, scientific language possibly contributed to the extreme hostility towards TT's practice in nursing, expressed by a number of vocal critics.[28]

Chief among a range of criticisms, these detractors accused TT's proponents of promulgating a religious practice under the guise of "pseudoscience".

A strong example of this repudiation of a secular, scientific basis for TT in nursing came from the prominent nursing theorist Myra Levine.[29]

> *The pretence of the healers that they perform scientific therapies is unconscionable. In our struggle to achieve academic recognition as a profession, we simply cannot afford to indulge in this kind of charlatanism. Therapeutic Touch challenges the validity of modern nursing research, teaching and practice. If its practitioners insist on their healing roles, let them honestly call*

themselves faith healers and stop claiming they are nurses who heal.

The above points to an important dialogue, where the stringent bounds of scientific ontology are being questioned, and where the deeper experiences of the spiritual explorer of healing are being brought into the domain of scientific inquiry. It is unclear whether there will be a harmonious meeting, where healing practices and their attendant worldviews can claim a secure place in secular society. Certainly TT, like all instances of spiritual healing, does posit a deep question to the assumption of a scientifically explainable material universe, upon which so much of the discourse in modern secular society is founded.

And my own suspicion has been that these perspectives may not be commensurate, despite the input of quantum mechanics and other scientific questions to Newtonian ontology emerging over the last decades. In my experience, Process Work values disparate points of view, which can bring relief to seemingly intractable conflicts such as have been described.

Much more could be written on this topic of the conflict in nursing around whether healing is a valid practice for nurses. My aim has been to give a flavour of the atmosphere surrounding this, as an important and highly challenging context for those nurses who are drawn to bring spiritual healing in modern healthcare settings.

The phenomenological locus of this book leads me mostly away from the conventional scientific outlook, into the depths of experience encountered by healers. I am uncertain whether such vistas on reality will ever inspire universal interest and respect, yet for me it is important to map these terrains in human experience, for clearly there are many, healers in particular, who are impelled to walk this way.

First principles

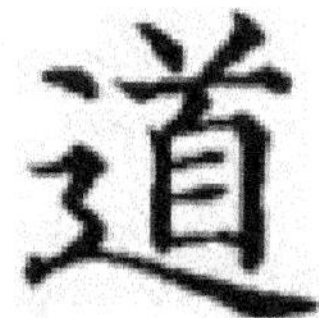

The Way that can be experienced is not true;
The world that can be constructed is not true.
The Way manifests all that happens and may happen;
The world represents all that exists and may exist.
To experience without abstraction is to sense the world;

Initiation

To experience with abstraction is to know the world.
These two experiences are indistinguishable;
Their construction differs but their effect is the same.
Beyond the gate of experience flows the Way,
Which is ever greater and more subtle than the world.

— Lao Tze, Tao te Ching[30]

To further illustrate the confluence between the experience of the healer, and that of the mystic, I offer a mapping, or a picture of this mysterious reality encountered by healers and other mystics — some personal interpolations, reports from healers, mystics and visionaries of various cultures. They amount to a kind of phenomenology of holism, more than a big theory of rational constructs. Such a take is in line with the phenomenological nature of this inquiry, as well as being aligned with PW's close association with Taoism and its phenomenological approach to unfolding experience.

Elementary phenomenology of holistic consciousness

I am not convinced that any conceptual schema can give an understanding of the reality that lies behind healing, for ultimately this is the Absolute, the Divine. As is often pointed out, aetiologically the word 'heal' goes back to the Old English *haelan*, meaning "to make whole" which brings the act of healing into alignment with the indivisibleness inherent in understandings of Divine reality.

Rational faculties are not adequate to comprehend or express this deeper reality. The opening stanza from the Taoist classic, *Tao te Ching* (attributed to the sage Lao Tze in the fifth-century BC) expresses beautifully this unknowable nature of reality. The Tao — Reality (or Ultimate Reality) is unknowable because knowing, in a simple rational sense, is a function of a completely differentiated individual, and knowing of Reality involves the awareness of the utter oneness of all. To be fully conscious of that is to "think" with the mind of the Tao, the mind of undifferentiated, ever-unfolding nature.

Voiced in virtually all spiritual traditions is the experience of oneness with everything. One powerful and beautiful expression of this human experience of the absolute appears in Hinduism, where the direct identification with the Absolute (Brahma) is articulated and practiced in the Advaita tradition. This yoga, or spiritual pathway with its roots in the Upanishads, is first found in the teaching of eighth-century scholar, Adi Shankara,[31] and has been expounded through the centuries by such seers as Ramana Maharshi.[32] According to the prominent contemporary spiritual teacher Bede Griffiths,[33] Brahman is "the one Reality beyond all phenomena".

In Advaita, the central truth is that there is never any separation between Brahma — "All-That-Is' — and any individual, except in the adherence to an illusion of separateness. The practice of Advaita, according to Ramana Maharshi, is the constant inquiry as to the nature of the self. "Who am I?" In any situation; the truest answer is "I am atman", which is Self — the inner experience of Brahman, All-That-Is.[34]

A way of expressing this is to say that the fundamental nature or "substance" of reality is consciousness, from which the mind of anyone cannot ever be truly separate. This is embodied in the words of the Brithadaranyaka Upanishad. "The Self is the footstep of everything, for through it, one knows everything".[35] This identification of consciousness as the basic form of reality appeared simultaneously in the fifth-century BC in Hinduism, as well as in Greek philosophy of Heraclites, and in the transcendent understandings of God of Jeremiah and other biblical prophets,[36] as well as in Taoism and Buddhism.

Consciousness in this sense is Being, and the knowing of one's being is not a rational operation, for the intellectual mind is always looking for some object "over there" upon which to settle, whereas Being is always "here", and can never be an object. The contemporary Advaita teacher Isaac Shapiro highlighted this in the context of discussing spiritual practice, or meditation:[37]

> *Ultimately, when you are doing some activity to get somewhere, even if it is to get silent, you are missing what is already here, because you are trying to get somewhere else. Truth is already here. The only moment you can know Truth is now.*

This is very difficult to accept rationally, and the very motivation of the person to rationally conceptualise reality may well present an impenetrable barrier to its apperception. This is, perhaps, because that which may satisfy the purely rational mind as truth must be an objective reality, and objectivity as such cannot approach ultimate reality (although it is held within it). In this sense, Reality is not objectively real, and is beyond rationalist or empirical verification.

Again, Bede Griffiths,[38] citing the *Mandukya Upanishad*, put this powerfully:

> *It is atman, the Spirit, that cannot be seen or touched, that is above all distinction, beyond thought, and is ineffable. In other words, one goes beyond one's senses, one's imagination, one's mind, and beyond word, until one comes to the Absolute beyond. And union with him is the supreme proof of his reality. One knows it by itself. One cannot know it by one's reason or by one's intellect, but only when one enters into it does one know it.*

Therefore, reality in this sense can only be known in consciousness — it is possible for human consciousness to be expanded to realise itself as the consciousness of "All-That-Is", the Divine, the One, the Source, Brahma. This is the Self, atman, the Divine reality of each person, realised in expanded consciousness. It is possible for humans to know their Being, to know what they are. This can never be rationally realised — it can only be ontologically realised, recognised, remembered (sort of). It is not the rational mind which does this, but the heart, and the spiritual mind. The nineteenth-century Native American Sioux leader, Black Elk,[39] clarified his Indigenous perspective on the role of the heart in knowing truth when he said:

> *I am blind, and do not see the things of this world; but when the light comes from above, it enlightens my heart and I can see, for the Eye of my heart sees everything; and through this vision I can help my people. The heart is a sanctuary at the centre of which there is a little space, wherein the Great Spirit dwells, and this is the Eye. This is the Eye of the Great Spirit by which He sees all things, and through which we see Him. If the heart is not pure, the Great Spirit cannot be seen.*

There is this paradox in the spiritual "journey" — where an individual seeks to have the "experience" of enlightenment, of realising their true nature, of attaining union with the Divine. And this seems the most intensely personal process. Yet in truth, as was pointed out by teachers such as the Buddha and Ramana, there is no individual, in the first place, to become enlightened. Self- realisation is not an experience taken by an individual and located in time — it is the recognising that all experience flows in the consciousness which is Source, from which human consciousness cannot be separate. That which one already is, and can never fail to be — Being — can not be attained, can not be achieved. Thus, it is not an individual who attains realisation of Self, but it may well be the case that it is Self (All-That- Is) who has decided before time began to now bring back to knowing the forgotten spaces in consciousness. This is what is known as Grace. The *Katha Upanishad* expressed this beautifully:

> *Not by much learning, not by the Vedas, not by understanding, is this Atman known. He whom the Atman chooses, he knows the Atman.*[40]

As some of the collaborators of this work have attested, the significance of the above for healers and healing is that truth is the healer and may, by grace, become evident when the heart is opened in compassion for the benefit of another. Put another way, healing is inevitable when the lie or illusion of separation is removed, and reality is remembered as love. I would maintain that knowing a specific healing modality (such as TT) is not necessary to healing, but certainly the practice of a modality like TT, as attested by authors such as Janet Quinn (quoted above) creates a space for this to be nurtured.

I have suggested above that there is in the act of healing an invocation of the Divine, because wholeness is by definition an absence of separation. As such, a healer may make no claim to personal individual "ability to heal", for healing must be a gift from the Divine, mediated mysteriously through the healer.

Process work and sentient reality

Arnold Mindell, the founder of Process Work, has long practised and taught the central importance to health and healing of accessing and unfolding deep altered states. He expressed this as "The Dreaming", influenced by his experiences with Australian Aboriginal peoples, and has also referred to this deep experience of unitary consciousness as Sentient Reality. Mindell has drawn on traditions such as shamanism, Taoism, Buddhism and quantum mechanics as he developed and articulated his ideas.

Mindell studied and worked as a theoretical physicist before becoming a Jungian analyst. In a number of his books, Mindell, citing pioneers such as Einstein, Heisenberg, Schrodinger, Wheeler and Feynman, has explored how quantum theory can help explain the human experience of wholeness, whilst also integrating teachings of Lao Tse, Don Juan, and The Buddha in suggesting methods to deepen awareness and solve vexing physical, personal, interpersonal, and world issues.[41–43]

Interestingly, Mindell was critical of some spiritual teachers' focus on Unitary consciousness to the neglect of more everyday experience. He described this as a kind of addiction to certain kinds of experience.[44] This is in line with Mindell's key concept of Deep Democracy,[45] by which he advocates that all states of consciousness, ideas, people, races, institutions, points of view, feelings, etc., are welcome, and not one should be prioritised over another. I write more about Arny Mindell's work and ideas below.

Multiple levels of reality

> *The egocentric psyche with its one eye fixed on wholes and unities may grudgingly admit personifying as a figure of speech, but never that the imaginal realm and its persons are actually presences and true powers.*   — James Hillman[46]

The above depiction of reality, realised in what may be termed "Cosmic Consciousness" or "Divine Consciousness", may not be the consistent experience of many people, although numerous individuals have been fortunate enough to be given intimations of such Reality. The above perspective on relating to the Absolute appears in all the traditions of human spirituality, and is present in writings which are relatively mainstream. The issue of multiple realities which present to healers is much less present in the accounts of spiritual philosophy or comparative religion, possibly because such an ontology seems to belie the unitary nature of Reality.

However, were one to see consciousness as the basic substance of reality, it follows that different states of consciousness might equate to, or reveal, differing realities, within the One. Clearly, those, such as healers, who devote themselves to exploring consciousness in its varying manifestations, might have much to report on this. Indeed, the accounts given to me by those I spoke with, and set out in the following chapters, are rich in such observations. Nurse healer and founder of TT, Dolores Krieger, wrote on this:[47]

> *A common perception among healers is that there are multiple realities, reflecting the multifold states of consciousness at our command. Which reality we relate to depends largely on the predominant facet of consciousness through which we choose to perceive our interactions with the universe.*

Process workers, some of whom do identify as healers, are trained and encouraged to work fluidly in three levels of reality, as we follow the unfolding processes of ourselves and our clients. These are Consensus Reality, Dreamland, and Sentient Reality.

Consensus Reality (CR) is the usual, everyday, agreed-upon reality of the culture; Dreaming Reality or Dreamland includes night-time dreams, synchronicities, odd, irrational, extreme or half- imagined experiences beyond the everyday; Sentient Reality is the undifferentiated, unitary reality such as is discussed earlier in this chapter.[48]

From the perspective of healers, the experience of multiple realities is highly significant, and sits as one of the biggest challenges to anyone committing herself to that path. This is central to the concerns of this research, for the actual experience of more than one dimension to reality raises enormous personal issues for the healer, who must grow herself through the implications of this.

Multiple realities

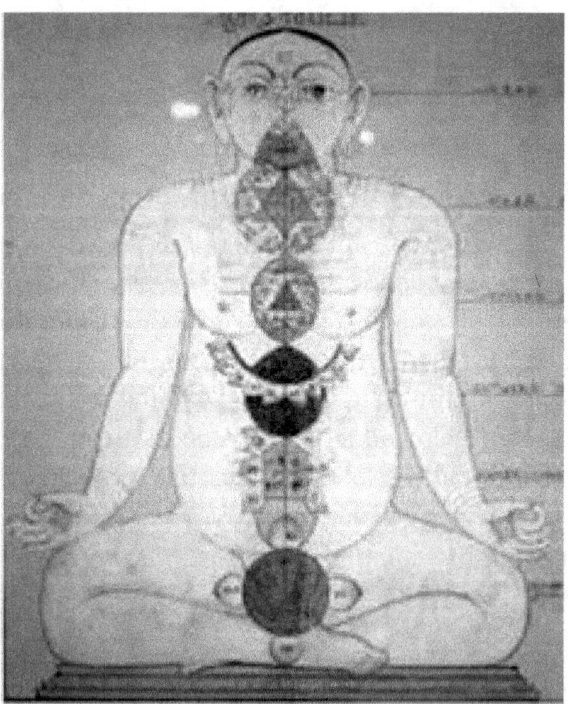

The chakras

Following is a discussion of multiple levels of reality, focusing on depictions from a healer, Barbara Brennan, reporting her personal experience. Notwithstanding her scientific background, Brennan's books on spiritual healing (termed by her "personal healing"), draw heavily in their language and construction of concepts upon Hindu esoteric spirituality.[49–51]

Observations of the human energy field

There are numerous writers who report these relationships amongst the human energy fields (HEF) (or "aura"), multiple realities and personal transformation.[52] The spiritual healer Barbara Brennan, who worked for several years for NASA as a pioneering atmospheric physicist, presents a particularly lucid and sophisticated account of this. In her book, Hands of Light,[53] Brennan details a schema of the human energy fields which she observed over a number of years practising as a therapist and later as a healer.

By Brennan's (1988) account, the physical human body is the densest (and most readily discerned) of at least seven co-spatial bodies comprising the individuated human being. Through having developed her Higher Sense Perception (HSP) (ability to visualise spiritual or nonmaterial phenomena), Brennan claimed to be able to discern the different layers of human form, which exist at different levels of being, or consciousness. Brennan saw these layers as being related to the chakras, the other major feature of the human energetic system, or "aura" (see the above image showing the location of the chakras on the body). In her second book, Light Emerging,[54] Brennan related these observations of the energy fields to psychological and other health problems.

By Brennan's observations, each layer is associated with a particular chakra, and deals with specific aspects of human functioning. The chakras lower on the body, associated with the denser, more easily discernible layers (or "bodies", as they are often termed), deal with the more corporeal aspects of human functioning, such as physical survival and sexuality, whereas the higher chakras and more subtle layers are associated with more spiritual and ethereal aspects of human functioning, such as love, life purpose, and relationship with the Divine.

By raising or lowering her own level of consciousness, Brennan reported being able to see a particular layer, holding the aspects of a human being existing within the dimension relating to a particular level of consciousness. The different layers or levels of the HEF, Brennan observed, became visible to her as she entered states of expanded consciousness, with the outer or more subtle levels visible to her only as she entered deeper and deeper (or more expanded) meditative states, often during healing sessions. Expanding one's consciousness into the more subtle layers, Brennan maintained, involved entering completely different realms of existence. She wrote:[55]

> *Each of the layers above the third is an entire layer of reality with beings, forms and personal functions that go beyond what we normally call human. Each is an entire world in which we live and have our being. Most of us experience these realities during sleep but do not remember them. Some of us can go into these states of reality by expanding the consciousness through meditative techniques. These meditative techniques open the seals between the roots of the chakra layers and thus provide a doorway for consciousness to travel.*

A conclusion from the above statement is that as humans we exist simultaneously in a number of dimensions, of which we are not always conscious.

Brennan emphasised the transformational process involved in an individual moving into consciousness of the higher layers and charkas of the HEF (human energy fields). She wrote cautiously of opening the chakras, and integrating the consciousness associated with the energy coming through the chakras:[56]

> *Psychological maturity related to each chakra is brought to consciousness through that chakra. Too much psychological material would be released by a sudden flow of energy, and we could not process it all. We therefore work in whatever growth process we are in to open each chakra slowly, so that we have time to process the personal material that is released and integrate the new information into our life.*

Bede Griffiths also wrote of the Hindu perspective of a human's spiritual bodies, and their association with spiritual transformation:[57]

> *In the Hindu tradition, there is a way of talking about this transformation which is in terms of bodily sheaths, or koshas, in which the human consciousness is involved, of which only the first is physical and the rest are subtle. The first sphere is the annamayakosha, the food kosha, which is the material body. Then there is the pranamayakosha, the level of the breath or life energy. Inside this is the manomayakosha, the mental body, or mind energy. In the West, this is generally thought to be the final*

stage of development, whereas in reality it is only an intermediate level. Beyond the manomayakosha is the vijnanamayakosha, and that is where one comes to the budhi, or intellect. Finally, there is the anandamayakosha, the supreme bliss consciousness. As one passes beyond all the limitations of the lower levels of consciousness, one experiences the bliss of the sahasrara, the highest level of consciousness, the anandamayakosha. At that stage one is open to the cosmic consciousness, the cosmic order, and that is where one becomes aware of the gods and the angels.

Writers in the field of transpersonal psychology and transpersonal studies, within which, it might be suggested, Process Work has a foot, also posit a multi-levelled understanding of reality, connected with levels of consciousness. Prominent examples are Ken Wilber's *The Atman Project*[58] and Stanislav Grof and Hal Zina Bennett's *The Holotropic Mind*.[59]

Finally, mention should be made of Carl Jung, whose insights in many ways inspired and funded the Transpersonal and New Age conceptions of multiple realities. He wrote in, *Memories, Dreams, Reflections:*[60]

The psyche at times functions outside of the spatio-temporal law of causality. This indicates that our conceptions of space and time, and therefore of causality also, are incomplete. A complete picture of the world would require the addition of still another dimension....

Transformation and experiencing multiple realities

Brennan's ideas (see above) regarding the psychological implications of entering into expanded realms in consciousness is very pertinent to this book. It is clear that healers, as they enter into these regions in consciousness in service of those to whom they bring healing, must take the time to process the emotional and psychic aspects of their being which come to light, or are stirred up, as they practice healing. It is inevitable that as a healer (or anybody else, for that matter) opens themself and enters these deeper (or expanded) levels of consciousness, they begin to become aware of psychological material which has been repressed from consciousness — much in the way that therapy can bring such material to light. The individual is challenged to come to terms with these unresolved issues ("baggage" as some call it), or will inevitably find that their progress through expanded consciousness is impeded. This is certainly my own experience. Thus comes the frequently heard exhortation that the healer must attend to their own healing in order to continue to bring healing to others.[61] This is explored in Chapter Eighteen.

And it is not simply one's own emotional issues which present themselves in the consciousness of the multiple dimensions of spiritual experience into which the healer seems to blunder almost unwittingly. The entities and thought forms met by healers in their travels in consciousness can be challenging to encounter, and are not always angelic in nature. Nor are these necessarily readily differentiable from the healer's own psychic or psychological processes. Some of the experiences in the unseen realms can inspire deep discomfort in the evolving healer, who may be challenged to develop in a number of different directions in response to these experiences.

Exploring the deeper realms is often characterised as somewhat hazardous, and that is certainly the case for those who are unwilling to or unable to process the material which is revealed to consciousness through spiritual practices. This is more powerfully the case the deeper one explores — to experience one's Divine nature brings forth to awareness psychic material held within, often at unconscious levels, which is in denial of This. In the face of that, many have entered disturbed states, including psychosis.[62] One form of psychological disturbance is sometimes called the "kundalini syndrome".

In one example from the literature, medical doctor Julia Hall discussed a kundalini awakening experience. She recalled:[63]

> *The day before I was to interview for an OB/GYN residency, I was in such doubt and so confused that I decided to go for a reading and a healing. This encounter finished the opening process which had been going on for several years. Within three weeks I was flooded with dream material and dreaming 15 hours a day. It was a total shift in my energy. Throughout the process I was confident that this was a spiritual healing and that something that was beyond me but was basically benevolent was in charge. But it was very, very disruptive. I developed what they now call "the kundalini syndrome". I didn't have flashing lights, but I did have a lot of uninvited visions. I could see energy between people and energies between charkas. I knew what people were going to say a second before they said it. This went on for two or three days. My spiritual eye was totally open. Along with it was a lot of pain in my heart. That period stays with me now and gives me confidence and conviction about this field of energy that most people don't see or validate.*

In light of the above, the process of personal revolution of the healer is perhaps inevitable on entering into realms associated with expanded consciousness, through which healing is conducted. The experience of shamans, found typically (but not exclusively) in Indigenous cultures, characteristically involves a transformational crisis at the start of the shaman's career.[64] Typically, this includes encounters with spirits or deities and, in some cases, involves journeying into other dimensions of experience (often called "the underworld") where the individual is dismembered, finally to awaken in the ordinary world as a shaman.

The quote from the Tavgy shaman at the start of this book is an example. This Indigenous experience of transformation is existentially, or psychically, very similar to that which is noted by Brennan and others writing about the experience of exploring deeper levels of consciousness. The shaman and writer Joan Halifax's words illustrate this well, affirming the sacred nature of the transition from sufferer to healer and spiritual intermediary:[65]

> *The opening vision for the shaman unfolds in a transpersonal realization resulting from a crisis of death and rebirth, a transformation of the profane individual into one who is sacred. For many neophytes, this realisation awakens in the dream-web when animal-tutors and spirits on the Other World appear. They come as emissaries of mythical beings, of gods and ancestors. And the candidate is doomed if he or she does not accept the instructions received in the dream from these presences of the Other World.*

Bede Griffiths pointed out that the understanding that there are a number of dimensions to reality is by no means an invention of Hinduism or the "new age". There is a ready precedent in the philosophy of ideals proposed by Plato. Subsequent Christian philosophers drew on Plato's notions to account for realms of angels and demons already present in Jewish cosmologies. For instance, Griffiths wrote of the early Christian mystic philosopher Clement of Alexandria's asserting that:[66]

> *Behind the physical world is the world of the angels. This as well … develops further in Christian mysticism, and exactly parallels the idea in Hinduism of the mahat, the cosmic order. Beyond the physical world is the cosmic order, the psychic world, and the world of the gods, and in Christian tradition that is encountered as the world of the angels.*

Plato believed that it wasn't possible for an individual to have direct experience of these other worlds of ideals, but the Neoplatonist Plotinus[67] is said to have had frequent direct experience of the other dimensions of experience that Plato wrote about, according to his disciple and biographer Porphyry.[68] Perhaps this highlights the difference between the mystic and the philosopher – the philosopher writes and thinks about reality, whereas the mystic, the spiritual adventurer, travels to those realms of reality.

The accounts of shamans have typically been brought to us within interpretations of anthropologists and theorists of religion from alien cultures. However, the phenomenologically rich descriptions of shamans' experiences in anthropologists' writings nearly always report experience of multiple levels of reality – journeying to the worlds of the spirits. This has been ever expected of the shamans serving their communities as healers and intermediaries of the gods and spirits.[69] In the immediately following chapters, the nurse healers co-creators of this investigation also give numerous examples of these experiences of multiple realities.

Process Work (Process Oriented Psychology)

I've mentioned earlier my deep interest in Process Work, also known as Process Oriented Psychology, a school of psychology founded in the 1980s by the physicist and Jungian therapist, Arnold Mindell. It is often referred to as taking a Jungian approach, although it has departed from Jungian psychology in significant ways, initially due to Mindell's focus on the relationship between dreams and body symptoms. In addition to its Jungian foundations, Mindell has brought to Process Work ideas from many places, including Taoism, quantum physics, field theory, communication science, Buddhism, alchemy and shamanism.

In contrast to analytic approaches to therapy, Process Work operates phenomenologically. Process workers engage sensory grounded communication signals, often nonverbal and unconscious, presenting in the moment. As such, Process Work in practice has a superficial resemblance to other dynamic approaches like Gestalt or Psychodrama.

Mindell posited three co-existent levels of reality — CR, Dreamland, and Sentient Reality — in which facilitators work and interact. These refer to the level of awareness through which a person, couple or group's process is unfolding, which is evident in their momentary communication signals. Process Workers fluidly track through these levels, and at each level the facilitator employs interventions based on specific skills and metaskills (feeling attitudes to therapy work)[70] appropriate to the level.

Of particular relevance here are skills and metaskills drawn from shamanism which are used in work on Dreamland and Sentient levels. Thus, "sensing the atmosphere" and "using the second and third attentions" — ideas drawn from Don Juan's teaching of Carlos Castaneda[71] are critical skills and metaskills employed in Process Work practice. Further, it is common to hear Process Workers speak of "shifting the assemblage point", also from Castaneda's writings, when discussing the transformations emerging from unfolding a process.[72]

At the core of Process Work is its eschewing of any fixed frame of reference to determine health or illness. Drawn from Jung's teleological concept of "finality", Process Workers recognise that an individual's process is always emerging — seeking to unfold — in ways that are ultimately useful, relieving and empowering. The communication signals of an emerging process are inherent in the presenting disturbance, be it a physical symptom like a headache, or a relationship or group problem, addiction or feelings of worthlessness or other psychological concern.

Like a midwife at a birth, it is only for the facilitator to accurately perceive these signals and support the unfolding process in the direction it is already going (usually unbeknownst to the client). Thus, disturbances mysteriously yield new growth, understanding and fresh ways to live life and relate to others. Whatever is in experience is somehow right and needed, this is central to the world view of the Process Worker, and informs their actions.

One area of sentient level work unique to Process Work concerns unfolding the processes of people experiencing significantly altered states of consciousness – "extreme states" — notably those in coma. Finding ways to pick up on and work with very subtle signals, as is the case in coma, requires great trust and sensitivity. The comatose or dying person is encouraged verbally and nonverbally to note changes in his momentary experience which may be very subtle. To work with such processes, the Process Worker must be very observant and attuned, responding congruently to these small cues within themselves and from the person they are working with.

In his book *Coma: The Dreambody Near Death*[73] Arny Mindell gave an example of working with someone near death:

> *I remember once being at the scene of a car accident. I was sitting near a severely injured man waiting for the ambulance. I suddenly had a vision of him leaving his body lying dead on the road. The next minute he stopped breathing. I spontaneously became very angry with him. "Hey," I said. "Don't do that now!*

Take your time!" He began to breathe again and survived. The kind of response you give to a minimal cue is important to the client. Your responses indicate that you have connected. He knows now that he has found you. Your responses also help him to become aware of what he is doing, and will help him to "say" more.

Process Work is often referred to as an "awareness method". In practice, Process Workers, like healers everywhere, work by paying very close attention to, and following, subtle signals within themselves as well as their clients. This requires the development of sufficient self- awareness to recognise what are their usual inner responses and experiences, and what is new and might be part of the field they share with their clients. In the moment, during sessions, Process Workers and healers follow and unfold their own inner process in order to in turn help their clients unfold theirs.

If asked, Process Workers may well identify the experiences of nurse healers reported in the following chapters as occurring in Dreamland or Sentient Reality, for instance. They may note the experiential channels they occur in and be curious about the level, or mythic themes in the background. My personal experience of PW as a client is of having my experience believed and honoured, and of having the flow of what is occurring for me in the moment accurately followed and unconditionally supported. Names and frames, communication channels and categories of experience are valuable tools for facilitation, but what particularly lends PW to the understanding of healers and healing is its heartfelt validating of all experience.

Summary

I have endeavoured to present a depiction of the reality or realities entered into by the healer. From the observation that living as a healer is a kind of yoga, or pathway to spiritual development, which reveals the healer to be a mystic, or spiritual adventurer in multiple levels of reality,[74] I have sought to orient the reader who may be unfamiliar with this area of experience, by outlining foundational understandings of these realities of the healer. I have presented a phenomenology of holistic consciousness, expounding the embracing of the fundamental unity of all-that-is in consciousness, or Being, is the basis of all healing. The transformational force of this understanding of reality is touched upon. Multiple realities experienced by healers is then discussed, which I have presented through the observations and insights of the healer Barbara Brennan,[75] esoteric Hindu teachings,[76] writings of the early Christian period,[77] and the shamanic experience of Indigenous societies.[78]

I sought to highlight the transformational imperative inherent in becoming conscious of these multiple dimensions experienced by healers, discussed by Brennan and others. I have noted the deep interest of Transpersonal psychologists and theorists in multiple levels of consciousness, and I have given a brief outline of Process Work as a valuable and sophisticated way to view and work with these alternate realities.

Section Two

I am being dreamed by Dragons

On my eyes those huge scales bask, and glitter golden.

Broken-hearted and stricken with untold greeds,

I dimly wander this world of ghosts and things.

But, yet, aloft on these leathery, indolent wings

All beneath is bright from hoard to sea.

I am beckoned by the gods and powers from all horizons,

And in my smouldering heart know every breath, ever.[79]

Dreamed by dragons: Tales of healing, destruction and transformation

Stories of Nurse Healers

Around the year 2000, I had long and deep conversations with eleven nurse healers. The following chapters are edited versions of the transcriptions of these interviews. Editing was done, first, to remove my part in the interviews, later, to turn them into more coherent stories or focused autobiographies.

There is, too, an account of my own experiences of coming to be a healer. I was in the highly privileged position of being able to sit down and reflect on my experiences, and add and rewrite as I saw fit.

It is hard to describe the great joy of connection I experienced in speaking with my collaborators; what a privilege it was to speak so deeply, on matters so close to all our hearts, with such bold and tender adventurers of the spirit.

Chapter Three

EMMA

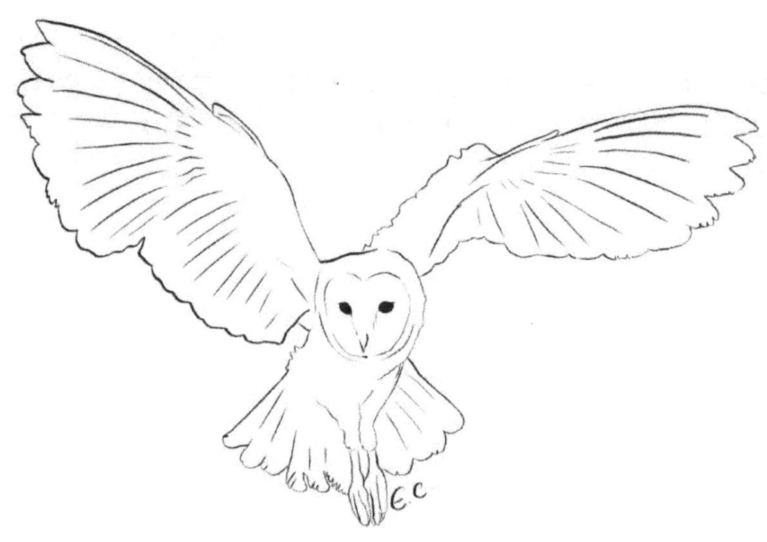

Emma

Emma and I sat down twice to speak, both of us enjoying our heartfelt exchanges which were, at the same time, comfortable and moving. We initially met because of her role as a teacher in her healing modality, and we were PhD students at the same time. She had reflected deeply — well before we met — on the unfolding of her life path towards being a healer. As we sat outside in the warm NSW north coast sunlight, she brought to our meeting the gift of a long feather, symbolic of the deep connection with nature she experienced in her ordinary life and "the spirit place".
I have felt blessed by Emma's deep and detailed disclosures around her sense of belonging, her evolvement in spiritual experience, and the challenges and blessings of living as a healer.

I think for many healers, and I know for me, some of the experiences of being wounded, eventually are the "coming home" experiences. As a child I used to spend a lot of time with fairies. Now, I don't know that I actually physically saw the fairies, but I knew they were there, though they weren't very responsive to this kid that used to sit in the tree; I got the impression they weren't really responsive to humans in general.

It was quite different from my experience going to church, and I was going to church quite a lot as a child (despite telling the priest I didn't want to be a Catholic any more). My experience of angels was very different — I had a strong awareness of angels' presence and I found them very loving, nurturing, and quite close.

The place where I had the most joy in angels was at the Salvos. I was about fourteen and though Mum didn't really think that was a good idea, I'd sneak off to the Salvos church, and there was the singing and the joy and I was aware of a very strong angel presence there.

But those experiences were always at times of pain. One of my reasons for going up the tree, and being with the fairies was to remove myself from difficulties between my mother and my father. Or my brother's asthma attacks. Once I knew he was going to be okay, alive, I'd be up the tree just to be away from the emotion of it all. Also to be away from my mother. The first time I really wanted to be up the tree was when my mother accidentally threw a pan of boiling hot water over my back. Once all the medical things had been attended to, I wanted to go up there. It was difficult, of course, because I had dressings on my back.

Those experiences of fairies, (when I was quite young) and of angels (later, when we went to live in the outback) happened at times of pain. We went to the outback because of my brother's asthma; also, I think Mum needed a break from Dad. But I was desperately unhappy. I was away from my Dad and my dog.

Emma

I was one of those kids for whom animals were more important than people in many ways. Even though we went to see my Dad in the city, I could just sense that the estrangement between him and Mum was getting stronger and stronger. In fact, they were both quite content within their own lives, and just meeting for holidays. I remember Dad took me to see a Western and I just howled and carried on about the horses — I didn't care about the Indians or the cowboys getting shot. So, being separated from my dog was a very big thing for me. The presence of angels was strongest around the most painful times.

I felt very much like the world of people wasn't a comfortable place for me. I don't remember any friends. I'm not saying I didn't relate to people, but I don't remember them. I remember being more in the world of animals, plants. The really good things around that outback town were the interesting plants. I found the trees really fascinating. And the salt bush — I spent hours examining the salt bush.

Mum very soon got me a dog. It was a way to help me have something to relate to, so she must have had an innate understanding. Often, though, I would drag animals home, saying they followed me. Cats with ringworm (I spent half my life with ringworms on my face) and dogs. Mum would get rid of the dogs but, quite often, the cats stayed. We ended up with quite a few.

I felt very different from other people. Very alienated. I don't know that I would have used the word "alienated" back then, but I certainly felt different. As though there wasn't a place for me in the world as it was. So having the company of angels was a very nice thing. I think feeling apart from other people did shape my life.

A person I really liked spending time with and who I did feel a relationship with, was my grandfather, Mum's Dad and my only grandparent who was alive. Though I didn't see him very often I was very close to him. When I was sixteen, I decided to go and live with him. I packed my bags and got on the train. I don't know where I got the money from, but I had enough for a ticket. When I look back, I think about poor Mum — I mean how hard it was to see your sixteen-year-old daughter just get on a train and go! Poof! Anyway, I got there, and grandfather said, "What are you doing here? Does your mother know?"

He took me to stay with an aunt, because his place wasn't really suitable. He made it perfectly clear to me that bigger kids weren't his cup of tea at all —

that he liked little ones. That didn't work for me, but it shaped that experience, I think even more, to watch out for the illusion of belonging. I think that was the big thing for me, the big lesson. It wasn't easy at the time, but I got caught on that roller coaster.

I ended up in Sydney. I wasn't quite seventeen, but they just had a thorough cleanout at Callan Park Psychiatric Hospital and I was looking for work. Anyone who was reasonably intelligent, who looked like they wouldn't hit people, was suitable to employ. The authorities didn't care how old we were, even though you were supposed to be seventeen. I was there for a while, but certainly wasn't old enough, emotionally, to do psych nursing.

So I left there and pottered around and did a few different jobs, and then ended up in another city. And that's when I started psych nursing. Through wandering around I found the niche where I felt I had something to contribute, the place that could be long-lasting work for me.

One of the things around mental health nursing, and I think that for many people at that same time, being different was okay. Being different, you still could have a sense of belonging to this group; it didn't impinge.

And in some ways, having that different experience or that differentness — probably because my experience was not different from a lot of other people's, that feeling of differentness, separateness in many ways — allows one to have a stronger understanding of people in that place. It has impinged on their lives and their way of being in the world much more than getting or having a mental illness. So it was a place where differentness was a strength. Maybe having ended up in the world of healers, it again is a strength.

I'm very content with that now. I do have a strong sense of belonging within my healing community; within the human place, and also in the esoteric — the spirit place. So all of these things have come together.

Regarding my coming to know the spirit place, my experience was much more a coming into it — a growing into it. I know for some people something very dramatic happens, and suddenly they have a very strong experience of the spirit place, or spirit world. For me it was more gradual.

When I was younger, I was truer to being a Capricorn — very sceptical; looking at things twice and saying, "Okay, how practical is this?". But I never lived that. Even though I thought it, I didn't live that. I had a dichotomy between what was going on in the head, and what was going on in practice.

Emma

In practice, it was more like, "That experience looks interesting — I'll go and work there". Or, "I'll go and be there". And it has nothing to do with the practical world of possessions, or of gaining deep respect, or those sorts of things. Building a career. It's like, "That looks interesting — I'll go and do that". So living in that space has made for a very interesting time.

When I look back, (and many people have had this experience) I know the intuition one uses in nursing was help and guidance from spirit. I have no doubt at all. And people would say things like, "I don't know where you get that radar from". And this was a time before intuition was fashionable — you know, in the sixties and seventies. It was safer to call it "radar", "antennas". "Your antennas are working well, today".

But that wasn't an awareness, now I look back. The awareness began probably gradually after my father died. My father was very special to me, and he died twenty years ago.

It was around then that I began to have more of an awareness of what I called "a parallel place", a place of spirit. Just before Dad died, a friend went to the spiritualist church where a healing session was happening, and I took my daughter along — she had a lot of throat and chest problems. I thought it was bronchitis. So I went to the healing service, and a spiritualist, Ralph, put his hands on her. "This child," he said, "has the most intense tonsillitis I've ever felt in my life!". I thought, "What is this man talking about? This child has bronchitis!". But of course when I looked down her throat, she had huge pustules for tonsils. So I became curious about how this man could do this.

That was when it really "began" began — began again, or whatever, in this lifetime. The awareness. I went to a few services at the spiritualist church and had some healings. That's when my awareness increased.

Dad died not long after that and I think it was the catalyst; helped me tune in more. This awareness that was just there — I could sort of see it out of the corner of my eye. But I think Dad's death did that — I could tune in and be a lot more aware.

It's interesting that my husband's death didn't do that. I have no idea why. And maybe it was because it was like... the last death, sort of thing. My grandfather had died, my husband had died, and then my father died. Like all the guys who were really important in my life keeled over one after the other, so to speak — in the space of six-years. Now I look at it, Dad's death was probably more like the last straw. Or the best straw, so to speak.

Emma

I didn't do anything with that awareness. I just knew it was there. And my daughter would ask me questions about grandpa, or about Daddy, like, "What's grandfather doing?", "What's Daddy doing?". I tuned in and I'd say, "Oh, well, grandpa's having a really good time". I wasn't making it up! I could really get a sense of what he was... or what, spiritually, his experience was and then translate it into three-, or four-, or five-year-old terms.

It felt natural to get that information. I didn't feel like I was speaking, or communicating individually with my Dad, or with anybody — with Grandpa. It was more like I would put a question out there, and the information would be given to me. It was much less personal than it would be now. I was so excited, the first time I had an individual conversation, on a spirit level. It was like, "Oh, whoopee!"

I think it's a part of this growing in, growing into — it felt really natural. That's the thing I look back on. It felt like an easy, natural way to be in the world. I didn't even think about or question it. And, now I look at it, it wasn't for me — it was for my daughter. That probably allowed me, or helped me feel more comfortable with the process. It wasn't, "Give me some information for me".

How was I able to distinguish information from imagining? I think this is one that all people who get information or pictures or whatever, need to think about, or need to have a sense of more than think about. As soon as you start thinking about it, you get into imagination and ego. The thing that happened for me was that my daughter would ask me a question, and the words would come out of my mouth. I didn't think about it.

I remember going to see a wonderful healer I used to work with, and she said, "You know that fine mind of yours?" and I thought I was about to get a lovely compliment. "It is a menace," she said. "An absolute menace! It gets in the way of letting the flow happen." And that's what differentiated the process; where I would say, "I wonder what is going to happen to me next week" and I would think about it, and imagine it. Without that "wonder" coming into it (like when my daughter asked me a question) the words would come out of my mouth. I wouldn't think. I wouldn't think.

I'd be feeling very peaceful, relaxed, and at ease. If I am in that thinking space, my body changes, gets a little bit tighter, because I need a tight body for my mind to work. I feel different, physically.

Emma

It's still a very similar process. But it can be much more individual, now. The first time I ever heard an individual, well, got a question from an individual — it was a case study for my healing modality course. The lass was pregnant and I was doing chakra work on her, and I came to putting my hand over the sacral area and a question popped straight into my head.

Oh, golly, this little... I mean, the soul wasn't there, but the little soul that was probably going to go into this body, had just asked me a question — "Am I still going to have the same awareness when I am born, when I'm in the physical?" I had to say I didn't know.

So the awareness can be much more specific and a feeling of an individual being close. Whereas in the early times (I mean, it was only twenty years ago — not very long) it was more like a sense of being supported. A sense of being supported and cared about, and helped through. Now, it can be much more individual — like a particular person, or a particular being in spirit. At times I certainly felt supported by angels' wings, or somebody's hand on my shoulder, or... So, that's more individual than a generalised sense of something.

I know that before I had any visual cues to what was happening with people, I still had a knowing. I could look at somebody and know there was a lot of red in their field. I'd say that was the skill that I was born with, like knowing that the baker's horse wouldn't stand on me, or those sorts of things. I maintained that awareness, whereas the others have developed over time.

When I first started working with healing techniques, that was very much the learning of the practical. It's been a steady evolution. The other senses developed over a period of time, and I think it came after the practical skills were there. It was like, "Okay, she's got all those. Let's develop the other aspects".

Now, as I've become more and more involved in the spiritual aspects, and living in that spiritual space, I can do that quite easily. The everyday humanness can be a bit of a struggle, and a challenge. The task is keeping that balance and seeing how this spiritual experiencing has communicated with my more mundane life. In fact, it's interesting, and I often quote Jung — to remember that we are spirits having a human experience — not humans having a spiritual experience. To remember that we're in this human experience to learn whatever it is we need to learn. And part of mine is the balance between living in the human everyday world, and living in the spirit world.

Emma

One friend said she could actually see me moving right into that spiritual space, and that I really needed to make a choice about whether I wanted other people to look after me or not. Because that's what I could do — and they would, because of my contribution to their welfare on a spiritual level. But, of course, the human side of Emma took over there. "No way, Jose! No way! I want to do it myself, my way!". And my friend said, "Well, you'd better make some choices then, hadn't you?".

It helped me come back to that place of balance. It's fine to think about what you're going to do on a practical level, but you need to put things into action. To say, "Well this is what I think I'll do, so I can pay the rent and eat, and all that". But that is still coming into balance. And it's just about there.

I think there are some great gifts in it for my mundane experience. Like when I'm working as a casual agency nurse with people in the mental health system. It is very positive and lends some richness to what I am able to offer to people in the system. Also sometimes, it's helpful for the staff, depending on where they're at.

It also allows me to feel at ease in the system. I've probably spent a lot of years with a lot of animosity and anger with the system, feeling it didn't serve the people it was there to serve. Now, I think there are things I could see done differently, but I don't feel the same angst, drive, anger and intolerance that I felt in the past. That is good for me, and is good for the people I'm working with. They're some of the very positive things.

* * *

Probably one of my major lessons is that the bigger picture is so important. This is the idea of not getting tied up with the little incidents. You go in, and are looking at the overall meaning for every individual in that situation, instead of what's affecting me, and you, and Mary. The lesson is more around the contributing where one can, and providing unconditional love where one can't.

I've talked about the positive aspects but also need to look at the challenging ones. For me, they are in the physical — money, providing for one's being. As the saying goes, "Before enlightenment — carry water, chop wood; after enlightenment — carry water, chop wood". The life doesn't change. I've just read, *After Ecstasy Comes the Laundry*, and it talks about the fact that even if we have wonderful profound experiences, it doesn't change

Emma

our everyday life. The laundry still needs to be done; there still needs to be money to pay the rent.

This realisation is difficult for me because of the illusion that being in a spiritual realm — or being in this place — seems to negate having to look after the other section. As if it's all taken care of. Now, I know on one level it is taken care of. But on another level I am required to actively participate in this human life.

It's not about grounding, I think. I probably see grounding as something being very different. The more experiences of spirit I have, the more important it is I remain grounded. Because what I wish to offer people who come for healing, or students, or people in my life, needs to be grounded grounded advice, grounded treatments, grounded teaching, grounded whatever.

Groundedness is really important, and I can be that when it comes to relating, or when I'm in that healing place. Then I'm in my work place. Now I think about it, maybe I become ungrounded when I'm thinking of, or being in my human place of living in this world in a material way. Maybe, even though I see myself, or know that I am grounded in many other situations, this material section is one when I'm not.

I think part of it is a belief. The more I have been involved in this path, the less I have, on a material level. Or the less I have around me, on a material level. Now I look back, I would cheerfully, say, I've given away at least half of what I had. I've never been a great one for possessions and I've always been good at clearing out. When my daughter decided to no longer live in the same house, there was no longer a need for many of the things I had.

For several years I was living as a contributing guest in a lady's house. That was very much an exchange of energy. The same thing with the next place I lived in for about a year — I paid the electricity, and did sessions for this person, and her father and her mother, and so on.

Connection with nature does touch me deeply. There is my experience of shamanism, although formerly I've never really felt a connection with the shamanic way of being. I just thought, "Oh, well, you know, the Native Americans from the US have had a great experience, and they're a wonderful people". And one of the techniques we use in my modality is a Hopi technique — back technique. So, it's been like a detached interest in shamanism, I would say.

Emma

But a friend kept reminding me, saying, "Your connection with the spirit of the animals — not just the physical being of the animals, is very shamanic". She even gave me some medicine cards, which I promptly gave away — I was probably resisting that. I tried some shamanic journeys, in a group setting and, while I thought it was very relaxing to lie on the floor, that was about the best of my experience.

When a few of my healing colleagues had seen a particular shamanic worker, and had very profound experiences, I thought I'd give it one more go. I found it a most incredible experience. The session put another piece in the puzzle for me, in that I had had a sense of animals being around. I had one cat who was the most difficult, obstreperous cat I might ever come across in my life and a few times I had a sense of him being around. I'd just say, "That was nice," and wouldn't investigate it any more. And so having this session with this shamanic worker just slid it into a place of, "This is another part of the journey"; it wasn't like it was separate, so it's bringing things together, pulling it, tying it all together.

* * *

After my shamanic session I spent time looking back at my experiences as a child and wrote about them and my connection with the animals. I thought that gave my experience as a child more perspective. It was the transformational journey, where the journey that you're going to have in this lifetime begins, but it's important for us to be able to see where it fits. And for me, that's where it fits, in that very strong connection with nature, and with the spirit of nature as well as the physical.

My power animal is the wolf, the teacher. I thought, "Oh, God!", a bit, but another part of me thought that the wolf would probably be the creature I looked to the most, as being able to be in the pack as well as being able to be alone. That's another important aspect for me, as coming from that place of feeling very separate and different, to now being able to be separate and different but also part of the group. I am part of the group, and the family.

A friend gave me a little bit of a razz about being so detached about shamanism, and I told her about having had a lot of experiences around an owl a month earlier. Interestingly, she said that she sensed a wolf cub around me and it was an indication of me integrating all those experiences as a youngster, or as a cub, or whatever, in being alone in the world. She says also that she sees me very much as a mother wolf — as the one who's protective.

Emma

I was also hearing owls a lot; I heard an owl as I was going to sleep. My night ritual is to read a few pages of a book, then lie down to sleep, and often do a meditation. And sometimes, I've ended up in a place like a celestial college. I can't describe it any more than that. I know it's a college, and it's very stark, and it's got lots of marble.

One time, I was in a room with the most magnificent writing desks and on each one was a pad and a lovely pen. I knew which desk was mine and, as I sat down and looked at the paper, I saw an owl — a little figurine owl — stamped in the corner of each page.

It was a monogram, like the very round shape that doesn't look like an owl at all. And I was told to write — write the book. Then I came back into my body and in the morning I heard the owl again. I thought, "I'll write that one down do some work with it, sometime". I'd say part of it was a prompt to get me to journal; part of it was about how quite some time ago I had the push to sit down and write my story.

So nature definitely does it for me. I've got lots of good stories. One happened in the US —in Alaska, a place I find very moving. I remember how excited I was flying into Anchorage — it was eleven o'clock at night, but it was still bright as daylight — and we flew in over the snow and the ice. I saw the northern star — which I'd never seen before, even though I'd been to the US on quite a few occasions. I think it was possible because it was such a clear night and I was looking out the window at just the right time. That alone gave me a great sense of connection to this place. Lots and lots of wonderful things happened there.

I stayed with a lady who was an Indian (not an Inuit — they live a lot further north). But — like many Aboriginal people here — she had only discovered her "Indian-ness" when she turned forty and was deeply proud of her identity. I was greatly privileged to stay with her and her wonderful husband.

One evening, I went to bed, and I had a great sense of loss — you know, being around these two people who loved each other so much. I had a great sense of being alone and being rejected because I took my husband's death as a rejection. I thought, "He doesn't want to hang around".

Another great love of my life, has also decided he didn't want to stay around. I felt very alone and it was interesting. It certainly happens for me that at

Emma

those moments there doesn't seem to be any spiritual support around at all. It's like you need to face the experience alone.

All the wounds, all those wounds of relationship were very open, and raw. But the healing came from nature. Again, I saw something I'd never seen before — a bald eagle in the sky. There was a fairly large window and I was lying down, asking for help to work with this wound. A bald eagle flew past, in what seemed to be slow motion. It was as if, at the time, the wound was keeping me earthbound. "I've got a wound, and I can't fly. One of my wings is sore."

And it was a warm healing balm of some sort — like honey coming into my etheric body but I couldn't feel it physically. It was more on an energetic level. And that was the beginning of that healing. Then the bald eagle was gone.

It was the beginning again and I remembered that all healing is a process. It's not like a magical one-off lightning and thunder experience.

I've been changed in that the prospect of relationship is not so scary. Before, I didn't consider the possibility. I remember hearing this healer say how all healers are going to be asexual in times to come, and I said, "Yeah! That's it, that's good! "

* * *

I think being able to bring a grounded presence to most situations that don't involve me — even though it's an external process — that ability to internalise, to be in that space, has been an important part of the transformation. Having such a strong connection to the spirit place has helped me to look at the bigger picture.

I'm certainly a lot less intense and more mellow. The word's not "patient" or even "tolerant", it's "allowing". One of my least favourite characteristics of myself was a sense of being able to protect people and doing it through controlling what happened to them. Now, there's more of an allowing way with people that I love. For instance, my mother broke her hip recently, and my brother rang me. Previously I would be there and make sure it was alright, that the hospital people were treating her okay, that she'd had enough pain killers, tra-la-la. Now, even if I feel very much this is my mother, and I know she's in pain, I know this is her journey. What I can do, I will do. But I don't need to be there to control it. That's certainly been a change.

Emma

People keep saying we have choices; I can't imagine not making the choices I've made — even though I do say it's the universe giving me a little boot up the backside.

In the beginning these were changes that weren't gradual, like facing the things that I feared, — not having much money working as a student general nurse, my concerns about my intellect (I saw intellect and education as the same). When I first went to university, I had a huge fear of not measuring up, not being intelligent enough, because I felt I wasn't educated. So these were some of the bigger fears, and the change was not so gradual.

Much of the rest of the journey has been gradual, and these choices have been mine. I've chosen to come to this part of the world and start this project and help nurture my modality's community in this part of the country. It was an active involvement in the process for me. Some of it was scary, but, "Okay, scary. So?".

There is, also, a sense of inevitability. Not so much about individual actions, maybe, but about the process. And it is that belief that we do make a choice before incarnating (I don't know about the word incarnation), or being, coming into this physical realm, or this lifetime, there are some choices that are made. I don't know that each individual experience is chosen, but the long-term things are chosen. And the lessons — it's more like the lessons are chosen. And how they come into being, well... that's the inevitability of it.

Still, it doesn't mean I wouldn't have had a choice to not do this. Now I can't imagine not doing it, but it doesn't mean I wouldn't have had a choice. I'm sure in previous times this soul has said, "Oh, I'm not going down that road – I'm going down this road."

And that's where we're back to the place of my mind saying one thing, and my physically doing another. The to and fro of, "That would be sensible, and that would be logical," and then doing something else. I hope I'm now getting the two to work in unison.

I don't think this journey as a healer is a tough road. I think it's one of great joy, and many, many blessings. I think I make it tough, sometimes, on that physical... the belief I alluded to before, that belief that if you're a spiritual being, then, you know, you can't necessarily be materially successful.

I do see hundreds of people being able to do it, and I know, logically, it can be done, it is done, and that there's nothing that states a spiritual person can't be materially comfortable. And I do like my comforts, so that's where

Emma

I think I'm the one who makes it tough — I don't think the universe is making it tough. I'm the one who is making it tough.

About the blessings. I think it's having that sense... (I'm getting a bit teary, here) of being blessed enough to have awareness of the spirit world; that knowing support of spirit in the work, in the things I'm doing. To connect with people on that etheric level. Being able to... say, for my Mum — being able to provide healing on an etheric level for her; some pain drain on her hip, and help her in that way. Previously I would have felt helpless, and hopeless, worried, and anxious. Now there is something I can do. That's a great gift, a great blessing.

To be able to meet with all the people that I associated with that have that same very strong sense of spirit, and understanding and willingness to listen, is a great blessing. My "family" with my modality is a great blessing — being able to relate to people like the leader in my modality. There are many blessings in this.

That's been very empowering. From that kid who felt a helplessness like seeing the "naturalness" of nature, where creatures can get hurt, eaten, left to die. And though I know the same things happen now, I don't feel that same sense of helplessness. Because I understand spirit thinks in thousands of years — not our lifetimes.

And the other blessing (though I don't always live it) is that grace — grace of being in that place. The other great blessing is being able to facilitate other people's journeys, in the teaching of my modality. That's a wonderful blessing.

And the same thing with being in a healer role. I've been empowered, to help other people to be empowered — if that's where they wish to be. And that, to me, is what nursing is truly about. So that's where, for me, the nurse and the healer is the same being — they're not different.

* * *

About the shadow. I think that there are some aspects of the shadow that help us clarify our journeys. When it comes up, it's important to explore it. I'm not going to go digging for it, just like I'm not going digging in past lives. If something comes up, then great — then it's time for me to learn that lesson. And that's been my experience of shadow.

Emma

There is some darkness in our world — it's not all wonderful light. I mean, how could we know the light without the dark? And I have experienced some of that — I feel it's been personally directed. Again, there's always learning in it. "Okay, what didn't I do? What did I do? Did I maintain a connection with that person, or with that situation, when?".

Recently, something came up around a person and a situation that I felt very strongly I was disconnected from. I was sitting at the kitchen table, talking to someone, and saying, "And of course, I know I really want to reconnect" — and I'd actually said it! So I knew there was a part of me that was maintaining that connection, thought it wasn't to my benefit. So, it was more of an unconscious thing.

So I think, for whenever those situations come along for me, it's a learning. "Okay, does there need to be more protection? Am I holding on to something here?".

Around the personal shadow — for me, it's been a very important part of the process, to be able to integrate the parts of myself that could be called the shadow. Maybe some anger. So it's important to integrate those things, and have them as part of the whole, instead of pushing them back and saying, "Oh, no, I don't want to be like that. I've got to be all goodness and light."

So what's involved in integrating? Well, first, being aware and acknowledging instead of saying, "Oops, I'm having a bad day today" and making it an abnormality. But rather acknowledging — this has happened; or I've behaved in this and in this and this way — and maybe getting some idea of where that might have come from. Not worrying it, like a dog at a bone, but saying, "Well, okay, this is an aspect of me. Where does it fit?". And the very positive thing is that integrating. For me, it was a part of accepting myself as I am — who I am. Being able to be a lot more tender, and accepting, and loving of myself led to more self care.

It helped cut across some of my difficult behaviour — I had a job to do and I'd keep going, and going, and going, and the job ended up being more important than the person doing it. By integrating that shadow side, it has helped lessen some of that type of behaviour that I'm not very content with.

The other thing needed is, that on the personal journey, on the moving through this life as we have it now, being more tender, self-loving, and self-caring. I believe that has helped me be more authentically caring with

Emma

others. Not because it was my job, or because the mother in me wanted or needed to be that way but because it was the more authentic self. That was what I wanted to say about those shadow aspects, because I believe it was a very important aspect for me.

* * *

About connection and protection — I think they are significant. It took me a long time, because of the belief that being grounded and centred was the protection; was all the protection one really required. I still encourage people at the beginning levels of healing practice to do that. And not just for protection, but for all aspects of their life, protection included.

I listened to one particular healer, who I have a great deal of respect for, who came to learn our modality, who works with that shadow side quite a lot — with entities, with (what would I say) discarnate aspects of the world and the spirit life. I went to one of her workshops, and certainly experienced some of the things she was talking about.

As I started working with other folk, this came up on several occasions, particularly around thought forms, which is something we use in our modality quite a lot. And there was a lot of personal experience of thought forms for myself, in being in a place, and attracting more thought forms of that type. If I was feeling angry, or discontent about something, thought forms of that nature might be there.

Something had occurred in our modality that I was feeling hurt about at first, and then, quite angry. It had to do with abuse from a person quite senior in the modality. And I thought, "Well, ta, ta, ta..." But during that time, my anger increased. It was out of proportion with the experience that I'd had. So I did some clearing work on myself, that I learned from another healer, and became really aware that a lot of thought forms had been attracted because of my anger, my place of anger.

My field was full of these thought forms. And that was before I had any visual experiences of a thought form. It was more like a sense of drippy magnets attached to my field, or within my field, attached to aspects of my field — particularly (being such a thinking person) around the mental layer. So I was thinking anger, and feeling anger. It was very interesting.

At times now — though much rarer than before, thank goodness — I get on the treadmill of thinking. "And if I said so-and-so, then so-and-so would happen, and such and such. And then they would say, and then I would say,

Emma

and tra la la la." At those times I will check my field, to see what's happening, because I think that thought forms are very attracted to that sort of stuff, and their presence just increases it.

Since I did that workshop, it feels a more natural response to situations. It's not so much that I've added a string to my bow, because one of the things this healer said was, "You wouldn't be here unless this was going to start coming into your practice".

I've had some experiences where I became aware of a shadow, or an entity, or whatever one would want to call it, with a person and I just told by my guidance that that's an awareness, and to leave it alone. This happened with a young man I was looking after, who had a closed head injury. His behaviour had been very aggressive; he'd even broken a nurse's arm. I was sitting with him on night shift, and became aware of this. And I asked, "What do I need to do?", and was told to not do anything. Told that it wasn't anything I could help with, or was intended to help with. So, yes, I have an awareness when around it.

I've referred to an inner guidance I have access to. I talked about the beginnings of this type of experience, but that's different, because that's more like outside information. This is more like what I would call a "higher self" information. Not even information — a higher self... well, "guidance" is probably the word (it's just that I hear that word so much, "and my guidance told me", and I think, "Whoa, yuck!")

One key experience around this was quite funny, and where I had an awareness of the individuality of my higher self. I have a friend who comes from this school that believes the higher self has a name. They call it a "breakthrough". And I was fascinated, because she's referred to her higher self by name all the time. I was working with this person and she gets guidance, which is really great.

Then another friend, who'd been to the same courses, had the same experiences. And all of these higher selves have very dignified names. I thought, "Oh, isn't this lovely? This is cute, it's very nice. I wonder if this could happen with me?".

And as I was sitting reflecting on this, I heard the line from a song, "My name is Jack, and I live in the back of the Greta Garbo home for wayward boys and girls". And I thought, "Now, come on! That can't be it! I mean, Jack is not very dignified". And there was this absolute joy, and laughter. The absolute joy

Emma

and laughter was of me, but not in me. It's a part of the aspects, all of the aspects of me, but it didn't come from within me.

So, to me that was a sort of breakthrough, but not like the one my friend talked about. And yet, I think that one of the things that hearing helped me to do, is actually listen a lot more closely and carefully — to even some of the everyday stuff, like, "Ring so-and-so"; or, "It's time you rang so-and- so". And the tone of some of the inner guidance has changed — it's more humorous.

There is process here, where I differentiate between my common everyday processes of consciousness, and something which is of a different magnitude, or order, or quality.

What's really interesting, is the fact that the healers I know who I feel "have it all together", speaking from other experience as well as personal experience — are grounded in themselves and in their work, and are able to articulate some of the differentiations. They are the ones who have had the transformational experiences; there has been a journey, as against those who have the sudden experience of spirit.

I think all of us — all of us healers, particularly me, get to a stage where sometimes there isn't a strong differentiation between ordinary thinking and guidance. As I was saying, sometimes I'd be thinking, "All right, this is the way to go", and find myself doing something else. I'm sure that was the guidance pushing me, but without me being aware of it.

So, yes, I do sometimes find that I haven't thought, "Yes, I'll do this, and then I'll do that, and then this will happen". It really does happen when you do that, anyway. I suppose that's because an awareness of that guidance is important for me, and for the way I am in the world.

I had an experience with a nurse healer who did numerology for me, and she said, "What are you doing?" I said, "Why?", and she said, "Well, you've got the Arrow of scepticism right through the middle of your numerology, so it's interesting that you're in this work". She then said, "But one of things about that is that once you're in it, you're in it".

And I understood that there isn't a scepticism, there isn't a lack of belief. I think it's because I've been very kindly treated by the spirit world, in that it's been a gradual process. So there hasn't been that major, "Oh, do I believe this, or do I not believe this?". You know, when I hear people saying, "And I heard a voice saying so-and-so and such-and-such, and I thought 'Is it my

Emma

imagination, or not?'" I've been very fortunate in that that's not one of my challenges.

I suppose my biggest challenge is not not being like my peers in nursing I never really wanted to be like all my peers, many of whom are very institutionalised — but it's feeling that very strong separation from them. As I went further and further along this esoteric road, the place where I had felt comfortable, I had felt a part of it. Belonged to it even though I still felt different. Ironically, the biggest challenge for me was that as I evolved as a healer I no longer did feel a part of that. I no longer do — even when I go and work in a ward area.

And, again, perhaps it's on the esoteric that I've become distant from my colleagues. As, for example, I feel that a lass with post-natal depression whom I spent a little bit of time with, that a part of the soul had just detached from her, during the birthing process. So, giving her all the medication under the sun, and having a regulated crying regime for this child, was really not going to do anything for either of them. I felt it was like being very different from what the traditional psychiatric scene was saying. So that's probably been a challenge. And even though I've laughed about it, how I overheard my colleagues once saying, "And she used to be so sensible".

That's okay, too. I think that was a challenge at the time. And it's fine, now.

Emma

Chapter Four

ANGELIQUE

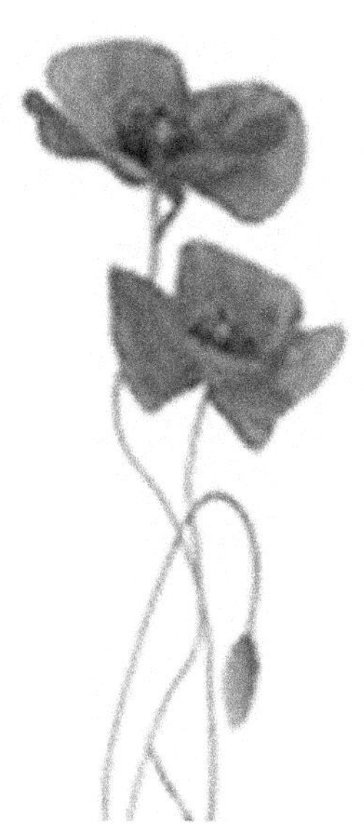

I have not met Angelique, although we connected deeply when we spoke. I found out about her from a flyer advertising workshops she had offered some time earlier, on inner journeying. I tracked her down online, and we spoke on an international phone call. I was struck by Angelique's sharing: how she was an explorer of many realities, how she was so focused on deepening self-knowledge, and by how connection, in its many forms, and finding balance amongst the different realities were central to her journey as a nurse healer.

In the beginning of studying nursing, I was also studying Sufism, and was very quickly involved in a Sufi healing circle where I received initiations into the healing art according to Sufi understanding. So being a nurse and being a healer were part of me from the beginning of my nursing studies.

However, I understood from the beginning that there was no place in the hospital for what I was learning in the Sufi healing school. It wasn't something I could apply. The mentality and the structure of the hospital were not receptive to it. I completely accepted that, even though some patients were already addressing things in a different way within themselves, and that would have been an opening for a different approach, alongside their hospital therapies.

The Sufi approach was one of very deep exploring, and more than healing. It also meant going into different aspects of being, specifically the phenomenon called reincarnation. It is part of something that's discovered and, very quickly, I may enter into areas that are taboo for some people. Yet, for others it's completely understood and accepted, even though many have their own interpretations.

I've been working, and learning about healing energies, and practising on people outside the hospital sphere. I might be touching someone's back, and be getting images. And when I'd relate those images to the person, it would make total sense to them. I would learn, in this way, that people have charges stored in their body that are connected to events. Those charges, or deposits, can be called to the surface, or called to our consciousness and, in that way, be released.

I've been discovering I have had lives before this one and I've received images from those lives with emotional charges or, simply, information. So, besides healing, this idea of reincarnation is only one of the next fields that come with it.

It was opening different things in my dreams; different layers. And some of the challenges I have faced — in this long, ongoing process — are to do with discovering that not all we see and encounter is of a benevolent nature.

Angelique

Especially with diseases — physical and mental. It resonates with areas that are in the astral fields. And in the astral fields there are many different energies that can behave in ways that may be very challenging — to your own health, to your own focus, to your own wish to be aligned with something that I would call "Source", or Christ, or anything in that direction. The challenges are right there.

I feel this ongoing story is just the nature of being on planet Earth, where different levels penetrate our reality. Sometimes we pick up on it; sometimes we don't.

I've been working as a private nurse in many different people's homes, and very often they've been old houses; maybe in the family for a couple of hundred years; in mansions, and castles and more simply, family houses. I have experienced, especially connected to people who are dying, a whole structure of demands that I've been able to see, and sense from the spirits around the dying person, who would want the situation around the death to be a certain way. Or that a dying person is describing what they are experiencing.

One particular example is a lady from a very wealthy family, who lived in a mansion next to a castle. Before she died, she saw men in black suits, dressed meticulously, and she understood that they were waiting for her. The presence of these entities (that's what I call them) would bring a feeling in the room that was not always comfortable to me. Having to deal with that as well as being able to take care of her, while shielding myself from parts of a very intense process was challenging; being present at the most extreme process in the human life — birth and death.

It takes a lot from a nurse to be so close to a person who is dying; there are a lot of energies from the unseen realms the person is processing, and working in an environment that does not appreciate the knowledge, or even the sensitivity to this, makes things difficult. I'm talking about the unseen entities relating to me in an adverse way, or a person demanding certain ways of doing things.

As a nurse you are already very flexible, but not to the degree that you have to completely let go of your own insights. So it's not only the patient you're dealing with. You have to protect yourself — often, actually — to be able to go on living your own life in your own authentic way and not to be of service in such a way that you lose yourself in your job. It takes tremendous

Angelique

strength. Besides the physical strain, there is mental and emotional and psychic strain and many nurses have breakdowns.

Often I have seen that when people die, I can sense loved ones coming close, and something like a landscape opens up, in a different world. I can sense whether the person passing over was going into a good field, or not so. I've been with a dying patient whose energy was very powerful after the death. They were a very angry person before they died, and that anger was unleashed over the whole house.

Sometimes I care for the bereaved if there is a partner left behind, but in this case, I didn't stay behind to support the deceased's partner, because the energy, and the very tangible anger of the woman's spirit chased me out of the house.

How I respond depends on the environment, and how far the environment is open for that. In this particular situation, the woman had been an extremely forceful personality, dominating her husband and the environment. After her stroke, she couldn't speak for three years, was paralysed and bed-ridden. She could not exercise any of her anger, desire for control.

So, in all situations, it's not just about learning the limitations of my powers (the limit is within myself) but this was a very clear situation I did not want to go deeper into. I knew my limits exactly — I'm functioning as a nurse, there to do my job, but nothing more.

There are other people who are open — open to receive a massage, or a foot massage, or even healing touch. It is an ongoing process, to learn where your boundaries are, energetically, for yourself. To know within yourself, to a degree at least, who you are, and what you are about.

Here's a more positive story from my nursing work. I was looking after two children whose mother was having a nervous breakdown. The oldest boy, who was three, was very smart, and had a tremendous temper. If anything didn't go his way, he'd bang his head against the wall, literally, until his mother gave in. When he was born, his mother had had a difficult birth with a tremendous amount of pain. What I could see was that this boy had a hole in his aura. And a lot of things — uncontrolled things — were moving in and out of that hole.

And I became aware that he was aware of that. And there came a point where we could both look at it and, very playfully, I started to polish up that hole. And it was like a ritual, for a couple of days, where we would polish up that big hole in his aura until it started to get smaller. He was starting to feel better in his body, was more at ease, and having fewer tantrums.

I've walked many paths. One that I've been studying with a lady from America and that has been extremely helpful to me, is "trance postures". I am also, now, teaching this. These are postures usually from pastoralists horticultural societies, who still were in contact, in harmony, with agricultural and nomadic life. They used postures — sitting, standing, or holding their hands — in a specific way. When someone shook a rattle, with a frequency that evoked Theta brain waves, it could invoke a trance.

You would go into an experience from your inner self, to discover more about yourself, and your psychic environment. Information through these postures has been tremendously helpful for me.

Earlier in my life I did go through difficult times. Being sensitive, there's always a challenge. Actually, it's a very difficult and sometimes confusing path. My sensitivity is about feelings, and also I'm very visual.

I've been meditating since I was sixteen — when I was with the Sufis — and before that with my mother. I meditated every day for an hour (half-an-hour in the morning and again before I went to sleep) and that's been a very powerful practice. I'm not doing that any more; life itself has become meditation.

When I work, many fields overlap, or intermingle. The difficulty I might have been experiencing is sometimes connected to not knowing my boundaries. The spirit, or inner vision does not stop with my body. I close my eyes and I'm looking energetically at my environment and my environment is moving through me. And I am in there. I need to be anchored to what I know I am. And, at the same time, feel and know that the doors are open. Sometimes the information I receive is clouded; sometimes, it's very clear. The lifelong path and practice is to discern which is which. My basic rule is, "When something does not feel good — be aware!"

I have been sharing this when I give workshops and I am able to create a field with a group. And within the field, is all the room and space to explore all this, and get a deeper insight. So, from being a loner, I have become a teacher. And I'm discovering a lot of people in the workshops have similar experiences; we learn from each other.

Angelique

Since I was a child, I have been known within my family as different. Even though, many gifts have come, have been recognised, from my mother's side, and from my maternal grandmother. And perhaps there is one sibling, or two, who is more open, and is inviting this in.

I've been pioneering, as I see it, on my own, without fear. I am not a fearful person, so if I see entities coming to me, good or bad, I don't run away, or go into psychosis, or… While I'm vulnerable, I'm also very strong and single-minded. I've been pursuing a path, and a calling. I've read a lot trying to gain an understanding for myself. Books by Yogananda were very helpful to me at an early age.

I am lucky enough to have remembered my own birth. And as a little child I would practise going back, maybe every week, or couple of weeks, into my birth — I wanted to remember it when I grew up. And also I remember my first dreams, when I was three or four years old.

Many years ago, I had a remarkable incident. I was in hospital with double pneumonia and was in a coma but the doctors sent me home, actually to die. It was my parents who kept me alive. As this was some decades ago, there were no suction systems at the time, so (be warned, this is not a pleasant detail), my parents would take turns sucking stuff out of my nose, so I would stay alive.

Now, despite the fact I was in a coma, I've been able to retrieve where I was in that time. I've been through a death experience, and have been making new arrangements, or new alignments for this life. So this sensitivity was supported by the inner worlds.

As a child, I had friends — invisible friends — and I'd play with them, knowing they were not from this realm. Also, my dreams have been teachers for me. If I look at the sequence of dreams in my life they are clearly instructive — about astral travelling, and eventually lightbody travelling, not only by myself, but also with groups. Step-by-step.

The sensitivity, and the path I've chosen is a challenge. But I'm absolutely not complaining. I receive a tremendous amount of support from the "unseen world", so I've not been so lonely. Though at times, as a mature woman, and very human, it's been very difficult in my relationships.

I was born in quite a small community. My difference from the other people around me was that I was more quiet, had a different temperament and played a lot by myself. The way I was born too, is unusual. The electricity

Angelique

went out at the hospital, at the very moment I was born. There were no nurses around, and I lay between my mother's legs for about half-an- hour. My mother said she could feel me kicking around, like I was dancing, I was moving my arms and legs, and to her it felt good. And I think that has been very, very important to me — to be able to come into the world in this way. And know I never hurt my mother.

On birth, for most, the first trauma is a slap. Well, after they discovered that I was born, and I was perfectly okay, the nurse came in, and there was panic. They picked me up by my feet and, as tradition dictated, gave me a slap on my arse to start crying. Still, I believe that because I'd had those minutes of peace and quiet, that has placed me in a different position in this life.

I remember around three- and four-years old, playing with my invisible friends. In the afternoon siesta time, when it was hot and most people were sleeping, I would be on the verandah and spirits would play with me. They'd rooch back and forward across the verandah; peek around the corner. We played hide and seek.

My parents sent me to a boarding school far away from home, when I was very young. I really missed my mother. My sister was at the school also, but I learned to care for myself emotionally, look after myself — through prayer and by talking to myself. Mothering myself.

As a child I'd visualise myself grown up, and my grown-up self would talk to me, and comfort me that way. I think of what a lot of people are doing now you know how when you've grown up, you're letting your inner child talk to you. I've done it the other way around.

I was lonely then. Now, looking back, I feel it was very Spartan, but I really feel it guided me in having to be strong. The strength, though, is deceptive. Over the last couple of years, especially in the relationship I have now, and in my work, people see my strength, and perhaps my power.

I know this and, sometimes, I show my vulnerability. But sometimes, people don't want to experience the vulnerable side. They might say, "Oh, Angelique, she's so strong" or be shocked when I'm vulnerable. And I deliberately want to show the other side, also, because it's not good for me to be seen as having only the power and support that I can give to other people.

I know my patients really like to have me around — I know I'm a very good nurse. And I feel it's a result of my background, of being alone, being lonely,

Angelique

and having to delve deep inside myself — to keep my balance, and to grow in a harmonious way. And I feel that's an aspect of what I can share with other people who are sick; to turn this into healing qualities.

About being in relationship... Well, because part of the time of my growing up, I did not have my parents around and, because the situation between my father and my mother at that time was not happy at all, I didn't grow close to them. I had a very dominant father and, perhaps, a victimised mother. So I had to discover a lot of things for myself about interactions between men and women, and sexuality.

Because I have gone through a lot of explorations in that field between men and women, I have come to really acknowledge my awareness of energies. And I think, part of that has translated itself in something like a tantric awareness, of how energies, how sexual energies affect one's psyche. How being monogamous really helps you to be more embedded in your own inner I AM. If you would be sleeping with many different partners, how that would affect the clarity of your own energy. And I think that people who are polyamorous (and I'm speaking of my own experience) tend to lose the pure connection with their inner I AM source.

And it is not only sexually that the energies affect you; it is also the environment you're in. Let's say, you spend time with a group of lawyers — your mind and your energy works in a different way than when you have a dinner party with, say, people who are designers. Your energy, your inner vision, your dreams move in a different way.

I think none of us are islands. I feel that to a degree, perhaps not to the same intensity all the time, we all are exposed to and are influenced by each other. I think that's one of the most important things to discover for yourself to what degree you are influenced by someone else's mind, or by a group energy. Also, at the same time, besides being able to be authentically yourself, discovering there is another energy that you can tap into when you're in a group.

I've been learning about that — having spent so much time in meditation by myself and also, in the last ten years, exploring the group energy. I've been feeling the tremendous power that's in a focused group — in such a way that you don't need to lose your own individuality. That's what I have been practising.

Angelique

Recently, I've been guided in the experience of the shushunga, the inner channel that radiates light. And from that light, when you sit in a group and everybody does that together, you're very much rooted in your inner I AM, but there's a field of light that can be consciously guided around. That light builds a consciousness vehicle. And I've often experienced, in my workshops, in a group of, say, fifteen to twenty people, that through the total of this light energy being built up, information of the planet, for instance, comes more readily to the individual. It's a benefit of working together in groups like that.

To me it is the way of the future. You know your boundaries as your own. Yet when we humans are together in that way we can access much greater power of focusing — of doing light work for the planet. Even into morphogenetic fields of war, to bring peace, for instance, to a particular conflict.

I had not been giving workshops for last two years but slowly the lightbody journey, starts; the doors are opening again. That has to do with remembering our soul journey. I've been taken, step-by-step, from 1978 onwards, over long periods of time through the universe, with very specific experiences.

* * *

There is a group of people — in America, in Australia, perhaps, and in Europe — who feel a connection with the Pleiades. It is one station in a soul memory retrieval journey that I've experienced. I've been taken to different places.

Some people feel they are connected to Sirius; and some seven or eight other stations. It is all a part of exploring who we are — who I am, and what I am — because I am much more than the body, and the life I'm having in this moment in time. That is connected to my identity — who I am, the "I ", or the "id- entity" that I am, deep inside myself.

This journey affects my everyday life because I have been able to have a clear boundary in my work. In my profession as nurse, I go "this far". In my inner being, I can be limited or unlimited. Most of the time I've been able to know exactly what has been required of me, as a nurse. But then, at the same time, I have a whole other level of information about my patients, and about my relationship with a patient in the moment, as well as what I need to learn in that situation.

Angelique

That is a whole level that goes parallel with this deep connecting with people I work with as a nurse. Sometimes, when I'm with a patient, I have a deja vu, and I feel it's existence telling me, "Yes, you're on the right track". Then, sometimes lessons and experiences keep coming back; then I know I need to move on, to move forward, now. It's part of what I like in my profession — I don't have to accept every assignment from the nursing bureau. I can say, "No".

As the moment, I have income from giving workshops. And, while being a nurse has been an important way I finance myself, I do want to move away from being a nurse, as such.

More about the boundaries. The way to understand them is through a series of exercises, well, more than exercises. They involve placing yourself, or stretching your consciousness — step-by-step — to such a degree that eventually your awareness is conscious of the whole of the universe.

It may not be detailed at first; it is a practice, and it's not been my path to expect cosmic consciousness. But I certainly had glimpses of it and experiences of the content of these experiences. I think it's very helpful; I think it is part of being human to experience, to know that there is a whole cosmos around us — and to know it not only from books and looking at it, but from within.

Think of it as stretching exercises — stretching and shrinking. When you shrink, step-by- step, it's almost like a fractal. When you're in full expansion, the whole fractal plays out in the same image of your own consciousness, and step-by-step-by-step you condense it, until you are within your physical body structure.

My experience has been that people who are on this path of exploration ("spiritual", or simply finding who and what you are) hold keys for each other. In that sense it is an egalitarian process — none of us is higher than any other. I hold keys for you, and you hold keys for me. And when we share that from an inner place, many more than us become richer and more aware and more conscious.

I do find that my particular journey raises issues or challenges in the more ordinary life that I live. And not only with other people — also with myself. I'm doing a balancing and harmonising act. For the last couple of weeks, this harmonising act brings me right where I am now, in my house.

Angelique

I'm changing my house, and looking through my stuff — a lot of stuff, from many journeys I've taken. I need to give it a place. And that's what I'm working on, so the issues for me are right in my own home.

I think I have developed enough sensors to know to whom I can talk, and to whom I can't. Also, how far I can go. I think I'm very aware of that, and I don't go into unnecessary challenges, with people. I can "talk shop" with almost anybody, but sharing the more esoteric or personal experiences is another thing...In my personal relationship, sometimes I seem to lose the ability to know what to talk about. While you open yourselfcompletely to someone you love, you're open to that person and, also, you give that openness back.

However, my deep inner spiritual experiences are not easy to share with him. I do make a few mistakes — that's part of my learning in the last couple of years. And that does make me lonely, and sometimes very unhappy. So we all get our share of learning and, when learning the hard way, pain. But, it's learning so that's good.

* * *

About issues of the ego: I don't believe that you must dissolve your ego, totally. I've gone to a lot of workshops, and met a lot of people. I guess it's something in me, something I radiate but recently I've come across the idea of ego, again.

It may be that there are things I learned, in other situations, that I don't have to flaunt, but I know that I may carry myself in such a way that some people feel threatened.

I don't think in this three-dimensional reality, the way our society's built up now, that it's helpful to dissolve your ego completely. There is a function and a place for your ego, but it should not be the ruling factor.

A few weeks ago, something related to this happened and I was completely flabbergasted. A person I knew from way back was teaching a trance circle. Yet he felt that he needed a clear statement from me that it was his circle, and he was in charge. I said, "Well, of course" because I was not — in my feeling, not in my mind — challenging his authority, at all.

I had, in fact, been in his circle three times; I felt I needed to be on the receiving side, and not always on the teaching side. So I just kept quiet most of the time, except when there was a sharing, when I was allowed to share,

Angelique

also. Perhaps it was the content of my experience, I think, that gave him the feeling that I was challenging his authority.

So I've had to be extra alert, and extra sensitive — without selling myself short. I have to allow for myself to be there — I cannot cypher myself away but if my experience is a bit powerful for other people, what can I do? I'm listening to other people's experiences also, so why can't others listen to my experience? Should I hold back because what I'm saying is powerful? I think that's really nonsense.

I'm not in an ego thing about it — I'm simply sharing. And maybe half the group really appreciates that I have shared it — because some of the women said we all are learning from each other. You share what you can share.

* * *

Anyway, being alert all the time is something that I have grown to accept. It is a vigilance, that is necessary as I move through my journey — I am growing to accept that I must be impeccable, to the degree that I can. If I make a mistake, I must be very compassionate with myself, because I'm also human. Exactly that.

The more I move into this journey, the bigger impact the small things have. It's good to ask, "What is small? What is big?" In summer, or spring, for example, I love to look into the hearts of flowers — and really hear and feel and smell what they communicate. And they're so sensuous! The flower may be small but it is such an entire universe — and so beautiful! Last summer, I was walking along a canal and there was a poppy in a green field. I stopped, and I looked at its exquisite beauty. That is an example of being what you are — I think a flower represents that, to me, in a way. If you lose the sense of who you are, have a look at a flower — a flower cannot be other than it is, with its own fragrance, its own qualities. And so I admire it, and the whole universe is in this poppy.

Appreciating the small thing that is also so large is simply an example. But it's also in the relationship, in a gesture, or in a look, or in the way you listen, or in the way you communicate.

* * *

I would love to live in a natural environment. I'm living in a city, here — not the worst of cities — but it would be great to live in a natural environment. It's why I travel so much. Most of the time, I work very hard and do this job

Angelique

well and I learn a lot. Then, I travel. I need my connection with the land, with the earth, with the elements. I need that for my balance. I need that for my spirit.

So as I'm walking my path I'm looking for a balance between all these worlds. It's a super-balancing act.

I travel many different dimensions. I achieve balance by using my intelligence to seek out what I know I need and do that totally. It could be the difference between accepting work, or being at home giving myself time to recover from having a cold. It's a case of really figuring out what I need from an overall picture. The challenges in achieving balance seem to be increasing, the challenges of this time mean I need to find money for a laptop, or a healing device to work with colours, light, for instance. Sometimes, I have to tell myself to have patience, to have courage. Sometimes, I need to work as a nurse and save, to do my workshop work.

* * *

The balancing act at the moment is financial, that's more of a challenge for me now. I've become really good at integrating and have integrated a lot inside myself. This is clear to me when I do private nursing. I might be four days in a row in someone else's house, sleeping in someone else's bed, someone else's room, someone else's psychic field. Yet every time, over and over again, I need to create my own "space bubble" and to clear the energy from the bed, from the room.

If I don't do that, I "lose it". When I'm very tired, for example, I might spend the first night in another environment not sleeping well, and I'm picking up all these things. Perhaps, the following week I have to go to someone who is dying. I've learned that if I don't take care of a few basic things the moment I walk into the space and the room where I'm going to sleep, I will lose my energy and get very tired.

If that happens, I can do my work on the outside, but can't balance it with my inside. So I simply get tired and become very aloof. That's like a defence mechanism but it's not good for my patients. While it is acceptable, because there are so many different people, and so many different ways of doing things, I do still make sure I do my job well.

At the same time, it's not pleasant to lose the sense of my own lovely vibration, in that situation. So, I need to remember it is a practice for me to

Angelique

internalise that which I am, and to really place it within me, claim my place and to hold my own feeling within the space.

In this situation I go into my inner light field, and sometimes in my inner magnetic field — and I let that energy come out of my hands. So I would sweep the bed — like I'm dusting the bed with my energy, because in the bed is a residue of other people's dreams and energy. If I don't do that, I pick up feelings — bodily feelings. They may be from a nurse who has slept in the bed before me. Or family members who have slept in that bed.

Sleep is a very private thing and so is dreaming. So I create space for myself to be there, and to be able to renew myself from my inner. I make sure to not mix it with other people's leftover dreams. It's a way of protecting my boundaries.

These are exercises it would be good for nurses to know, because when you work with patients you are very present within yourself. Also, we need to know we have picked up things. I think everybody, especially student nurses, asks when they are exposed to a disease or something, "Do I have this? Do I have that?". It's important to clear yourself, mentally and emotionally, from what you've been exposed to, and to return to yourself.

* * *

There are beautiful sides of being a healer. When you're able to see that someone is getting well, and that life force is returning to them, and the disease is leaving them, is one of the most beautiful things. A wonderful gift.

Even when you witness someone dying in peace. Or someone simply feeling better after you've washed them. Things like that are so gratifying and fulfilling. There are very beautiful sides about nursing people back to health.

Something about the sensitivity of the healer attunes one to these processes and enables us to be in support of that. I know that many nurses have this ability — otherwise they wouldn't be, or survive, in this field. When you feel good within yourself, that's the time you can do your work. When you lose yourself, you must take time for yourself. It's more easily said than done, because I know that many hospitals are understaffed, so there are a lot of things that would be beneficial to restore yourself, that you cannot do.

But I feel we need that. Let us appreciate ourselves for what we do, and what we have been doing. It starts within ourselves. I know that a false sense of modesty can be very destructive. So we need to honour what we

Angelique

do. Very much so! We need to show that towards each other; to appreciate what someone else does. In that way we energise ourselves and each other.

Angelique

Chapter Five

CHRIS

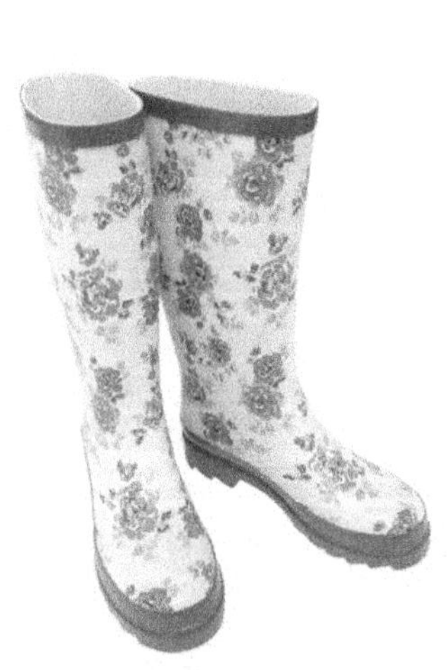

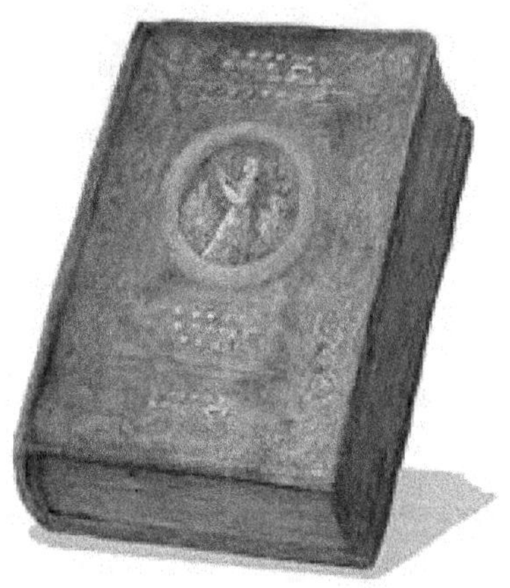

Chris

I met Chris through her contact with the university faculty where I was studying, having previously encountered her academic writing on healing. What was striking in our exchanges was how her experience in the world is so connected to her "languaging". Her process of speaking, of conversing was so much how her connection as a healer comes forward. Chris called herself a "gabbler", but it was such a deep pleasure to share conversation with her and hear how she used speech to "knit up" the breakages in people's bodies, minds, psyches. I found it hard to "un-knit" (break down) her account into themes. Nonetheless, I see how her big mystical experiences and the lineage in healing permeated her childhood and meant she struggled in functioning well in CR and how the wounding earlier in life profoundly influenced how she evolved as a nurse healer in her adult life. I loved her insightful and quirky reflections on healing and the nature of being a healer, and found it fascinating to hear how hard it is to speak about these in a way that depicts what really happens.

I'm reflecting about my memory of driving quite close to home, probably within about a 10- mile radius of where I lived. There were elderly people who were known and named as the person you went to for rheumatics, bone problems, when the dogs were off colour. When the calves had scours you'd go and get a drench from somebody. So there was not a differentiation between animals being cared for and humans being cared for.

I grew up in a farming area and in a farming family where the picture as such was nature. You were, all the time, looking out and feeling, sensing what's going on with the weather and what's happening with the plants and the grass, and then, of course, the animals. Life would be the relationship with weather, with the cows, then dogs, then grandparents, then parents, then kids, then chooks. It was a hierarchy of relationships.

And when Dad went and did this transaction we would get dressed in our Sunday best, and sit in the back of the car and wait. He usually took a bag of potatoes, or some produce, or meat, in exchange. And there was this sense of silence, with a big S. Something was occurring, was shifting around us.

We were aware of that; we all were. And I think it was just the way that people sat with it, and would say, "That plant's telling me it needs a drink", or "I can hear that cow, it's just not happy there". There was always that level of communication that was acknowledged. And then the response. There wasn't just, "Oh, I see or hear this". There was the action that went with it.

I felt I had, as a child, that big cosmology framework. And then I did the varsity stuff, and that was just expansive and had lots of things in it. But my nursing training had a shape that (I realise now) I didn't have much of a capacity with; I've had to grow the capacity in myself. That's been the lesson for me in becoming a nurse and being able to let nursing work through me.

Chris

I guess I went as a serious kind of person into being trained as a nurse. And I just loved it, I was fascinated. I was in my mid-20s and I'd been farming for years. I'd been milking all the years I was growing up. My dad became ill and I finished varsity and I went home and worked on the farm with my brother for three years, milking. And then, there came a moment when I just had this sense, you know. "Go nursing."

You ask me if, before I went nursing, I thought of myself as a healer? The answer is no. And I still don't. I don't think of myself in that way at all. If people seek me out, we don't tend to use that word in our conversation.

The way I understand it is the way I've been brought up in my family. As an eleven-, twelve- year-old I was having visions; I was seeing things, both in the past and things in the future. My sister as well — it wasn't uncommon in our family — everybody was very fey.

I remember my grandmother (staunch Irish woman) saying to me that I mustn't say anything unless somebody came to me and asked me. That was amazingly helpful, because I'd see things and then they would happen and then I'd think, "Whoa, oh dear, what am I going to do?"

* * *

Except for comments like that, like not saying anything, she guided me, silently, really most of the time. I've always held to that guidance. So, I've only ever gone and spoken where people have invited me to go and speak. If people think the things I talk about make sense, in terms of putting words to what healing is, then it's because I do stand absolutely clearly in this sense of nursing and midwifery as expressions of the life that belongs to human beings. In societies.

I live in a certain community, and people in that community know me; know there are certain things that I can do. But they also know that I will say, "No, I can't do that," or also say, "I know exactly what you're talking about, and I know somebody who'll be able to help you". And if I can't do that, I just say, "Leave it with me," and I do what I saw happen in those days. You would think something, then maybe you would ring the person, and they'd say, "Leave it with me," and then you go away.

I can remember hearing a phone call come, or remember Dad looking at Mum across the table and saying, "I think today's the day I should go and see so-and-so". They would be picking up on the wavelength that that person had come into knowing. It's a very precise thing. There was no need for great

Chris

assessments, or fancy conversations at all. This was what was happening, and this was what was.

When I work with someone, often we'll meet on the beach, or somewhere by water. Because it is absolutely clear to me that I am, to some extent, inconsequential in it. I might be the elemental form that is at that point of interconnection really, but I have a sense of something. I have a sense that within each of us, within myself that we do have the spark of life within us, which is a correspondence with the nature out there. I've had to learn this through a life threat. We've somehow got this weird idea that we're separate. Of course, we're not. But if you take Jean Watson's idea, or some of those, Margaret Newman [80]... their idea that the soul has a body, then for me that helps me realise that most of my nursing training actually flipped it the other way around. If I say the soul has a body, it is more like how I was brought up. And that's the soul's nature.

What I find now (and I think, "Can it be this simple?") is that if I am just how I am, in nature, and the person is with me in that space... there can be a healing. Sometimes I yabber on and we have a full-on passionate conversation but we're just walking along the beach. Or if they're in bed at home, or they're in hospital or a hospice or whatever — then if I've been outside, and I'm in it — in a sense that it's in the images, and it's in the talk. Or we're touching or holding something. So it's like, I do have this strong sense that when a person reconnects with nature — their soul — then this alignment with their deep inner healing force happens!

* * *

I was born prematurely, and in a tricky circumstance. That was my first life threat. And I know I was conscious of choosing to be born. I have a clear memory of that, before I was born. Not of being born, but then immediately afterwards.

I think for me, the healing the memory of the memory of my birth, where I nearly died, was making the connection that I'd have a huge, "Oh no!" whenever something wonderful was going to happen in my life and then I'd then think, "It's all right... now where does this come from?" I realised I had to separate what I call the "birth story" from the "death story". When I did that I thought "I'm going to live to be an old lady!" And prior to that I thought often that I'm not long for this life. Once I separated those stories, and thought, "No, I'm breathing, I'm fine," I put the death story to the side.

Chris

And my second experience of a life threat was getting cerebral malaria. Afterwards, I had to learn to read and write — get myself going — from square one. As an adult. I could stand but, initially, had no memory of how to go to the toilet. Or how to feed myself. It gradually came back, and I remember just having to sit. That's all I could do, I could just sit. I remember the day, somebody gave me a pen to hold, and the realisation that there was nothing between head and hand. It did not register.

What happened was really interesting. I remember thinking, "This is exactly how it was when I was born"; I had his fearsome determination, or, "This is what life actually is". You know it when you see people like that, and you see babies who were born in an impossible situation, who've got this boomf in them. And I felt it. I remember having that as a baby and it was happening as an adult. Though everything else was falling apart, there was this energy. It gelled as if it was... it was me, but I had the awareness of it. It was like a force-field type of awareness. It was like hanging on.

When I was starting to go unconscious from the malaria, as that was happening, I remember calling up the sun and the moon and the wind and the stars, because I was going. I put them around me and slipped unconscious; I remember slipping away.

I was in my early thirties and nursing in Papua New Guinea when I got malaria. It took me about three years to get myself going again. But I remember reflecting on this, and thinking, "Yes." I had a sense of... it was determination, but I didn't have any names. It was just a spark of something.

Did this make a big change in the way I approached life? No, because you see it had always been there. I think I had always nursed with awareness of that spark in other people. I'd worked a lot in ICU and coronary care and neonatal units and paediatrics ... always in intensive situations, with people who were in that fight for their life. In that situation I had a powerful awareness that you used your life, you put your shoulder to their life to fight, because without you doing that, they would die. I wouldn't have survived without other people doing that for me. And I mean people had clearly done that when I was born. I think that story is within you.

* * *

I have lots of maps in me. And when people who come are talking, when I'm most aligned with nature, there is a sense of a huge expanse. While I'm twiddling around in my intellectual mind, as they are talking, images come to

Chris

me out of my own maps which alert me to where they might be in terms of their storying. In those moments, I find I can softly just push in on the edge a little bit. Soften it.

I know to do that by how I see. There is an invisible process going on. Visionary. Images. To do with images. It is the soul, it is the language of the soul, in images. I don't put that into words; I never put it into words and I don't frame it in terms of past, present or future, or anything like that because that slows it down.

It's getting out of the way, which means getting my intellect out of the way, but being 100 percent present. So I'm 100 percent subjective, and 100 percent objective. My biggest challenge has been learning to shut up, because I'm a real gabbler. I'm learning better now how to use the talk to

knit a whole... If the person's come to you and they're broken; if their heart's broken, their soul's broken, and their body's broken, then no amount of touching or quietness is going to fix that, really, in the amount of time you have. If we've got an hour, I might knit them up with story. And in that, I'm using my hands, and my voice becomes like patches and I know precisely what I'm saying, and how I'm saying it. So I have now lots of stories. Big stories, little stories.

And sometimes they're a long way away. You know, the meat and bones are here, but they are like, away up in the trees a long way away. They may not even know where they are.

And so I'm always talking to their soul. Wherever their soul is. And I don't go looking for their soul... And that's a real key thing, because what happens is, they might not have seen their soul for a long time. They may not have lain down with their soul laying down in them which gives them a quality of sleep.

And so I have (it just happens) a sense of speaking with the essence of them. I mean, I believe it's somewhere, because if it wasn't around, they'd be dead. So it has to be somewhere. It's just that, they've forgotten, or lost it, or put it somewhere. Well, I think souls, they have to get together and talk. I really do think that. And why would we be coming together anyhow? There is something happening. Maybe their soul will come. I don't know. And I don't go looking for it. I sit here. And so I have to be within my own soul being.

Chris

I don't talk about myself as being a healer. I tried out lots of labels for myself: "independent nurse practitioner", "nurse healer", "lesbian". Lots of labels, you know. This was many years ago. I actually thought to myself at some point, none of them actually express me, or who I am. And every time I used the label, people approached me in a certain way. And I'd think, "Oh no, I'm not like that!". So I decided, probably about twenty years ago now, not to use any titles. I would just use my name. For that reason. Yet you and I know that we have this absolute passion about healing.

* * *

When I'm at home I don't identify myself in any particular way, because people know by word-of-mouth. People often ring up, or come to the door and say, "So-and-so told me that I should come and see you," or, "This nurse said, you're the one I should come and see".

And we don't then have a big conversation about what they said and what this person thinks they need, or anything like that. We just know that we know. And then we step into what I call "the not knowing". The space of living the moment of the meeting actually brings something out of the potential. Calling myself something would get in the way, because then the person can be thinking something, and I can be thinking some bullshit thing, and then also, you get into playing around with words.

I don't think at this point people would necessarily say at home that I'm a healer. Because I think we're moving into something else. It's like that old term lingua, the language of the moment. And I think, the difficulty for me talking about healing as a healer outside of moments, is that I would then have another language which is an intellectual gobbledy-gook language. Which isn't actually the healing talk that I use at home with a person or with a family.

I suppose that goes along with not wanting a label, but also honouring the fact that other people in the community say, "Go and see her". I don't put out a shingle or anything like that. They don't have to name me or their illness or themselves as a problem. See, if you start doing that, you are defining something that then you've got to unpick and, energetically, that wastes time.

* * *

I have an ability with touch. Before I started to use words, I always was able to use touch. And so, when I began to nurse, people would say to me, "Oh

Chris

your hands! Your hands!" And I knew. I thought, "That's nice — my hands are good, my hands can do something". So, probably for the first fifteen years of my practice, I did hone in on the gift of my hands; I developed that. It then created a framework for me to know how to manage myself in relation to other people. In a really ethical way.

Also, in that time I read a lot of the literature to do with massage and so forth. It was fascinating and interesting but, I thought, came nowhere near what was really happening, in relation to hands, skin-on-skin.

I think it's interesting when you say, "What is the journey?". Having been born prematurely, and having been cared for, and having those experiences... premature babies do have a certain response to touch. So it was no accident, when I looked back, that I was interested in touch. I had grown up in the cow shed with cows using my hands all the time, gardening and so forth, that my hands were a vehicle for me to grow myself, and then grow my interactions with other people. But one of the big things for me then became letting other people touch me. And allowing that skin-on-skin process to occur.

I was a child who was quite fey; there would be some people who'd say, "not very grounded". But I was very grounded, and very practical. Very much in the gumboots. But I just had a big map in my head.

So my learning was how to not let other people reframe my reality, and turn it into a negative or pathologised space that I would move into, or would frame me up as being in that. Not let it affect me in very much a "power over" way. And to be able to use my nursing, my use of touch, and the ideas that I had, in an open, honouring, honest, quite simple way.

To be open to people in the community saying to me, "I'm not going to come back if you don't let me give you some money," or "You need to do this". So that was the community tapping on my door saying, "This is what you need to do". I'm summarising things that took quite a lot of angst.

Within mental health nursing, when I first started creating a practice in the community with a group of other nurses, we were caring for people who were schizophrenic and extremely ill young women. We were trying to care for them in the community and in a home environment rather than in an institution and were working with people who were totally disintegrated at one level.

Chris

I was fascinated at the way their world was framed. The reality was that they were standing within the world, seeing in the way that I could see, but actually completely unable to manage themselves or their lives and keep themselves safe. It's a shock when you first see that, and you haven't met anybody in that space before. You think to yourself, "This is interesting — I have the same kinds of experiences that they have; I'm not a schizophrenic, what's the difference?". As I had done from when I was a teenager, I went to books to find answers for these things.

As a sixteen-year-old I stayed with a Jewish family for a time and they had the sacred Jewish texts. I remember finding these books and thinking, "Oh my God, it's written down! These things are written down. How amazing!". When you have a big map of things where you see things, and then you see it actually written down in a text, or you see something that the words are not dissimilar (they belong to the Jewish tradition) yet I had complete comprehension of what was there in the text.

People talk about the (Akashic) record that spans… well, when I was young, I would go there, or sit in the space. And have a sense at night that people would just bring volumes and lay them down. And all the years right from when I was about four, I had a sense of being awake at night, sitting up in bed, and being in this place, somewhere else in the world, of course, but just being in this place where people would bring these big books, and put them down in front of me.

And I never talked about that until I was in my twenties really. There were about three school teachers during my primary school, in these country schools, who would just look at me in a certain way. I'm sure that these people had an awareness, and there were probably other people in the class as well who had an awareness of these kids who were just being there, you know.

I didn't feel as though I was living in different spaces, because I was living in an environment in my home space where this was all congruent. It was the school education and the curriculum in the school that I was trying to bend my head around. I thought, "I can't do it". I couldn't do sums; couldn't do maths to save myself. And do you think I could do English comprehension? No! The things I didn't learn then, and the things I haven't learnt now… I was trying so hard to get these things right.

Yet, there was this other. I remember, at a certain point, being shown a whole… well, all the names of a lot of plants. I thought that if I just sat here

Chris

and let this come into me, then I would know the names of all these plants. And there were so many other things going on. I had to get up and milk, and I was tired, and thought it was such a loss, to not be able to just sit there and let it come into me.

* * *

I think the other sadness was when I thought, when I had cerebral malaria, that I couldn't remember. It was a fascinating time, because there was nothing to think with. I had to wait until things started to come back to me. Which is what people with head injuries say. Having to just wait until your brain organises itself again.

It was very exciting when I found it all written down in the Kabbalah. It leapt from the pages. I remember thinking then, "So it's in books!". That was pretty amazing and began my love of books.

I read everything. Anything. Many esoteric ones. And I would think, "How do we write things down?". Because there are a lot of books that are just people's ideas of how things work. I hadn't known these kinds of experiences could be put into written words. When I saw an article by Rene Weber — the philosopher who influenced Dolores Krieger — her story was beautiful to me, because it was not dissimilar to my story. Knowing as a child, and then being a philosopher, and philosophy squeezing her out — she could never get it right in terms of the text. She trained as a doctor, and then as a medical technologist. It allowed her, she felt, to finally say it how it was. I'd made a decision early on, that if I had enough courage, I could just write. That's what I would really like to do.

I haven't followed up on it yet. The things that we're talking about now, are the things that would go into the story, the one not yet written. So, I'd write and be reflecting on what's gone on, but it probably makes people think, "Oh, she's for the birds, she's a bit in the outer space department". Whereas, actually I'm immensely practical, pragmatic, and very down-to-earth.

The other thing for me is — somewhat of a dilemma — is about writing down my esoteric experiences. My family have always very much supported me, but my grandmother was very unsure about whether or not these things ought to be written down. If they are written down, they are in the text. Like the Bible or a sacred text. I now respect that. She was a very wise person. She was not educated, but had that ancient wisdom in her.

Chris

You would be hard pushed to say that many of our nursing textbooks are like sacred texts. Which is sad, immensely sad. I'd be hard pushed to say that a lot of my tutors regarded nursing work in that way — as sacred — although there were moments where you could see that that was how it was.

* * *

Challenging things don't really arise, for me, on the unseen levels. It's quite a simple thing. I have more struggles doing things socially correctly. For me that's been a bigger challenge, to not blow it socially. In my twenties and thirties, that was a dilemma.

I was very shy. Feeling different doesn't worry me. I love how people are and know that everybody's different from each other. If people ask, "What are you interested in?" or if they ask a simple question, like the price of fish, anything... I would go into a great long speech about something. It took me a long time to realise it may not be what they were asking and they'd go, "What's Chris on about?". It was like I'd missed the cue. Sometimes I had to pick the moment when I was going to make a speech.

* * *

Regarding the experience of expansiveness, you have a choice. I had a choice. I could treat it as a curse, or treat it as a challenge. As a teenager I knew I had to absolutely say, "I'm going to do this". It was as clear as that. Either the expansiveness was going to be a flipping nuisance or I just live it. When you're young you tend to be considered either a dreamer or away with the fairies — you know those colloquialisms people use to describe it. I wasn't; I was milking and, you know, we had young kids in the family and we were physically very into it. And I did a lot of tramping and surfing and things like that.

But by the same token, I had a sense that people would talk with me, and think, "Where is she?". I think that happens when maybe you've got the edges of your perception a bit bigger. You know when everybody was looking at the eclipse the other day, it had a massive effect on them. Everybody was in a big space. I thought "hooray". They were talking about it.

"Ah yeah, this is interesting," I thought. They had gone out and looked at the moon, you know and were talking in a really expanded way; it was amazing. Yes, it was a magical moment.

Chris

Chapter Six

GABRIELLE

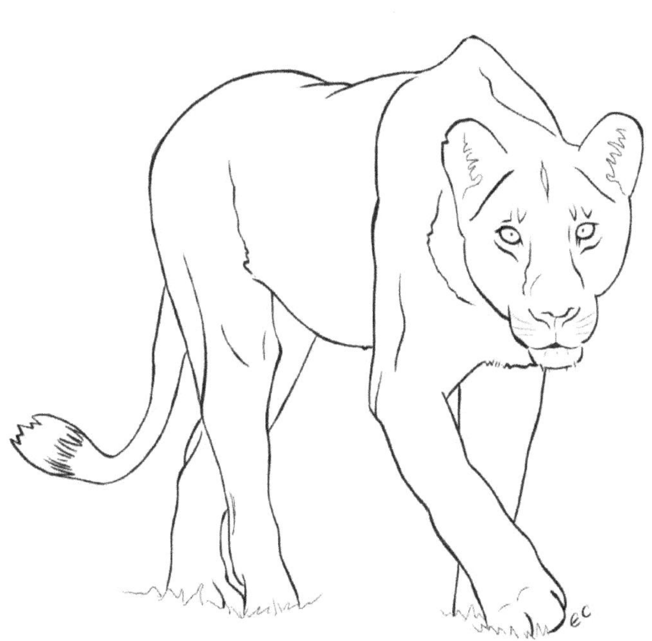

Gabrielle

I met Gabrielle at a nursing conference; I already knew something of her reputation as a writer on healing and we met twice at a café. I loved her deep and, at times, emotional disclosures, and her challenging inquiring mind concerning my project. Gabrielle told me how central connection to people, to spirit and to her heritage as a healer was to her journey. She talked of the challenges with her demons and her woundedness, and blessings of awakening in spirit.

I'll begin with what happened to me when I did a shamanic journey for myself, a little while ago. In the shamanic journey, I was shown my ancestors on the female line on both sides of my family. On one — the Irish side I wasn't too surprised. But the other was a great surprise. These were Yorkshire women from a more puritan background. Married to butchers. That was my background.

What I was shown was an inheritance of women who've been, sometimes, witches or at least called witches; women who've known about healing, have been healers, been midwives. In that process they have, at times, suffered. Not just burning, which I suppose we're all aware of, but more subtle sufferings: being ignored, thought mad, not understood. The consequences have been depression, alienation, all those sorts of things.

The experience in that shamanic journey revealed my personal connection to this. And it wasn't just my personal connection in my life, it was my inheritance. Just as I've inherited a certain kind of nose, and a certain kind of eyes. It was that too, and those women have passed it on to me. I had a real sense they handed it to me. And that's very new for me.

I was shown that some of my fear, for the next step in my journey, related to that. But I was also shown that it was my deep inheritance. That somehow and of course, I can feel the tears coming because I always know the energies around it — what I am to do now, and have been doing, is accessing something that's deep within me and beyond me and part of what I have inherited.

In my own experience, my journey to become a nurse healer started when I was eight when I read a book called *Jean Becomes a Nurse*. It's about a nurse in a British hospital, and very much "Era 1" nursing.[81] But it caught my imagination. And all through the years, I had wanted to be a nurse; never a doctor, which has been interesting.

I remember the next step in my journey clearly. About six months into my nursing training, at St Jerome's Hospital, I was driving home in my little red car, dressed in my little stripey white and blue nurse's uniform, with my

Gabrielle

white apron, and nearly bursting with joy! Joy of being able to nurse people, to work with people, and help them to feel better.

St Jerome's was a very profound experience for me. I learned there about being with people, and I was taught it by "sisters" as we called them — often the ones who worked the evening shift. I learned from their sense of love for patients. And I was taught, shown the significance of simply being with people. We were told off if we were standing around the pan room during visitors' hours and there was a patient without a visitor.

Six months into my training I got rheumatic fever, and I was very sick for a few months. When I went back to work, I had eighteen months which were pretty horrible. I could only just manage to work, and go home. I would go home sometimes to my parents, and cry. Now I would understand what happened differently.

I had a wonderful doctor, who looked after me, and when I went to see him, he made me feel like a queen. He was a small man with glasses, who said to this nineteen-year-old, "And how are you?" and mean it. He suggested once that I give up nursing, and do something else. At the time I gritted my teeth, and said "No!" So, I had to go back into nursing. And I have to tell you, on the other side of nursing I was given no quarter for the fact that I still wasn't well and, in fact, wasn't well for a further eighteen months.

I've just wondered, not very long ago, what would have happened, and whether that was the call to stop nursing then and do something else. I don't know. Whether I would have gone into another form of healing? Perhaps I'm talking about a metaphysical meaning of my becoming sick. I suppose I'd have to say that's the other track in all this — God. For me, brought up as an ordinary old Anglican, I've always had a very deep connection to my God. Tears again...

When I was sixteen my mother nearly died. I'll never forget the call from the doctor who said, "We're taking her back to theatre (she was bleeding); you'll know in a couple of hours if she's going to survive". My father was devastated. I remember going into my bedroom, closing the door, and crying, (I'm teary now) and having, I suppose, an experience of the numinous. That was a sense — though the pain was still there, and the dreadful fear and all that stuff — that I was not alone. I was really aware of that "not alone-ness". That was very special. But you couldn't talk about it much, because people... I wanted to tell one of my friends, but she doesn't believe in God. Never mind, I've learned about that...

Gabrielle

So, the same year, or not that long after I got sick and was in hospital, and I was in pain. And I called to God, and He didn't answer. I felt, He wasn't there. I just remember that, and I remember the nurse who told me that I had to wait for more pain relief, because it wasn't time yet. And I remember the way she told me.

I suppose that other theme (when I'm talking about my spiritual experiences, that's where it's come in) is as a nurse and a healer there was a real sense of "that's what I've been called to do". So when I look back on it, it was quite a wounding, all that. Particularly the rheumatic fever and what it did, not just to my work, but the fact that I had no other life for so long, at the time when most people are having lots of fun. I missed out on having fun, I think. I was just beginning to learn about fun, because I was a dreadfully serious little girl.

* * *

Regarding my evolution as a healer, I have to say that a lot of it was very ordinary. But always it was like the poem "The Hound of Heaven?" by Francis Thompson. It's about being followed, trying to run away, and always... He says, "Up the years, and down the years..." or something like that. And you hear the feet behind you.

* * *

I think that I've always had that sense of being with God. There's so much of the story that's ordinary, and yet not ordinary, and I think the things that stand out to me, particularly, are the people. The people that reached their hands out and spoke to me. That was the spiritual. My first tutor, who'd been a nun. My first midwifery tutor.

Years later, when I had difficulty at work in the same hospital, I went to see her. Now this was an occasion... Because I'd been passed over for a charge position, and I had the sense (which in some ways has been part of a theme) of never quite fitting in. I came to her in pieces, and she put me back together again. Just by listening to me.

So it's been a learning out of everyday things — people who do things like that for me. The mixture of the loneliness of never quite fitting in, and the other part of me that always wanted to put things right — fix it up. That meant I stood out, and said things — looking back on it, not always wisely.

Gabrielle

All that was part of the crucible of what's made me who I am. It's like asking "Which bit in the crucible, which bit of dross is the most important?" and I can't pick. There are some significant stages on my journey, and some were very wounding. Wounding from my own profession. If I was going to say what the spiritual thing was, it was my own profession's wounding me, dreadfully. I loved and hated it and wanted to transform it. Wanted to minister to it. But it wouldn't let me, and still doesn't.

This has transformed me, yes. Out of it, when I went to uni, I was pushed into doing the Masters — I didn't want to. One of the significant women in my life made me. Met me in the tearoom, and asked the question, put me on the spot as my boss. I said, grudgingly, "Oh, all right" and I went off and did an accelerated learning course. We had to do an affirmation, and my affirmation was, "I feel good about myself". I realised that it was, "I feel good about myself", with a bracket around one of the Os — "I feel Go(o)d about myself". "I feel God about myself." It was very powerful for me.

I went off to uni, worked with a man who wrote wonderful things, taught without teaching, and transformed my way of teaching, my understanding of teaching, my understanding of healing. He introduced me to Jung and all that archetypal psychology. I wrote my thesis out of that.

If I was going to use one word, I would call it "relationship". For me, the concept that I came across when I did Jean Houston's work, from her book *The Search for the Beloved*, really encapsulates it. It's a deep longing, inside. I think, for me, the whole thing is about being sought out and invited to be who I am.

About three years ago, I did a five-day workshop around using sound. In the middle of one of the activities, I had an experience which was the most terrifying of my life. I don't know how to describe it, except I had a sense of being called by the divine. The sense was a female sense, and the word that comes to mind is "Siren" of the soul, and the call was piercingly sweet, and utterly frightening. All I could say at the time was, "Fuck off, God!" I was so terrified by that siren call, I said it out loud to the group.

The other great discovery for me was of labyrinth. I'd been travelling round Europe with my husband and I met the labyrinth when I ended up at Grace Cathedral. I walked the labyrinth three days in a row. On the first day, I was admonished. "You have failed in love." And I had to wear that — I had. The second day, I walked the labyrinth to the sound of the Magnificat being sung.

Gabrielle

And the third day, I was asked (tears) if I would do, "Something". I wasn't told what it was, but I was given the choice. "Will you do it?" I said, "Yes".

So, my journey since then is learning to keep saying, "Yes". It has taken me into my own fear. Into my own doubt. Into seeing how I devalue and disintegrate myself. How I put up blocks to the flow of grace, and to the flow of "Self", and to the flow of healing, for myself and for others. At the moment, it's doubt. Doubting who I am, and being very scared of who I am. And finding that difficult place between being who you are with humility, and ego. For some reason, often that fear comes up, and how much of that is now, or whenever, I don't know. I just know it's there.

I suppose the other part of the story, is of learning about myself. The second time I ever walked the labyrinth, it spat me out, because I wasn't paying attention. I was an academic in a university, I was writing about caring theory, I was teaching it. I'd learned Therapeutic Touch… blah blah blah. And for a year-and-a-half, I was getting more and more depressed. And then, one day I got so angry with someone that I decided to leave. I was spat out.

That's five years ago, and the big journey for me, the emotional and spiritual journey, is of learning about myself, going to different healers myself and finding out more and more about who I am, who other people are and where I am to be and go and do.

One of the things I do is I have spiritual companioning once a month — I go and speak to a wonderful woman, and also have other care myself. She said something which meant a lot to me not long ago. You see, I don't have very much income at the moment, and so I'm actually learning about trusting in money. We have no money past Christmas. And it'll come. So, it's a lot of learning, a lot of learning.

It's learning to trust. But not be stupid, it's not about sitting there waiting for it to happen — it's about learning the flow, about learning when to be still, and when to act. It's about learning. I think what I feel is the whole process is being taught, you know. A lot of ego — a lot of responding out of my own fear and doubt, and closing people off for that.

I'm seeing it. Watching myself do it and my two ways of responding. I see someone doing something very good and one part of me sees it and says, "I'm no good, because I could never do that". The other part says, "Bullshit! You've got your own thing to do, and what they're doing is great. It's

Gabrielle

glorious, enjoy it". I shift between the two. But at least I know, now, that's what I'm doing.

I did a journey, had a healing with a very special Healing Touch woman and in the healing I was told to stop putting myself in the ditch. It's something I still do — it's around doubt. I hear about a patient who hasn't come back to see me, and I think they should. Or something else happens. And I throw myself in the dirty water — "I'm no good, blah blah blah". That's my demon, one of them. It sounds a bit dark, but it's not really.

There have been all kinds of amazing things that I've seen and discovered for myself. Learnings... I was doing a Therapeutic Touch workshop, in a big city hospital, working with people. It was a lovely and just as we were working together, I had this sense that the pussy cat that had been with me for fourteen years was suddenly there, in the middle of the workshop. Just in front of me. Amazing, because he had a horrible death — a lot of pain — a short time before the workshop. It was like he came back, and said, "I'm okay". Then he went.

Another amazing story is doing the recent shamanic work and finding out that my power animal is a lion. I've always had cats, and people keep giving me pictures of cats. I didn't think I was that catty, but, you know, I've got lots of pictures of cats. Apparently that's one of the features of... you can tell your power animal by what people give you.

So, this is a story about claiming. When I did the recent journey, the first one, we had to become our power animal. To my horror, this power animal was a female lion, padding towards me through the long grass, pad-pad- pad-pad-pad. Then, she was on the kill! And there was a big bloody piece of meat. I was going, "Oooh! No, this isn't the kind, nice thing to do, to tear things apart". So, that's still something I'm working on, something about power and being tough. And ruthless. So that's one story.

Since that workshop, I'm different because I'm learning to know what it is when I'm in my power. Just lately I've been in my power, and I know the feeling when I slip into it, and when I slip out of it. I know that when I'm in it I glow. I know that you can't stay in that particular power state forever. You can't sustain it. You are not meant to, I don't think. But there is an underlying state to it.

Something about that process is very interesting. It's about knowing when to go in for the kill. And when not. Lions spend a lot of time resting. Cats spend

Gabrielle

a lot of time resting and sleeping. When they are awake, though, they know what they're doing. They're very efficient! When I talk like that, it feels much better than it would have done before the workshop.

* * *

When I went to learn Therapeutic Touch, and did other modalities, they all began talking about their guides. Red Indians in the corner, and this and that and God knows what else. I thought, "Shit a brick, what's this?"

Part of this journey has been a profound challenging of my spiritual beliefs, and a realigning with them. So I'll tell you a story.

I think one of the themes of my story is that of a very good, very square, very serious little girl who always did things right, learning to be very different, and finding out that, actually, she was extremely different all along.

A part of my journey was to find that what I've done in my life is to take on some of my father's pain. He'd never spoken about it; it related to his experiences during the war. I still do not know exactly what it was, but I have a very good idea.

Part of my growth healing was to do work with a particular person — this special man, who sits and listens. That's all he does. To realise that part of who I had been as this good little girl, I had been out of love; taking on my father's pain, which he could never express, but it was tied up in his body. And (tears again) one of the loveliest things that happened for me was to know that, and to do that inner work. Then, about this time, two years ago, I went to walk a labyrinth and I was told that my father was healed, and that I'd done what I needed to do, take on his pain. I'd given the gift.

My father died seven years ago. I think that children often do that. We talk about wounds in childhood and all that sort of stuff, but I wonder how often small children, out of love, take pain on for their parents and carry it for a little while. Then the learning is to let it go; it's been a most profound experience for me.

Attached to that was nursing him at home with my mother for five days before he died. It was magic. I'd done my Therapeutic Touch workshops with Dolores Krieger, and while I was in Adelaide we heard he was very ill. Two

of my dear friends were in there with me. We did a distance healing for my dad. Then I flew home, and he'd had to go to hospital, palliative care unit. Of

Gabrielle

course, I'd only seen him a month before, but he looked ghastly. He was terminal. Well, his body was.

I was sitting in this room, and suddenly, suddenly I felt, "There are angels here!" There were two, I suppose you'd call them cherubs. I didn't see with my eyes — it's a seeing in the head or wherever. They were golden, and they were hovering, and they were (more tears) rejoicing in him. Just rejoicing in this man! His beauty because he had had such a tough time, for a lot of his life. I couldn't believe it! I just observed — they had no part with me.

We brought him home, and we cared for him and that wasn't easy. I had to be the nurse and the daughter. I had to stand back a little bit. That was my gift to him.

The family and friends came and there was a sense of being enfolded and encased in love. My mother said to me, "Some people wouldn't understand this, but this has been a most beautiful and wonderful thing" and we just stayed there, because he didn't want to go! He wanted to do it his own way, and was pretty cross.

The night before he died, I was standing in the shower in the funny old bathroom, and the angel of death was there! The angel said to me, "Only those who need to be afraid of me, are afraid". And Christ was there, standing in the distance.

I went to bed and I spoke to my father. I said, "It's okay". And at four o'clock in the morning, this wonderful nurse, who cared for him and us, came and said to me, "Gabrielle, your father has died". So we went upstairs, and she had cared for him. He was lying on his side all curled up, so cosy, and so cared for, and so at peace.

She said to us, my brother, my mother and me, "Around three o'clock, I had the feeling that he'd decided to go". She was sitting with him; he didn't want any of us. "And when he did, the whole room was filled with blue lights and a most intense feeling of peace". That was the great gift from that nurse.

Then, another gift came in, from a friend who'd told me the story of her sister dying. From it I knew that my father's soul would still be there in his room. I didn't tell anyone else, actually. So we moved in and out of that room. We all went in, took our own time, said what we needed to say. The funeral director came, and he said, "Do you want us to take him?" We said, "No, it's not time". He went away, and half-an-hour later I went into the bedroom and thought, "Oh, he's gone! He's gone!" I just knew, I didn't want

Gabrielle

to be in the room — it was just a body. Well, not just a body — dad's body, but, you know My mother and brother had the same response. They didn't know what I had known. So, we said to each other, the old bugger! He was hanging around to see if he agreed with the funeral arrangements, before he went". So we had a lot of laughter — he had a wicked sense of humour. We had a lot of laughter, at the same time.

That whole story for me is the story of when things numinous came back... coming back around from the time I thought my mother was dying. Now, when I think about it, that's a cycle, a circle, isn't it? It came back to me and was the first time I became aware of angelic presences.

That experience has just meant I've... the word that comes is "awakened". I've been able to know now, something like that. And over time, sometimes I'll be sitting, and think, "Oh, yes!" I'll just have an awareness. I'm sure there is a lot of stuff there all the time, and each of us has a different time when we become aware of it. So it allowed me — this happens quite a lot when I do healings — to begin to integrate it into what I do.

There's a lot of flakiness around this type of stuff and I think that's another part of my journey. How to work with this sort of thing, which is taken and misused. I don't talk a lot about what happens, unless it's appropriate for the person.

In particular, two words have come up for me around who I am as a healer out of all this — I wrote a poem at that workshop, about being a bridge for people to walk over to find what they need to find. And being a mirror, so people can see who they are.

But I'm still finding out who I am as a healer. One of the parts of my journey is to try different modalities, but to know I don't belong to any of them.

When I try to belong, it doesn't work, and I get a big lesson, as in this story around a healing modality.

When I was studying this modality, in the intermediate levels, I felt very threatened by all this guide business and stuff, and spent the classes encased in a little bubble to keep myself safe. (I can laugh now.) I'm making no comment, it's just where I was at.

I was creating a sort of psychic protection, because some of it was about people abusing other people's realities. Someone told me that Christ wasn't who he said he was, and I was affronted. I thought, "How dare you say that about another person's truth!" You know, one's truth is one's truth! (Again, I can laugh now.) It was a good learning.

Anyway, at another level, I learned the techniques and I use them, and they are great. At the penultimate grade I was told in a meditation that I was not to continue as a person identified with this modality. I could use the techniques, but this modality was not my path. Before that grade, you've done a whole year of being closely supervised, you've done innumerable healings and all that. I was told not to. It wasn't my path.

Was that my inner guidance? I'm very aware of that bloody word "guidance", and guides, for some reason. I was told! By God, I suppose. I'm Anglican, you see. I come from this place, where I don't need an intermediary. It's been an issue for me that it's me and God. If an angel comes along, or something else … whatever, it's because we are both in the service of God. I think a lot of people put the angels and the guides in the middle, and forget about who they are. We all serve, we all express…

At the end of the grade, you get a certificate saying you've done the whole course. Unless you've screwed up and done something dreadful, you can call yourself a practitioner. The next step is to get certification for which there's a very rigid process. I did all that, sent it off, spent probably nearly $300 doing it.

They knocked me back. They said, "You haven't done this modality, this is not right, you need to rewrite all this stuff," which meant weeks more work. In my view, the assessment process was flawed, because the processes were not consistent. So, instead of toeing the line (there's strong pressure in that organisation to toe the line) I refused to. I wrote back and gave my position, asked for a review, and got an answer. "No, Resubmit." So I said, "I withdraw my application".

That was a huge learning. That modality has given me so much — friends, contacts, wonderful healing techniques; challenges, that I needed to be challenged on, all sorts of things. And now this lesson. I thought, "I'll just finish this off. I'll just finish it off. I like things tidy". But I needed to listen carefully, because I pushed.

I went against what I was told. I wasn't told forcefully; it was just a knowing, more a knowing than a telling. Sometimes it's a telling — like the labyrinth. I knew that was where I wasn't supposed to go, and I was knocked back.

Gabrielle

How would I like to wrap it up? My spiritual companion has said to me — she looked at me one day, and said, "Gabrielle, you have been so faithful to your journey!" It was very nice to be acknowledged. "Yeah," I thought. I think that's what it's about — it's about being faithful to your journey.

Learning to listen, learning to play, learning to dance. Learning to not be too serious. Learning to have fun. Learning to not take myself too seriously, which is a great fault of mine. Living with uncertainty and doubt. Getting cross with God. Trusting. Trusting. Trusting. Trusting. Trusting. Trusting. Trusting. Trusting. That's about it.

Gabrielle

Chapter Seven

HELOISE

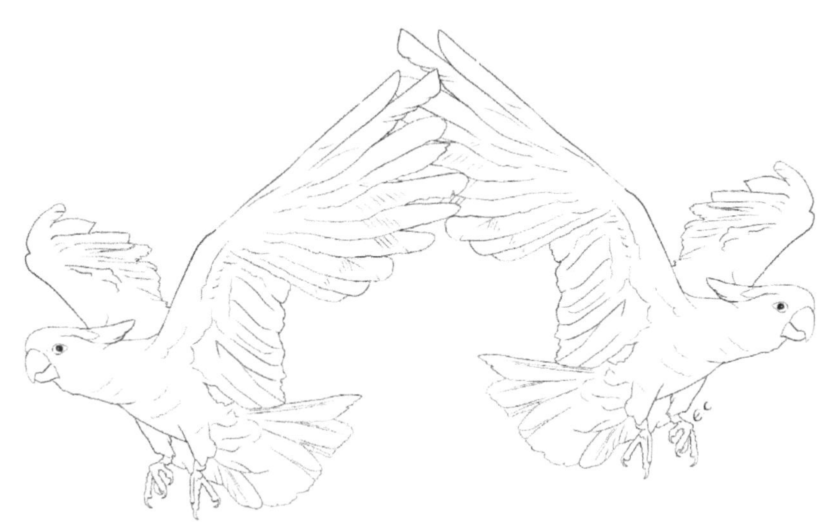

Heloise

Heloise met with me in her home, about an hour-and-a-half's drive from where I was living. I vividly recall the quality of her voice as I transcribed our conversation, its holding timbre and how it was both warm and lyrical. She spoke with me about formative figures in her childhood, about her spiritual experiences and insights, and also about her subversive healing in her work in mental health settings.

When I was in general nursing, I discovered that the system and the training for being a nurse, was not enough. I didn't do university training and so I certainly didn't have the awareness, the communication skills, the self-understanding that people have now. I was eighteen had come from a fairly spiritual background; grown up to be an individual.

When I went into general nursing, I found it demonised a spiritual perspective, and was depersonalising and pretty scary. I went into nursing because I wanted to help people, be there for people, and look after them when they were not able to look after themselves. But I found everything reductionist and mechanical.

I got into trouble one day, for talking too much to a woman who was very distressed, and anxious, who was going to theatre for some exploratory abdominal surgery. She had a husband, a couple of young children and was incredibly scared that she had a major cancer. Nobody would talk to her about it. She did go to theatre and came back. Later, she came back to consciousness and, within some days, started to be really aware of things.

Somehow, she managed to jump out of the third floor window, and killed herself. I think the anxiety drove her to it. I think that her emotional needs weren't recognised or met — a great failing of the system.

It was a huge shock for me. I think the grief process — the anger and the pain — all came after that. It was so dramatic for me, an eighteen-year-old, in hospital where people are supposed to be taken care of, to be present when someone jumped out of a window!

What's more tragic is she ended up not actually having anything life-threatening. That was the biggest glowing evidence for me of the failure of the system to look after people adequately. It didn't deal with the emotional aspects, at all.

* * *

I don't know if it's because I'm a Libran, or I've got, you know, seven air signs most of them in Libra — but being in relationship is a big thing for me. I don't think that you can have an impact on, or help, or be there with anyone else for any process, if there's no relationship. I learnt that very quickly, through a shocking demonstration. I knew that if someone had spoken to that woman, had sat with her, had asked one of the doctors who probably had the pathology on his desk for days, to say, "Hey, come and speak to this woman, she's very anxious," it might not have happened.

I really think a holistic health approach is needed.

I've got a long background in psychiatry now, and the same thing happens in psychiatry — just in a different way. We're so obsessed with the mental, that nobody looks at the emotional, the physical, and the spiritual. I realised that to truly help someone, I had to bring myself; after I'd brought myself, I brought whatever skills I had. But unless I brought myself, my Self, as authentically as possible, relationship was not really happening. And that also means, for me, having to drop any professional persona.

So for me the journey of healing is a journey around relationship, and relating to the person as a whole — all aspects of who they are. If they have a mental illness, it means also looking after or facilitating what's happening in the physical. I think unless the four realms are balanced and recognised, or in awareness, illness is going to happen one way or another. I know a lot of people have awareness of spiritual, or a concept of God, and they know about their bodies, but they don't know about their mental, or they don't know about their emotions. You know, those in psychiatry, only deal with mental — you can't talk about spiritual in psychiatry, because you're then considered to be delusional or, "As mad as the patients".

It's not comfortable or even permissible to relate an experience. Like the time I went to the mountains and looked over a cliff for a while, then turned around and walked back up through the bush, and saw yellow auras around one bush. "Oh well, it's my eyes, it's my sunglasses, it's something," I thought. I checked it out with a few other people, who said, "No, I can't see it — but great you can".

I have had experiences where I know that other things are possible, and we're quite limited, really. I don't tend to talk about those ideas in psychiatry. I did share some experiences once, and had a psychiatrist say, "Oh, it was an optic nerve spasm" or tell me there was something wrong with my lacteal duct. I have had colleagues go, "Oh, here she goes again! I really think you're quite delusional, Heloise, with these spiritual ideas".

If you have, as I do, a concept of spirituality and energy healing and psychic phenomena, or other things and live outside the limitation of a lot of

Heloise

medical practitioners, then new ways of doing things become important. Now, I know synchronicity happens all the time and I will quite often experience it. One experience happened after I'd done Reiki One and Reiki Two. I did Reiki because I wanted to be able to give more than I was giving to patients, without inviting the criticism or the judgment of people around me.

It meant I could be talking to someone, and put my hand on their shoulder; or say, "Gee, you've got a headache. Let me just hold your head, and see if I can find any tension there," and I could do Reiki at the same time, and nobody would know. I guess I did it to become a secret healer — to save myself from some of the uncomfortable responses — not so much criticism, but more being made fun of. There was a fair amount of, "Oh gee, you've got wacky ideas". "Heloise's crystal ball gazing," because I used to wear a crystal inside my uniform. Mostly when I was working in psychiatry, I wore a rose quartz down my bra, because I just wanted to stay grounded in the love, and not get suppressed by the energy of the system, and the judgment of other people. I did Reiki a lot.

Usually, though, I don't use it secretively when I'm working. It depends on the person. In mental health I have to be more careful than I probably would in general. But with someone who was acutely psychotic, I probably wouldn't tell them. Interestingly though, I might say to someone I work with, who is okay about that, "I'm just going to do a little bit of Reiki, and see what happens". But I find it amazing, how just using it, and not talking about it with the person, can help. Mostly I'll ask for subconscious permission from the person, but not vocal. With this, their energy seems to solidify — come in, not be so scattered, and ground more.

Reiki was my first possibility, and it was my first opening into "secret healing", or "non- judgmental healing". After I did Reiki, a remarkable set of synchronicities began to happen, particularly with one person.

On one day off, I was playing tennis, and had a conversation with my friend who advised me to warm up. "Ah, I haven't got time to warm up! Just hit those balls," I said. It wasn't a serious game, anyway. Well, I sprained my ankle. I was an hour-and-a-half out of the city but I went back in, and went to work. I couldn't get up the stairs, so hopped down the corridor. I sat down behind a desk and soon one of my clients — Phil, with whom I became very close — turned up. He couldn't see the bandage on my ankle but said, "Oh, well you should have listened to your friend and warmed up before you played tennis". Surprised, I said, "How do you know that?" He replied, "I know". Now Phil was somebody with a diagnosis of schizophrenia!

He did that all the time with me. I would come back after some days off and he would know what I had done, or say something about it. I got a bit interested in this phenomenon. One day, I had to give him a Modecate injection, and couldn't bring myself to do it. Phil used to talk to me about prophets and saints, and energy. He'd point out people on the ward and say, "That woman over there, she needs love", or, "She needs joy," or, "She needs to be bad — she's been good all her life, that's what's wrong with her. You guys won't fix it".

I'd talked to the psychiatrist about the experiences I had with Phil; who answered that I was either delusional or it was a one-off thing (despite my telling him it had happened four or five times). I said I didn't want to give the injection; I had a huge conflict with that, in myself, because I thought what he was expressing to me was from a higher level of awareness. The psychiatrist suggested I take some stress leave for a few days, because I was losing my judgment. I certainly didn't give Phil the injection.

After those experiences, I got more interested in energy medicine. I'd been interested in crystals, but certainly didn't use crystals at work. I did use bush flower essences in a fairly big way; was even making my own, because I lived in the national park which was a perfect environment — no telegraph poles, and quite energised. One New Year's Eve, we were drumming and playing the didge in the park, and I saw a couple of spirit figures dancing. "This is a perfect place for essences," I thought. "This place is really alive at night!". I started using the essences, in my work, with people who were depressed, though certainly not much with people who were psychotic.

I had a client — a woman with a very troubled background, who was from Kosovo (this was about six years ago — before what's been happening there recently). She had cancer and the doctors were not optimistic about her survival chances: "Lung cancer, that's it!" It was an apex cancer, and I was talking to her about that, and she was very scared to leave her two young children, who were in her custody as she'd separated from the husband.

She had depression though the doctors diagnosed schizophrenia. I didn't think it was the right diagnosis. The more I got to know her, the more I realised she was a healer in her own culture. On one occasion, I was really upset — someone I knew had died — and she cut a little square of red satin; fringed it, then put some white stitching on it, and pinned it under my skirt.

Heloise

It was to protect me, and keep the good connection with that person till they passed through — they'd died suddenly, so it wasn't a lingering death, and had only died a day earlier. And it was to stay connected, help them move and go, and protect me from anything else that was coming in. I never ever thought of her as psychotic, but she did talk about how she could see spirits. The doctors, on hearing this, would say, "Schizophrenia — definitely!".

She had people from her community come to her place for tea leaf readings,. (I don't think people come for guidance if they think you're crazy). In the wider community, not many believe in tea leaf readings or any of that stuff. I asked her about bush flower essences, and we picked out some bush flowers together, that we thought would be good for her.

I was talking to her about the essences on the ward; showing her how to use them. She was crying and hugging me. And I left them with her, and I pulled back the (so-called) privacy curtain and bumped straight into a doctor. "Oh no!" I thought. It had been such a nice encounter with her, and she was in such a great space with me. We were acknowledging that there are all kinds of healers, and saying how true healing doesn't rely on an intervention by a medication — you have to have other things in place.

And when I saw the doctor I came crashing down. "Oh, God — he heard me. Now I'm going to get it!" I thought. It wouldn't have been getting told off, because I was a senior charge there, but rather the disparaging, "wacky!"

This man was a mature doctor; he'd been a GP for years. So I said, "Hello. Eavesdropping, where you?". "No," he said. "I wasn't eavesdropping". Then he asked if he could see me in his office and I was somewhat strong in my response. "You know what, Paul?" I said. "You're new here, and I know you're a GP. But I really don't want to hear — I know you heard what we were talking about, and I really don't want any criticism about it. I don't want you to, you know, go into that psychiatry mode of thinking I'm a bit nutty, and maybe I shouldn't be feeding into people's delusions."

"No, no!" he said, smiling. "I just want to really acknowledge you. I've done naturopathy for a long time you know, and I'm so happy to find a like spirit around here." That was a great thing for me — it was almost like a healing of the first incident when the patient jumped out of the window. In time, Paul and I became "colleagues in subversion" in the system.

In my time, I have had experiences with people who have spiritual emergencies, or existential crises, or crises of their beingness. I've seen

Heloise

some who have funnels of light coming out of their head; or funnels of light going into their heart; those who are burning up with energy; or those who can see auras or can hear voices. It's hard to differentiate, sometimes, between what is a psychosis, and what I think is something else — that can be managed as something else.

One man I worked with had light pouring out of the top of his head. He felt like his body was bigger than a city; and it could contract, and be smaller than an ant. In my understanding, they're all spiritual states of energy and being. I think the expansion is anima, and contraction is lagama. Those two states — as transcendental techniques — can be present all the time.

The medical officer I was with wanted to get him scheduled but, of course, the man resisted vigorously. Looking at him, he was a reasonable person; the type, I'd say, who is going to have a more spiritual crisis. He'd had a significant background of body cleanses, had been trekking around Tibet, Nepal, and so forth; had done a fair amount of meditation and practised one of the peaceful forms of martial art.

I suggested, before he was scheduled [detained under the Mental Health Act], I'd have fifteen minutes with him. The medical officer agreed; it was just to stay there, be quiet, and assist. So, I got the man to lie down, put my hands on his crown chakra, and got my co- worker to hold his feet. I got the man to connect with his breathing, and breathe consciously rather than automatically. I created a circle of light around his body that included us. I spoke about being grounded, being contained. I gave him Reiki on his head, and then his throat, and then his heart. And after about fifteen minutes he was absolutely fine. He told us it had been a "blowout experience", and he couldn't wait to tell everyone about it.

As for my own experience... I definitely can see auras around things. Sometimes it is shining energy, a bit like the little flecks you see moving across your eyes when you meditate.

Sometimes I have a profound sense of being "the right one" for a particular person and I know that if I hadn't been there in that situation, something else would have happened to them; they would have been medicated, or put in the system, or...

Sometimes it's not so much that I make a difference to that person, that I fix them, but that it's the combination of them and me, the sum of us being together, speaking together. I'm there, doing my job, and they come to see

Heloise

me because of some experience, or something getting a bit too much for them and then we come together.

When someone comes in and tells me their experiences, I think, "Great!" It's like my world isn't mundane any more and theirs is normalised. More like an exchange of energy — or a sharing of something. A mini darshan, if you like.

When this happens, it makes a profound difference to my day. A blessing in my day. Or a test to see that I stay open. I don't have that sense every time, but when it does, I feel expansive all day, my heart feels open. It's not in a saccharine way, like, "Oh, my heart is open to everything," but more a physical expansion.

When I have that experience, everyone else who comes in after them, and every crisis that presents, gets solved quickly and easily. For example, someone will come in after that, and go, "I think I'm really cracking up, I think I should be in hospital". And I say, "You've got too much awareness, so you obviously don't need to be in hospital". "Yeah," they say, "I have!". So I become a reminder for them about how they can cope, and and are just not listening to themselves. It becomes a crucible for the truth. Now, I'm not the truth, and they're not the truth, but the combination of what we talk about allows the truth to emerge. If they come in crying, thinking they should get locked up, they go away laughing. When they leave, I cry, feeling that an amazing thing has happened. How does that happen in this space called a "mental health crisis room?".

Let me tell you about a sweet young man, about twenty-three, who had been to a ten-day meditation retreat in the mountains. I don't know exactly what happened, yet when those at such retreats flip out, the organisers like them to leave.

This young man had left after eight days and come to the city on a train. I'm not sure how he managed to get on that train after such intense days, but he did. When he reached the city terminal, he was picked up by the police, because he was just walking up to people and staring and acting very weird.

He was in a paddy wagon outside the unit. We couldn't see him, and we couldn't take him into the unit because there were two paddy wagons outside the unit, and a big drama happening inside in another part of the unit.

I was in the community area nearby his paddy wagon and said I would go over and stay with him. They were about to give him 100mg of Largactil, or some such medication — without even interviewing him! Anyway, he was freaked out by the time he reached the unit, and the police were with him. He was making himself tiny, and shaking in the back of the paddy wagon.

I asked them to let him out, because we couldn't go inside the unit. I spotted a piece of lawn nearby and said, "Come and sit on the lawn with me. I'm Heloise, and I'm from the community. And I'll make sure that's where you go". I meant into Community care. "Don't worry, you won't have to go in there," I said, indicating the unit. "Where have you been? It was to the meditation place, right?". We both lay on the lawn, and spoke for about five minutes. Then he went into a foetal position again.

As I watched him, I thought, "This guy is having a spontaneous rebirth — I can do this, so let's have a look". I told him what I thought was happening, and how through the meditation he had opened himself up to some cellular memory that hadn't been integrated. I asked him if he was willing to allow me to give him a bit of Reiki.

He said, "Oh yeah! Reiki — I love Reiki! That would be great!". I gave him some Reiki and started to get him to connect his breath. Within some time, he released that his trauma was due to being sexually abused by his grandfather and, he hadn't dealt with it, but he had become conscious of something previously hidden. I think the meditation brought it up.

He was calm enough to go home; we got a friend of his come and get him. It was a good result because he was another person who would have been admitted, definitely medicated, even been IVd.

He came to see me the next day and arrived with a beautiful crystal. "Oh, you're like a light! A light in the madness out in that world!" he said, "but wasn't I cool to create you, being there, at the end of that, for me!". Yes, I think he was cool to do that.

It was a very good experience for me; I might have gone into my usual response which was to keep going with what I had in front of me — I had three crisis assessments to write up. But something told me to go over and see him. It's not like a voice — it's like a knowing that says, "Well, go over". Every time I listen to that both of us go away feeling good.

* * *

My own spiritual evolution? My father's brother, Charlie, was a minister of religion; a mad bugger who was big, fat and a comedian — he wore his "dog collar" backwards; really not what you'd expect a religious person to be. He was fun, and funny — he could have the whole congregation laughing and laughing. At primary school we all had to go to religion classes. I went to Sunday school, because I had to be confirmed. I didn't do it because my parents were religious (my father was a hedonist and my mother was into Egyptian mythology) but for Charlie. He was my godfather.

He gave me experience of religion being something that wasn't obvious anywhere except around him. He was passionate about God; loved God. Charlie was political as well; strongly involved in unionising the painters and dockers. His words and his actions lined up, he was prepared to put himself out. He was involved in fighting for prisoners' rights. Charlie also went behind the Iron Curtain — loved Russia and went twice a year. He had a profound love for people — all nationalities.

He and his wife were deeply generous. Often, we'd go to their place on holiday and just as we were about to eat, there'd be a knock on the door. It'd be someone needing money, food, somewhere to sleep. They would be invited in and get to have a shower and Charlie would give them clothes. Then they'd join us for dinner. One of us would have to sacrifice our dinner. But we always got something else.

It never felt like being punished; it was always intended for us to recognise the value of serving. To learn how giving up something you have, or sharing something you always have would make a profound difference to somebody else. Being around Charlie had a huge impact on me. He wanted me to be a nun! His own children were out of control and I was, the "good girl". I was quite a bit younger than his children so I was "his hope".

When we were kids, and we'd stay, he'd say, "Oh, get in the car, we're going out". When we'd ask where, it would be to see someone in hospital. He'd make us go with him. "Oh, this is someone dying — so you'd better come and have a look, so you know a dying person when you see one. And so you know how to be around one".

Charlie would take us to the morgue, or the local funeral parlour. "This is a dead person — that's what they look like". We'd go to a baptism, to a wedding. He made the whole circle of life a part of everyday life. Charlie was able to be with all of that and see the bigger picture.

He was able to give comfort, and he was able to make a difference. With him, being spiritual, being religious or loving, or working for God — a fairly

Heloise

big concept, that you could actually be on God's payroll — could be joyous, and lots of fun.

* * *

Do I feel like I work for God? I'm not conscious of it all the time, but sometimes, I guess, I do feel like I have. Because when something happens that could have gone another way, I feel I have been blessed, another person has been blessed. I don't particularly feel like I cause it, but I feel the blessing came through.

Sometimes I feel like the combination — me and whomever I'm with — is bigger than just us. There's some other presence there and we were brought together because I was the right person for that person's life to go a different way.

Sometimes I might not be working intake, but minding it for a short time, and a guy comes in who wants to talk about his mother who's psychic and he's experiencing all these phenomena. Somebody else might have thought he was crazy and scheduled an appointment with a psychiatrist. But I'm familiar with the things he's saying.

Sometimes when I have that feeling after something's happened — someone's come, and we've talked, and they've left joyous, saying, "Thank you so much. I don't know how I got you". I say, "I don't know, either, because I actually wasn't supposed to be here".

Sometimes after that I get a very expanded sense. I don't know if it's God — I suppose God's a good word — I do feel like God orchestrated it. Sometimes I feel God's happy with me.

Sometimes after I have that feeling, when I go outside, my perception's different. Instead of seeing how dirty or noisy or how seedy it is; how many alcoholics, drug addicts, rude people, bossy people there are, I see an expanded place, of light. It used to be a very hard energy to work in but now, I don't know what it is, but I might be walking down the street, and down the other end, walking towards me, is some energy that's really light. Like an aspect of God. And, rather than lose energy going out there, I get renewed.

That allows me to be different, when I'm out there. As if I had an elevation in consciousness or something. Sometimes, I am in the flow of "everything is perfect", and really easy, and though it might be a troubled environment,

Heloise

and there's a lot of aggression and deprivation out there, I seem to skim across the top of it. I feel protected.

* * *

I've had a couple of experiences where I was nearly killed at work. Once a woman lunged at me from across a lift, and put a knife to my throat. The knife just stopped just short of my throat — it was as long as her reach could go. She could have kept coming, but she didn't. I felt really protected.

I was with a friend of mine once and we were in the country. My friend was friends with an Aboriginal man, who was head of a remote tribal community. A very old Aboriginal healer called "Nosepeg" (with a bone through his nose) lived there, too. People from that remote community occasionally came down to the university so their language could be recorded. Nosepeg was down there, and had only been out of his area twice in his eighty-year life.

Some time after this, he died up on my friend's land. I don't know if this is customary, but in that group, certain leaves were lit to help a spirit leave once they had passed — particularly if the person had not died in his home area.

I didn't know any of this and was up at the land one day, and I was walking around out in the dark with the dog. Now, no kidding — right in front of me I saw a figure — an Aboriginal man with white hair sticking out, fuzzing around his face, with a peg through his nose. The hair on the dog's back went up, he yelped and ran home. I was so glad I had the dog with me because at least he saw it, as well.

I raced back, and was babbling. I couldn't talk. "Da, da, da, da, da," were the only sounds coming out. My friend, who was pretty smart, said, "Are you all right? Did you see something?" and I said, "Da". "Did he have a bone through his nose?". "Da, da." "Ah." Scurried around, found a photo. "Did he look like this?". "Da."

Once up in a gorge, I saw an electric blue snake in the middle of the air — not on the ground, but in the air in front of me. "Oh well, I'm going crazy," I thought at first and then, "No I'm not". I don't have much trouble integrating it; it's a fraction of what is possible, anyway.

* * *

Some of my most amazing experiences have been during rebirthing sessions. One time, I was lying on the verandah of a house we had when a flock of white cockatoos flew over me, and left. Between their wings was the finest powder, and I could feel it coming down, I could rub it between my fingers. Fine wing powder fell all over my body and I felt totally smudged — as if my whole energy was cleared. Then I felt big — I was bigger than the verandah; my feet were over on the headland. I was so expanded that I felt a knowing of everything — not the knowing of knowing it, but a feeling.

I've had lots of spontaneous past life experiences in rebirths. Somehow, I also know that I'm a healer, and some experiences when I've been having massages. Once, it seemed it was going to be rather ordinary — some oil and couple of rubs. But as I lay down I saw a woman standing at the end of the massage table, with a big shield. The shield was like the one I was given by Uncle Charlie after a trip to Russia. It was a big piece of brass that had been a table, from Turkey. Another woman came and joined the first one, next to the massage table; the women looked different, but had the same shield. I heard a clink when their shields touched and, I felt protected by — I don't know. I call them "the sisters of the shields".

* * *

About disconnection: If I was working in a violent, aggressive or really confronting situation, part of my intuition might tell me to contract. I don't disconnect totally but my openness changes. Sometimes I flatten my chakras I get a hint to shut down psychically, so that I don't take in all this stuff. It's like a toxic overload — you want to be sick, want to vomit it up, to get rid of what feels, in a way, like evil.

I remember once seeing a man — a very ordinary person and he was telling me how he'd gone bankrupt, and had left his wife and children. He'd been a top executive and had lost his job. He did not seem to have any obvious mental illness but his reaction of deep humiliation, and shame was so severe, it was not in balance with the situation and, likely, something from his past.

He began to tell me how he could understand bombers. He spent a lot of time in the library, researching how to make bombs. And he planned to plant bombs in major public places. His aim was to kill as many people as possible.

"Oh," I said. "What about children? Little innocent children, or babies?". He told me that nobody was innocent. Everybody was part of the evil that goes on, and the death of children was really important — it brought more focus to what had happened, and it raised the profile of evil.

Heloise

I was working on intake, where you're supposed to see people fairly quickly but we talked for about an hour-and-a-half and I got locked into some shadow psychic space. He wouldn't talk to me with the door open and, ordinarily, I'd not shut the door unless I felt really safe. I felt safe with him I didn't think he was going to do anything. But I did open the window, because the room couldn't contain the perverse evil way he was talking. He spoke, after some time, about having been abused by brothers in a Catholic Church boarding school. "You know," I said, "there are ways to address that, now. Address your pain, and do it legally".

But he was insistent that calculated, ruthless multiple bombing was the only way now that the world would listen. He said he was a huge fan of the bomber of a kindergarten in Scotland, where many children had died. The more people like that bomber, the better, he said. I felt as if some great big black thing started eating me up; I felt really sick. When I said I would need to talk to someone else about him, he quickly said, "Oh, no, you're the only one I'll talk to — if you go and get someone else, I'll leave."

In the end, I said I had to get a drink of water, and I would have to talk to somebody else. I ran out to the toilet, feeling very sick — totally toxic with this evil energy. I was close to tears in the presence of that. I've been around other evil things — people having murdered someone when they were psychotic, but I think that man's ideas were the most disturbing thing I'd heard for a long time.

The idea with someone like him is to pull in as much of yourself as possible, so... well, that's what I thought, anyway. That way, you are just a sounding board for them, hoping it might defuse their intention for a while, until it builds up again and they go and talk to somebody.

I felt there was not very much of me at all present at the time — just somebody trying to survive till he had had enough ventilating to be all right again, even if just for a while. Until he needed to do it again. That was actually what I set up — that when he needed to talk, he would come in, and talk to people about it. Because my experience with it was so toxic, we had to arrange for two forensic people to talk to. Otherwise, it was too disturbing.

I had bad dreams about it for a while, as well — it was an energy I don't think we get exposed to that often. Of course, we read stuff in the paper, and see stuff on the TV, but being present with that energy is very unnerving. I remember feeling really small and really contracted — certainly very cut off

Heloise

from anything spiritual. Like there was no space. It was also difficult to breathe; I felt if I breathed too fully, I'd take it in!

I've had experiences around people who are remarkably violent, but that's a contraction, as well. And certainly if someone's yelling, "You're a whore!", "You're Satan's daughter!", or, "You're the anti-Christ!", or, they've got you confused with someone they know they've got to kill, I can manage that, and not be affected by it. I do that by withdrawing energetically, or shutting myself down, or putting a blue cloak around myself, and I'm still able to be present to it and try to impact it energetically.

Mostly, I don't think it's something I have to do, to shut down or withdraw. I think sometimes there is evil — there is pure evil, for whatever reason. And it's very poisonous, and it's toxic when you're in the presence of it.

* * *

Now I'm working in a different area; I'm in rehabilitation rather than emergency. Some days when I go to work the day is just fantastic and every day is easy. Every day I can see the impact I'm having in a really empowering way for other people. It's all just happening with this ease and grace. I'm getting addicted to going to work, now, and it's pretty good. It's a lot more grounded for me now.

Now, in this job, I don't have such a great investment about hiding what I do from anybody else. That's very freeing; I don't have to hide it, because it's obvious, in some ways. Interestingly, yesterday, about five people commented in the morning meeting, that they'd noticed a dramatic change in the "bomber" man. I was acknowledged by one of the other nurses for having done this work with him. It was actually work I had begun with him, but I had given him the tools to do it himself. And I think that's the best work you can do with anybody, anyway.

Now, because they're certainly not orthodox, everybody was saying, "This is awesome, this person was so chronic. This is a miracle! How is she doing this? How did this happen?"

One man said to me, "Heloise, I know this is happening because of you, because of the tools you've given me. But it's a miracle, because my psychiatrist has told me that this is a chronic condition, and will never get better".

Heloise

I just said, "Well, that's an opinion and, you know, I've got an opinion on everything! I live in a sea of opinions, but that's all they are — opinions! You know, that's only his opinion. You paid him for it (that may be unfortunate for you), but it's not the truth!".

When I can, I use a bit of everything I know. This is my great day at work yesterday. To start off, I used Reiki on someone who was having a burning stabbing pain in their chest. It went very well. Then I used some breathing techniques, some Alexander technique and a few bits of cognitive behaviour therapy with another person. It was something along the lines of, "Well, this is what you think, and it's automatic. Thoughts are automatic, so have a look at what you think and then see if it's actually true." It's sort of belief system awareness.

Then I use a self-confidence meditation. I used a yoga nidra tape. Now, what else? I use a lot of humour — because it works very well. You always know, if you're talking to someone and it's serious and you're challenging something about them, and they laugh, the game's up.

They know that it's... they just do it — they know it's not real, and they know you know.

Heloise

Chapter Eight

JAMES

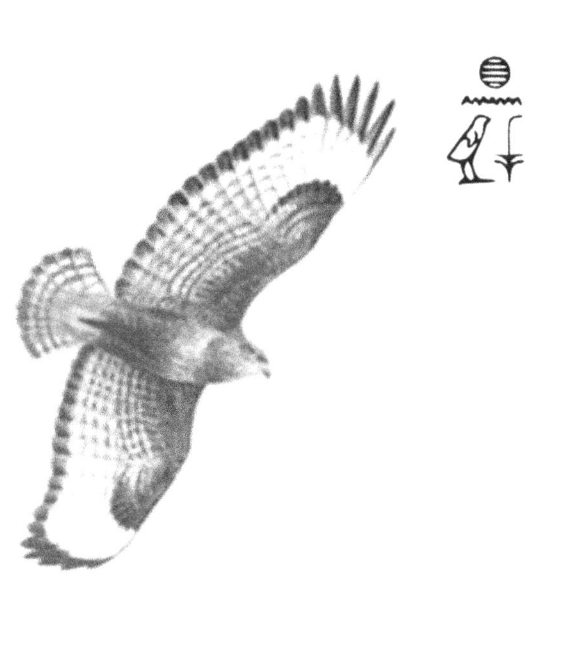

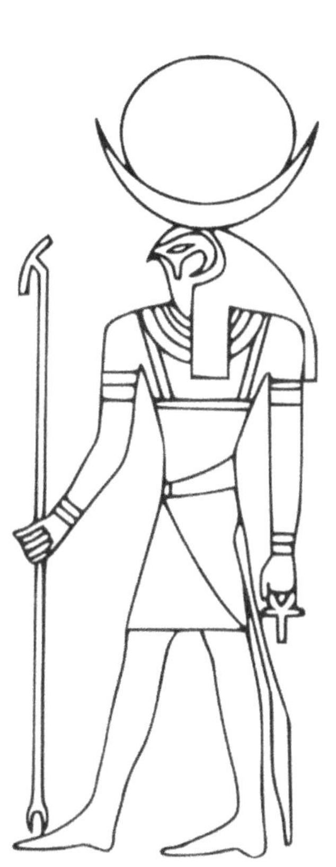

James was a formidable presence. Speaking with me in a motel room during a nursing conference, he was together warm and ruthless, broken, outlandish and impeccable. He detailed the remorseless nature of his awakening to be a healer - of its terrifying powers and tender blessings. He spoke about his spiritual teachers, how he was lovingly guided by them through the challenges of a dramatic spiritual awakening.

First of all, I don't think I'm a nurse healer. I don't think I'm a healer. I don't think anybody is. I think we can participate in healing, and we have certain skills, intention, consciousness, that we bring to a healing context. I don't doubt some people feel they are healers — that they either channel healing energy, or feel they're doing it to people. But my suspicion is that what's taking place is much more complex than that.

There are the limits, limiting ways of our rational mind to understand it. We put a label on it. We perceive ourselves to be channelling, or we perceive, "I'm somehow doing healing". But in practice, in reality, I think something deeper might be taking place.

However, if I accept the title as nurse healer, as a working name, as per the research question "My emotional and spiritual experiences associated with coming to be a nurse healer... " I would say that for the best part of forty years, twenty of which were in nursing, I saw myself as a very conventional person, with conventional approaches to nursing and health care. People had diseases and diagnoses, and you solved their nursing problems associated with that. Fairly simple, well-structured models. I did not consider myself to be a healer.

Around the age of forty, I began to experience a number of changes, that would have been concurrent with a shift in view of what nursing was all about. I could see that if it was personal, then, for various reasons, I'd have had to take a long hard look at myself and the way I was in the world. See what was making me happy and unhappy and, indeed, sick. And out of that, over the next four or five years, came a gradual shift and it took me away from my previous lifestyle.

The other side of the coin would have been a sense of, "I'm not sure if this stuff works when I'm nursing people". It was a sense of limitation, a sense of boundaries that ought to be challenged. A sense that there had to be a better way. As I say, at the time I was working within a very conventional system, in an acute medical unit for elderly people. So, both the personal and professional perspectives were under challenge.

James

When I was coming into my late thirties, some things — not least the complementary therapies — began to interest me. Now, if I ask myself why, I couldn't tell you. I was very conventional, or saw myself like that. But I attended a workshop on "Energy healing" with a woman called Mary. To this day I couldn't tell you why I went there.

Through my veils of cynicism, I did learn something about energy healing over the two-day program. I was still sceptical, and my way of dealing with that would have been to ridicule whatever it was that didn't fit my world view. I now know why I ridiculed it. But, at the time, it was my way of keeping away what I saw as too flaky, or odd. It didn't fit my view of truth. I had to have very clear ideas about truth; about what was true for me. It's interesting, then, that a shift in terms of what I was prepared to accept professionally was concurrent with an internal or personal shift.

In that two-day program, I experienced things, which, as I mulled it over weeks later, couldn't be put down to changes in room temperature, or the influence of a teacher. I know, in working with a couple of individuals, when learning about energy healing, I felt things in my hands.

It was an interesting experience to use my hands in that way. I'd never done that before. Though I do use quite a lot of touch when I'm talking to people and when nursing patients; I was always fairly easy with hugs and things like that when people were distressed.

* * *

This behaviour is in contrast to my upbringing — very touch-deprived. The family I grew up — average, working class family — was one where people didn't touch. The only time you got touched was when you got a whack.

Other expressions of feeling, except for anger, were rare. Loving feelings were few and far between. I never heard anybody say to anybody, "I love you". The word "love" was never used in my family; never used or expressed, verbally or physically.

There are certain instances in my childhood where you can see, in retrospect, there was love. But doing that makes you realise how important the expression of love is in a family. Particularly for children. And the expression is vital; not just the understanding that it must be there.

James

I can't say I ever thought of myself, until probably my forties, as being particularly spiritual, as I understand spirituality now. I don't think my world was particularly God-centred except for a while, when I was a teenager.

Throughout my early twenties, 'til about forty, I had no strong sense of a holistic universe, or divine entity, or anything like that. I had some rough beliefs, but they were well drowned in my hedonistic, and workaholic, lifestyle. This lifestyle would ultimately have been very destructive.

At around forty, a time my rational mind was dismissing as mid-life crisis, I described to my friend, a holistic doctor, what happened to me. I was dramatically bounced around. Almost everything I'd come to believe was important — in terms of my emotional health, my well- being — was challenged and undermined. My physical health, my work, and my relationships at all levels were challenged. Nothing seemed to be on firm ground.

And my friend said, when I look back at the individual incidents happening then (what I would now call a spiritual awakening) "You were possessed". It was a possession, in the sense of something gripping and beginning to shake me out of...

How can I unpick this story? I had grown to a point in my life that was filled with certainties and they were reinforced by the culture I lived in seventies economic rationalism, aspiration for success, individualism, everything.
I went for that fully. I was in the top league of my professional organisation; big house, all that stuff. Lots of money. Worked my rocks off. Writing, books, publishing. Everything I would think a lot of nurses would dream of having; would be seen as success.

Then things began to shake that. It was interesting, when I look at where fear lies in me, (tongue-in-cheek I would say in "lower chakra" terms) it would be things around basic security: money, health. And if those two wobble, they produce real discomfort for me. I would dismiss breakdown in relationships, I would not be concerned with all manner of things that bother other people. I had no great sense of artistic appreciation of my work, and all those things. My core needs, which in psychological terms came from my childhood, were rooted in money. Money was important, it was security, you had to have a roof over your head. But, at around forty, my core challenge was felt in my physical health.

James

I was speaking at a conference overseas and I passed out. The organisers managed to get me off the platform and I was, eventually, okay. Two weeks later it happened again. And I thought, "There's something wrong here".

I went to my doctor, convinced, "This is it". I "knew" I had a brain tumour, or something like that. After he checked me out, he said, "There's nothing wrong with you that six months in a holiday resort wouldn't cure". "What do you mean? I'm stressed?" I said. "There's nothing wrong with me? Check again. You must have missed something. Can we have some tests? Can I go for a brain scan, or something like that?".

"There's nothing wrong with you," he said, "except, you've got to stop. If you don't stop, you'll die". I was in a state of physical crisis and, at the time, was working in a unit where I'd done a lot of work recognising how the staff were under stress and the resulting strains in relationships with patients. I met a psychotherapist, who I invited to come and work with the staff.

We were in my office one day, around about this time of ill health and I was feeling generally bad. As usual, I had arrived at my office with a trail of secretaries behind me, and umpteen telephone messages; was barking out orders, and throwing on my white coat to dash into the ward and do something significant! He was sitting behind me, and I heard a voice say, "Who's looking after you?" I turned. "What do you mean?" I said. He replied, "You're doing all this stuff, who's taking care of you?"

I quickly said something like, "I pay you to look after the staff. Don't start doing therapy with me!" And then he gave me the name of a person he knew. I've no idea, to this day, why I went to her, she was a psychotherapist. And, 'till then, my whole upbringing in fact, I believed, "You don't talk about yourself to others. You don't talk about personal experiences. You don't talk about family, or anything like that. You don't do it. You don't share your deepest emotional feelings." I didn't even know I had any, to be honest.

Though I wasn't able to recognise what it was, or where it was coming from, I was having lots of emotional difficulty. Since my divorce ten years previously, I could count many episodes of depression. At that time, I didn't really know what depression was — and it was definitely something other people had. But there would be long periods of feeling really in a dark place. I put it down to being affected by other people, and would actually often turn it round and make other people's lives unhappy because I was feeling bad. So all that stuff was hanging around.

James

The being "possessed" continued for several years; continues to this day. It is a sense of things happening in or with my life that, even now, I cannot say I made decisions about. Some other drive put me in that psychotherapist's room. Some other drive made me black out. Some other drive said, "Turn".

* * *

I look back and ask, "How did I end up in that?" because who I thought I was then didn't fit with what was happening; didn't fit at all. So "possession" I understand as the sense that something within oneself, be it one's own soul hunger, or God intervening, was beginning to push me. Some part of me was not prepared to carry on in my life in the way that I was. I know, looking at physical symptoms and other things, had I not made changes, I wouldn't be talking to you today.

There followed two years of therapy, which freaked me out. I got sicker, which people often say you do and the more I worked on my inner stuff, the more I would have episodes of quite serious illness. It was almost to the point of pulling out of therapy. There was a direct correlation between my episodes of therapy, and getting very sick and it was often associated with chest problems.

Chest pains, and a lot of chest infections, one after the other. Until eventually, I had one that was so bad, I became pneumonic. I was not responding to antibiotics, or anything — I just got sicker and sicker and I was losing weight. That, funnily enough, was all at a time when I was getting into some heavy duty stuff in therapy around my parents, and what had happened to me as a child. It was almost as if there was some part of me that was driving me forward, there was some other part that was saying, "No, stop this. Stop this". Even to the point of, "If you don't stop, I'm going to stop you and, actually, physically kill you".

As I look back now, I think what was going on was some part of me that was pushing outwards, determined to be born. And something else determined "No, this stops". And one could look at that in psychological terms as ego and super ego. But I know, this was a painful soul birth taking place — that the deepest core of my being was simply no longer prepared to go on being controlled in the world by who I thought I was — this persona I had invented, or had invented for me is, ultimately, a destructive path, at the physical level if nothing else. There was no way a body could have sustained what I was doing to mine; in terms of not paying attention to myself

James

physically; in terms of promiscuity; in terms of drinking — I'd go through two or three bottles of wine at a sitting; I smoked heavily. The works.

Probably the same year as I went into therapy, I had the Energy Healing session; the same year as the workaholism was reaching its peak. I think I'd done the Energy Healing and had an interesting experience. As soon as I came back from the course, people close to me said I'd changed. Everybody said I looked different — calm, rested. I didn't seem to get as angry, or as frustrated. That lasted several days. People asked, "Oh, what's happened to you?".

But after a while, one falls back into a normal working pattern, you know, the endless stuff that one was doing. What I also found — this stayed with me for about four or five years — was there was an episode of a deliberate, sometimes not so deliberate, working on changing what I was doing, in this reality, to make it more heartfelt. But I still had the old stuff, because that's the way I made a living.

Another pressure to keep doing that, apart from that's the way I made money, was that fed also the fame and the fortune stuff, all the ego nourishing things. And another pressure was people saying, "What's wrong with you?" or "There must be something the matter with you. You don't seem to want to do this any more" or, "You've become boring, because you don't get drunk any more". A lot of friends fell by the wayside about that stage. My spiritual teacher said, "Expect that to happen".

And so, over about two years, there was an awful lot going on. But at that time, I can't say I put my finger on things as happening. I can't say, "This is what's taking place". It was a time of confusion, sickness, disruption. For some reason, then, I got back into Energy Healing and got to know the principal teacher (Mary) very well.

If I had thought Energy Healing was flaky, I should have waited to see the things that Mary was into; even more weird. I ridiculed the woman. I was terrible; would do it publicly. She believed in the interconnectedness of all things. She believed that one could use things like the tarot, or the labyrinth, to get deeper insights into oneself. At that time I dismissed it all as complete bollocks.

But by chance — if chance it be — I always seemed to end up on Mary's doorstep. We worked together, and fought together. Fought really hard. Her way of being in the world was different from mine, and I was utterly

James

dismissive of it. She wasn't attached to material possessions. She was — is — a deeply spiritual woman, with profound insights. So, I kept going and I kept having conversations with Mary.

Around that time my therapist invited me to a meditation meeting one evening. I sat, arms folded and stuff like that. But the guy was a very sensitive teacher and I got into it. Through the meditation work, through tarot and things like that, funny things began to happen.

I'd passed through the phase of being really physically sick, and reached a point where I was being in the world with reasonable equanimity; more than previously. Then I noticed new pains arriving. A sense of things that I'd once valued not meaning anything to a part of me any more. The car, the house, the clothes.

There was still a part that it mattered to, but now it was in conflict with something else that was very strong, and able to expressly say that all this stuff didn't matter.

Other things began to happen where I thought, this is what madness is all about. I'd begun to hear things, and, when I was with people, to see things that they couldn't see. I would see colours around people. Or, would be with somebody, and have a sense of knowing something about them.

It was really a strong knowing; sudden — a really possessive thought about somebody. Yet, because I thought it was madness, I'd find manipulative ways to check it out. I didn't want to ask, "Are you currently being treated for liver cancer?" Or something like that. I would have a sense of, "Why are you saying this to me because I'd know that you're telling me a lie, and actually you're really thinking that other thing that I am somehow aware of".

So, I'd engineer conversations to check it out. It would have been too flaky to say, "I've just thought this, were you thinking it too, and is it true?" But there were weird things like that going on. They seemed weird because they were spontaneous. They didn't arise from anything I could put my rational mind around.

So as this was going on, I had a sense of my world falling apart. The world I had previously believed to be true and important was actually untrue and unimportant. And that was causing disruptions, in me, in relationships. This phase bumbled along for a while with regular episodes where I would try to ease myself back into my world as I always had it. And whenever I did, I would feel as if I was being knocked back.

James

This is where it felt frightening; I wasn't in control of it. I became frightened of speaking at conferences; knew I wouldn't be able to do it. I would begin to feel physically sick or afraid I was going to pass out again.

Other things began happening. A book I'd read as a teenager and never understood — Jean- Paul Sartre's Nausea — came back to me. He describes a man in middle life. I understood. "This is what it is. This is what it feels like." And when I'd had this nausea, it could arise in the middle of a conversation. Somebody would come and talk to me about primary nursing, for example, and I'd feel sick, physically. Oof! It would come over in great waves.

Someone would ask me to speak at a conference about nursing models. They'd mention the pay and travel and I could see the temptation. But as soon as I'd begin to say, "Oh, yeah, oh, great!" I could feel the nausea again. I might be at a conference, and somebody would come over to talk about nursing, and I'd feel nausea. I just didn't want to know. It was as if, again, some part of me, the rational part, was saying, "Oh, you're sick, there's something wrong with you".

But there was something else. The nausea was there. If I'd begun to go along my old path, it was pulling me back in a different direction. That's where the notion of "possession ", as I said earlier, comes in – somehow it was against my will. And it got more and more intense.

* * *

One day, and I still don't know why I did it, I took drugs with a woman I knew. Now, apart from alcohol, or tobacco, my whole life had been about control. Tobacco and alcohol, in any case, are not drugs that open you up; more like suppress things.

This woman had worked extensively in shamanism using mind-expanding drugs and I trusted her. Apart from that, she did say, "You're ready for this, you need something, because if you carry on like this, you're either going to crack up or die".

So, on a sunny summer's day, I took some MDMA (known as ecstasy). The drug didn't work in the beginning; my fear was stopping it. I became aware how much fear I had in my life. It wasn't a case of popping pills at a party, which I'd seen friends and others do. This was a sacred ceremony — I was prepared for it during the whole course of the day. I'd fasted. I was surrounded by sacred symbols. Music, preparation, and I wasn't on my own.

James

I was guided and nurtured through the whole process which lasted about half a day. No, I could probably say it lasted for days. The peak was the first part.

So, within the space of a few hours, my whole life was changed. Because what the MDMA had the effect of, was the final lurch away from whatever it was, that I was desperately hanging on to. It was the stuff that I felt sick about every time I moved back towards it.

When I woke the next day, I said, "Jesus, my life is full of so much shit! It really is. Almost everything I deem important is actually unimportant. What I thought of as real is no longer real". But then, of course, as the weeks and months unfolded after that journey, my rational mind came back in. I then no longer trusted the experience, because it was associated with chemicals.

I also got caught up with, "I really want to have the experience again". These are all very useful teachings. Very useful teachings, very useful later on in life, both for myself and others. That provided more stuff to work on. But again, a new vista, new way of seeing the world opened up.

On the first occasion, probably for several hours I was in fear, in a great struggle with letting go of anything. Then, as I gradually breathed through it and began to let go of my fear of not being in control, and trusting this stuff, all kinds of things began to happen. Because I trusted the person I was with, who helped me just breathe through it, I began to have profound visual experiences. The interesting thing was, the teacher was in ecstasy herself, because there were things happening which she could see — vast flocks of birds flying around the garden. Kestrels, falcons, the type of birds that don't usually arrive in a suburban back garden. I kept saying, "Can you see what I'm seeing?" "Yes," she answered, giggling helplessly on the lawn as flocks of birds arrived.

Last, but not least, I could hear a bird calling from what seemed far away. I could see the shape, and it was calling, this plaintive cry. It was a buzzard (English hawk) and I really wanted to go with it; I wanted to fly up with this bird. And I couldn't. I could hear the bird speaking to me. "Come with me. Come to the west, come with me".

Later, when the drug had worn off, I had all this stuff in my head. Now, every time I see a buzzard, I'm in ecstasy with it. Some years later, when I learned some shamanism, the immediate connection was with the buzzard. It was my power animal and still is.

James

This experience was me being kicked into an altered state of consciousness. And I knew when I finished the journey, it would have to happen again. Part of me was eager for the next one, but my teacher was careful. "No, you'll have to wait now," she said.

Three months later, she took me through it again. This time, there was no fear, and a long process of ceremony leading up to it. It was just pretty amazing. There was a complete sense of union with the divine. Total loss of... well, so many things, you would need fifty recorders to capture it all. That's just my story; my experience.

The important thing was that phase — which lasted three or four months was the watershed. Despite my occasional efforts to go back to the old way, when the shadow would reappear I'd have to deal with it. Temptations would come, and each one, I know, was an opportunity. I'd began to see them as opportunities to learn, rather than things to have a fight over.

For about three or four years from then, I felt like an iron bar that was being bent and made to go in a different direction. And there were long episodes of physical, emotional, mental, spiritual struggles. The whole thing is a spiritual crisis lasting several years in which almost everything — my values, my ideas, my knowledge — was turned on its head. It was terrifying.

* * *

I didn't know where things were going. It was so against my psyche, my whole makeup all about money and control and the certainties of life. And within the space of a few years, they all fell apart. A lot of it was awful. A lot was wonderful. I was awakening to wonderful things in my life. Like the love I have for my partner, my children — it transformed my relationships. It was what love really was. People said I was becoming more available; more present with them. They noticed I was less caught up in my stuff.

This came with challenges. Let's say, you know people like you, but now, it's in a different way. I've had to learn to take care of myself differently, as someone who's more available. Otherwise it's just, you know, I can't heal the world. But somehow, if you become more available to others, then you're like a moth to a flame. More people come to you. The great demands on me ten years earlier had been, "You've got to do this, James; you've got to speak here James," and it was all over the world.

But I was damn near killing myself doing that. I wasn't able to set limits. Also, I didn't want to — because I wanted all that power and stuff. Now the case, has become, "Help me, help me, help me". That is something of a test to pass yet, because in a few cases I was getting really quite exhausted from being so available. And I had to take care of myself, and go off into retreat.

I realised this was the other side of a similar coin. At a phase in my life, everybody I knew was in crisis. There were marriages breaking up, businesses going bust, serious illnesses for so many — my kids, my former wife, my partner —and they were all at my doorstep looking for help. I'm talking scores of people. My phone would ring and I would think, "Who is it now?" Part of that process had to be learning, seeing the other shadow side of power, which is just about also wanting spiritual power. Being able to be the great teacher, the great healer.

I'd say, for the last ten years, it's been a rollercoaster ride and it hasn't finished. It may never finish. I just learn to deal with each part as it comes up, and appreciate the teachings.

* * *

I think there were two most powerful healing moments for me. One was when Mary, who I'm very close to, is a great teacher and guide, and who I keep informed of how things are for me, said, "You need to meet Ram Dass". She knew Ram Dass — he's this guy in the States. He is a brilliant, brilliant man. Beautiful man. She said, "because so much of what's happening to you is what he's recounted". Mary was an acquaintance of his. This was around the time of all my experiences, about the buzzard, and my hearing, "You must go to the west". Such signs went on for months. I'd get signals, or calls, or hear from people I didn't know who'd say, "Go west".

So we went west, to America. Mary phoned Ram Dass, and he agreed to see me, which was a rare thing as he doesn't see people one-on-one. He sat and listened to my story in all its detail. And he shocked me in two ways. First, he said, "You're in danger. You do this, you do this, you expect to be terribly right and happy." He told me three things I had to do to take care of myself. He could see my hunger; I wanted more drugs, I wanted more experiences. There was not a question of addiction, in a physical sense; it was the desire, now that I'd moved, to move faster, and quicker. It came from that place in my ego that wanted it all.

Which wanted all that before; now, it wants all this.

"That's a danger to you," he said. "You'll get justice, you know, it will kill you. Because you will want to take drugs more." And he added, "You must have time for integration. You must stop". He gave me three very clear pieces of personal guidance.

One was, "Stop the drugs. Just don't do them any more for at least a year". The other was, "Pull back on any spiritual practices. Just spend time taking care of yourself. Stop meditating for a while. Just be ordinary. Ground yourself". The third was to give myself time — at least three months — of being very ordinary, grounded, growing vegetables. Without that, something could go wrong.

I look back and think, "All these coincidences, where do they come from? How did I end up at this man's door?". There is a sense that something was putting me there. Then the question is, "Why? Why is this happening?". I didn't see. Another fact could be just that one looks back and sees what was once a muddle of events is, actually, a picture. You know things seem to be connected now. Whether that could be an illusion for the benefit of hindsight, I don't know. But my feel, I feel that there is a pattern that was deliberate, that was guided.

Now where that came from, I don't know. I remain in a state of unknowing. Which is a measure of whatever happened to me. Had you sat in front of me ten years ago, and asked me a question, I'd never have said, "I don't know". And yet now, I don't know. I don't know who I am. I don't know why I'm here. And I'm happy not knowing. I don't need to. I don't need certainty over and above the few certainties I have in my life.

One of T.S. Eliot's lines fits the point you reach in your spiritual practice. "And what you do not know, is the only thing you know". And so I am now in a place in my life when I'm just dancing with this uncertainty, and not knowing. Watching everything as it arises. Watching whether to go with it; to stop, or to go. Almost every one of these questions is a test, an experience, a chance for a new learning. New growth (not sure about growth as it implies a lineal process) or a new expansion, perhaps.

In the process I'm talking about there was a sense of things not being cyclical, but a spiral. Which is an interesting coincidence, because all my symbolism was around spirals. I was dreaming spirals for years. I went out to America chasing a spiral, and got caught up in these things. There is a spiral vortex on the land where I live. I happened to be working with the tarot, where my symbol is the chariot, and the chariot is a spiral symbol. So that's the big step. Sometimes it feels as though you've gone back where you started, but it's never quite the same and it's just kept spiralling along.

James

Sometimes up, sometimes down, sometimes you feel you're going nowhere, sometimes you're going everywhere.

After the end of my meeting with Ram Dass, Mary left the room and we just continued our conversation. I was opposite him and he sat about a metre away. I had a strong desire to sit on the floor in front of him which I did. (If I hadn't, I would probably have fallen off the chair.) He carried on talking about why he'd given me the guidance he had, which he said he didn't normally do, and that I could come back and see him any time. He said something to the effect of, "Because it's not your will, here. What you want doesn't matter". And then gave a quotation from the Bible — it was the one on my mother's grave stone. (Now, I don't believe in chance any longer. Nothing is chance). He said, "After all, it's not my will, but Thine. Not my will but Thine."

I can see it now. He raised his right hand up, his eyes rolled in the top of his head, then, his head came down. I thought he was passing out and wondered what was happening with him. I was ready to reach out to him, and then he zapped me. Next thing I knew there was a blinding flash. I couldn't see anything but I could feel a tremendous sense of heat, my skin was flushed and red; I could barely sit.

The moment passed and I got up, he held on to me. I just gathered myself to say, "Thank you, thank you, thank you." He told me I was a lovely man; nobody had ever told me I was a lovely man before and it really cracked me up. And then, I left him.

Mary was there and she took me up into the hills. She said, "What's the matter with you? " And I'd just sat on a hillside watching deer coming out of the woods. Deer are one of my shamanic animals. And there were hawks circling in the skies. So it was a really powerful incident.

After that time, I've seen him many times. He might tell me off, but recently he is mellow, soft; it's like a gentle sun bathing when I'm with him. A sense of what might loosely be described as energy, passing, or being brought down by one being for the other — what in Hinduism is known as "shaktipat".

Part of my meditation practice was hearing about Mother Meera, and going to her. I'd go to Germany, twice a year, and sit in the forest there. Each evening we'd go into meditation with her and go for her darshan. When she touches you on the head, and looks you in the eye, it is a great experience.

James

The picture is of an average middle-class, middle-aged white Western man, kneeling on the floor in front of an Indian girl. It doesn't come easily, initially. There are so many teachings just in that; it goes against my whole upbringing and cultural background.

Being there, however, was deepening my meditation practice. And just being with her the first time, I was sitting there thinking, "What am I doing with all these fools here? When do they come and ask for the money?". And then I realised, "I'm one of these fools, because I'm here!". Then I thought, "Well, I'm so embarrassed now, I can't possibly walk out of the room, there are 200 people there".

All my judgmental thoughts came in. I was afraid. I don't know how I ended up there, on her doorstep. A calling, if you like, again, to go there. As I sat in meditation I thought, "I might as well meditate. I can just drift off, go somewhere. I'm not going to sit here for two hours like this. I'm not going to sit in front of this woman. I'm not going to go up to the dais". I sat, watching these people kneeling in front of her, queuing up to go forward.

I kept meditating and had an intense vision of my father — the way he would deal with me. I could smell his hand; could see his hand in front of me. I could smell tobacco in the room. I remember vividly the scar on his hand and the way he would try to suffocate me.

I think I came out of meditation in this posture. It was that suffocating that he used to control me... hold me down and rape me. But I came out from that, and all I could think was, "I forgive you". It was a culmination of therapy and things like that. I may even have said it out loud. "I forgive you". It was a powerful moment.

That was when I knew I was ready to go forward. I knew it was my time. So, I sat in front of her, and I came back and carried on my meditation. It was a healing moment for me. I just let go. I'd gone through all the therapy, and I'd done the drugs and everything else. And here I was, sitting in a quiet room, about two months since I had seen Ram Dass; like everything had brought me to that point. It was a tremendous release! But I wasn't crying, or anything like that.

Everything seemed clear as crystal. As if some great dead weight that I had been carrying around, dragging along, had left. It was gone. Because it wasn't just, "I forgive you", it was also, "I forgive me". I forgive me about feeling guilty because I'd talked to my therapist about what my parents had done. My childhood talk said that you never talked about what happened in the home.

That was a great releasing moment. A classic example of "healing the wounded healer". It's all part of the stew, the casserole, if you like. I felt I'd been casseroled for months. And somehow, all this stuff that had previously been me — these compartments and bits — had all been put in a pot. But now, the ingredients had produced a different meal. The meal was not just the ingredients.

* * *

I wouldn't say it was a linear process, and often it was a confused time but around about that time I think I made a commitment to get rid of this stuff. The old nursing stuff. I was going to finally let go; it didn't nurture me. It hurt. I would commit myself to deepening my practice in Energy Healing, in meditation and other methods. Because that was now more important. That was now a truth for me.

I spent a few years, then, getting it together. But it was grudgingly, not easily. Sometimes the old thinking crept back, and little tests would come. Somebody would say, "James, we must have you for this. If you don't come and do this we will get so and so, and they are not as good as you... you're so wonderful". And I'd be thinking, "Oh–oh!". The little voice, the ego stuff was there again.

The ego's here now. He's never anywhere else. He's an interesting companion, and I really appreciate him. Because part of the forgiving process is, when looking back, upon terrible things that happened in one's life, and looking back on them now with appreciation — one loses the anger. Part of forgiveness is that you don't see events as terrible things through which you hold anger, or victimisation, or anything like that. You let them go. It's the alchemical process. One turns lead into gold. You look back and say, "Oh, wow". If that hadn't happened, I wouldn't be here talking to you now".

* * *

It brings a dimension to my work in healing. I have an understanding of the shadow, and how it works — both personally and transpersonally. I have experienced the shadow. My God! It's not something I share with people. I think the shadow or the side of consciousness manifests itself in very interesting ways.

James

But there is, still, a very strong rationalistic part of my brain that needs things validated, otherwise I'm never actually quite sure. With drug experiences, for example, I only began to believe this stuff once it started happening without drugs. I realise one can get as high without the drugs and bypass that process. Still, I see them as a valuable kick, as it were, at that time.

Like a drug addiction, however, one of the shadow sides of this spiritual awakening is it's like an addiction. It becomes a wanting of more experiences.

The other side; what it has taught me is that those teachings must have a purpose. They feel purposeful. For some reason I have been woken up, or have woken myself up. Whether it is purely to be, just be me, whoever I am, or whether that purpose is to be, in some way, of service to the world, I don't know. But I am inclined to the latter, because of the signals, the things that go on around me. I had to check whether that is the ego stuff? Is it the, "I want to be the great healer, an important person," stuff, playing itself out again? Right now, it doesn't feel like that. It feels like there is a purpose, a destiny. This happens to people and, I believe, if it's for any reason at all, it is service.

What I have learned from those many shadow experiences, is how it is not possible to work with this healing stuff without bringing up the shadow. One of my shadow sides is impatience. When I hear people swanning about, talking "love and light" and stuff like that, I really feel that's not "it". I don't think we can be as fully available in service, with those in need, unless we recognise the shadow in ourselves — in them, in how it works, how it is playing itself out.

The healing process is about transforming shadow into light. And so I think if one is more aware of that — that's one dimension of the experience of shadow, if they serve me in some way, it's to make me more aware when I am working with people, of a degree of humility. It's not me whacking light into somebody. There is something going on here, of which I am but a servant.

One personal experience was being in a shadowy place, which I would have rejected as an illusion had there not been others present with me — both witnessing and feeling what was taking place. Also being scared spitless by it themselves.

James

One evening, Mary and I were in a house with someone else and it was just a perfectly affable evening, drinks and a meal. I didn't have any alcohol, I just had tea. As we were about to leave one of the men said, "I'll show you around the house". As we walked upstairs I began to realise the symbolism lying all around the room — sadomasochistic imagery. I looked at Mary, she looked at me. We both got a sense of, this guy is making some offer here. The way he blocked the stairs on the way out, all this sort of thing.

I was firm, got myself and Mary out. We both told each other we were glad to get out. It was pretty obvious what this guy was into, and what he wanted. I think was making assumptions that we would, in some way, be interested in joining him. We left the house.

But, what was a fine evening suddenly turned into a thunder storm. It was pitch black outside. No lights. When we got to the place we were living, there was a chain across the drive, and a black motorcycle parked there. We were in the middle of nowhere. The nearest house was at least a few kilometres away and, where we'd just come from, was on top of the cliffs at the coast. It was the middle of the night and we saw no reason for somebody to park a motorcycle, a black motorcycle, with no registration plate on it, in the middle of nowhere.

"Oh," I thought. "Is this a burglar or something?". The house was down the drive and rain was lashing down, I got out of the car to undo the thick lock on the gate chain. It was thicker than my finger and the key wouldn't work. I could sense Mary getting afraid. I was getting scared, too. Those psycho-horror films began to pop through my mind. Eventually I snapped the metal sheer off the lock. Normally, I don't have the strength to break metal but my rational mind said maybe I was able to break the lock because it was flawed. But I did. Then I threw the chain away and drove on down the drive down to the house.

Part of me was trying to be, casual. Be "normal" and say things like, "It's time for bed, see you in the morning". But, we looked at each other and Mary said, "You can feel it, can't you?". "Yes, I can do more than feel it. I can see it!" I said. It was like darkness coming over. Lights kept dimming and I went into a catatonic state. I couldn't see or hear clearly what was going on. I could hear Mary's voice in the distance, and she was doing and saying all kinds of things to take care of me.

I saw an image of a man and I began to fight. I unveiled the shining hero with the sword, going into the darkness and doing battle with this stuff, and

James

driving him away. This is all imagery and symbolism. When I opened my eyes, it was a perfectly ordinary room, but with flashing lights in it and things like that. They could have been the thunder storm affecting electricity. Mary was seeing things and feeling things too, and it went on for hours and hours that night.

The more I fought, the more this dark thing advanced; I could feel hands gripping me. I was searching for answers. "Did you lace my tea? Is this a bad trip? Have I'd been given drugs?". It went on for hours until I reached a point of collapse. All I would say was, "Can you help me? I can't fight this any more". The more I fought it, the stronger it got.

* * *

The lesson of that story for me was how to deal with darkness. You don't fight it. You don't, however good you think your motives are, use the very weapons it uses. You don't use violence, aggression, anger, no matter how noble you think you are. Because it would itself tap into dark. And, there have been many incidents like that since, each one a test, each one frightening. Some people would see it as psychosis. Had I been on my own I would have thought it was madness.

Yet, by chance — if chance it be — there have always been others present, varying people. Once it was a devout Christian minister with me. And this type of semi-visual manifestations, if you like, are also moments in which one learns a huge amount. That's if you pay attention.

They could merely be my personal shadow manifestation; I believe actually, there is a greater shadow. The personal and the transpersonal at work, in the universe. There is a struggle between the light and dark and there is that which is beyond that. The void, the place of total safety, beyond that.

Meanwhile, these forces are at work in this reality. We work with them. But how do we choose to work with them? I think the way is not to go into battle with it, however, one does that and then sees battle taking place. But you don't turn light into dark that way. You walk away from it; refuse to have anything to do with it; do not use its tools.

That has influenced my work in healing — in watching that going on, and being aware of how, when people are sick, at some level the shadow is at work in them. In shamanic terms, it's soul sickness, or loss of soul. An entity has moved in.

James

I'm using words and labels now, which I really don't like using. This is stuff I know and I feel and experience yet, in translation from the inner knowing to the outer knowing, something is lost. I believe it is not possible to put what is essentially non-conceptual into the conceptual. The ones who get closest to it are poets. They can play with words to stretch their meanings. In normal conversation it's very difficult.

So, while one has terrible experiences — frightening, dangerous — there is meaning and purpose in them. They are offered to us as teachings. I've talked with many wise people about this, all people I trust and theydon't dismiss these as illusions. Ram Dass said that to me. "The more you unfold, the more you are challenged — so, where the light is strongest, there the darkness grows strongest too. That's your work, and your spiritual practice is how you work with it."

There are countless occasions where my shadow would really love to work with this, and become powerful. Occasions where I could be tempted; could have done this or that. And I still am tempted! But I know what I learned. Though it is an opportunity, when one is challenged by the shadow, it is also a risky experience — in all senses. In being challenged by the shadow, an advantage (if advantage is right) is that one learns of it, and how it works.

Because you know your enemy — you understand the workings of your worthy opponent.

It influences the work in my everyday life in the awareness of what goes on in people when they may be sick, when they are troubled. I'm not talking about spooks and ghosties and that stuff, But, when I 'm working with somebody who is sick, for example, part of my work is to watch that I don't get caught in my agenda for them. Be it, "You have an illness, I want to make you better". Or something else. It's me going into the dark with the healer's shining sword to do battle and that's not the way it needs to be.

I mentioned the time I was saved from that dark experience when I surrendered to God, to Jesus, whoever it was and I saw a mountain with beings on it. The moment I surrendered, something happened. There was a tremendous vision of an Egyptian God, Horus, who in my shamanic work I am associated with. In a moment, the darkness just went. Mary saw it too, because she was in the room with me. "It's gone," she said.

What I sense is that if people are into the shadow side themselves, they act just like a focus for it to be manifested more deeply in the world. It channels,

James

if you like. I don't think it's that intentional, that some beast with horns sits there saying, "Here's one. If I get this one, I can get these others". It's more subtle. But the work is becoming aware of the shadow side in oneself, and how it manifests.

I guess what I'm getting at is, if one wishes to work in healing ways, there are no short cuts. One has to do the emotional work, to work on one's own shadow. It is not possible to say, "I'm just going to stick with light and love, and I'm going to do this, and I'm going to send your diseases away". That is a bastardisation of the healing potential.

Those people are not ill-intentioned, and I'm even cautious about dismissing that way, because I'm sounding very judgmental. At holistic gatherings I've bumped into such people and it's always nice when people are wishing you love and light.

And I do believe in the power of non-local healing — I'll take all I can get, thank you; I'm very much for prayers. But at the end of the day, there is also the shadow, and I'm wary of the collective denial that this nasty stuff has to be dealt with.

I don't think we can be fulfilled as healers unless we have worked both on our own shadow, and we are realised enough, awakened enough, to see how much our stuff can get in the way when we work with people. When I'm working with patients and clients, I know a significant part of the work is me watching me. Not watching the client; watching me. Asking myself, what am I doing here? What am I getting caught up in here? So it can even get caught up in one's natural human compassion — to see another one relieved of suffering. "I really wish I could take the breast cancer away. I want it to go away for you". It's tough to pull out from that and not get caught up in it and come at it from a place of, "Not my will, but Thine".

I'd had many experiences with patients and clients. One example is a man called Alan. When we come together, he bows down at me "the great healer" thing, He has a laugh and he's learned to say this tongue-in-cheek. Now we are working together in session of energy healing and, halfway through, we pause. If I can see something he knows I'm seeing something. I say, "What's happening with you now, Alan?" and he describes what I'm seeing. It's the same. I've got his image almost perfect. This has begun to happen with many clients, now.

James

So where does teaching end, then? I have moved beyond, perhaps in energy healing. Ten years ago I had to have the structure, energy fields and the hands, and everything else. And now, I'm just there, and stuff is happening. With Alan, for example, I was working with him a few weeks ago, when he was having his toughest time ever. He was off his Valium, off his anti-schizophrenia drugs. He wasn't drinking, so all his props had gone. He wanted this. He's worked on himself with such courage, I could cry for him sometimes. This man has had a terrible life. Everything you could throw at a man has been thrown at him and he is still standing.

We were working away, doing energy healing and I felt him settle and relax. Then the image started. We're so into it now and I was saying, "Oh, George's back". George, his dog, had died some years back. He said, "Yep". I said, "Where you off to?". He described a scene and I could see it in my head. I said, "Well, okay. I can see a wall ahead of you. I have a sense. Go towards that wall, that stone wall". He took the dog to that stone wall. "Can you see the hole at the bottom of the wall?". "George's digging in the hole," he answered. I said, "Good, let him dig. What's he digging for?". "He wants to get something for me." I can see it in my head — George wanted to get something for him. So here — the consciousness thing is in play and we're both in the "pool " together. That's what's happening. I don't think it's telepathy, and I don't think it's projection.

The dog digs and brings up a bottle. I know there's a message in the bottle. Alan says, "There is something in the bottle". I say, "Open it". Alan opens the folded paper. I can see a piece of paper; even tell you what the words were. "Don't give up now". He opens the paper. "The words say, 'Don't give up now'."

Am I giving him something that he's just adopted, taken, you know? I don't know. Is he giving me something? I don't know. We're trusting it. Just going with it. See what's happening. When he opens the paper I think, whose writing is it? His dad's writing. He says, "My dad's writing". Now, Alan had a terrible relationship with his father but now, that father has been transformed into someone who helps him, not somebody who beats him. He's gone through that phase. "I know I've not got to give up, now. When I'm in this really bad state and I really want the drugs again. I know I've not got to give up".

"There is something more," says Alan. "The dog's still digging". The dog carries on. Brings up another bottle. I know this is the moment. I said,

"What's in the bottle?". I know there's nothing in it. He says, "It's empty". He says, "That's it, isn't it, James? That's why I'm like this. Because I'm afraid, I'm afraid of what's in the bottle". Now, Alan is in a terrible state of anxiety (which is why he came to me that week). He is so afraid, because he knows now the bottle is empty. The doctors won't give him any more drugs. He's committed now. The bottle is empty, and he's no more props to lean on — they're all gone.

I could feel the shift in him. In energy healing terms I felt his energy field shift and it was a healing moment for him. The point was, he healed himself at that point because he had insight as to where his fear was coming from. Because he could see where it was coming from, it lost its power over him. It lost its power.

Now, is that energy healing? Am I doing it? Is he? I don't know and the answer is, it's none of those and it's all of those. One enters the sacred space.

* * *

Recounting these things helped me to affirm some things, that I feel right about. One of them, because I witnessed it recently, has to do with the case where people feel certain about things. They are certain they see angels, or that this is going on with somebody's chakra or something. I don't doubt their honesty, but I'm really not certain and I'm not sure certainty is helpful for people. Maybe some clients need certainty, when you're with them in healing relationships. But I think what I'm certain of, is that I'm really not certain.

While I personally experience things, visual things, fluctuations in a patients' energy fields, my hit on that is that I'm witnessing something that has filtered through my mind, which struggles to put a rational explanation on things.

Therefore, if I experience something, like a light around somebody, or the presence of an angel, I am cautious with it. I wonder how far it has been culturally embedded in me. My culture knows about angels, I see this thing, and therefore it is an angel. Rather than be aware that one is experiencing a sense in the healing space which is the rational mind struggling to understand or find a label for it.

For me, there is a wariness of what I, rather judgmentally, call a new-age fluffiness — talk of angels and energy fields and spirits and stuff.

James

I know some people are gifted with a sense of certainty about things.
I understand that. I share it; it happens with me many times and I hold that
in the context of healing. But what I have learned to do, right or wrong, is to
keep my trap shut. Not say to patients, "This is it, this is what I see, this is
what you've got, this is … I know this, etcetera". Rather if it is discussed at
all, it is done very gently.

If a patient says to me, "What did you see, what did you experience?" I will
always have caveats. "Well, you know this is just my perception. It's limited.
I can tell you this, and I'd like you to use that to interpret, to work with the
ideas; not take it as a definitive diagnosis. I will tell you on condition that
anything I say may be just complete bollocks, or it may be deep certainty".

Only rarely, probably on three or four occasions, in the past seven or eight
years, have I put aside tentativeness. This is a teaching I received from Ram
Dass, because of the way he was with me the first time I met him. There are
occasions where you have to put aside tentativeness, when you feel
somebody is in such deep danger that you have no option but to say, "You
must do this is. I really want you to do this".

I liken that to my experience as a nurse in a psychiatric unit where a patient
says, "I'm throwing myself out of the window". Do I let him do it? No I don't,
I stop him. And I think there is a point you reach with somebody, where you
weigh all the things in the balance, take all the bits into account, and have to
say, "This is what you must do. I believe you are in danger, I am concerned
about this".

It's very much a two-level experience. One is, I could say, the raw
experience, which is in a realm different from the rational world. Then there
is the way you make sense of it, and bring it into the world, and ground it in
practice.

* * *

Somebody sent me a birthday card, when I hit fifty, a few years ago. A
picture of a long grey- haired bearded man, halfway between a wall; he was
walking through the wall. There were two distinct worlds on one side. She
said the card was for a man who truly walked in two worlds. In my existence
now, my life is one of being in two worlds simultaneously — ordinary reality,
and non-ordinary reality. I walk between both; I've a foot in both camps,
permanently. Sometimes I'm more in one than t'other, and sometimes more
in t'other. But most times, it's just moving backwards and forwards.

James

A primary challenge with this, in this work, is the risk it brings to you (and to others) if you're not gentle with yourself. If you don't rest a little bit easy, and be tentative — not get caught up in certainties of things. It's relatively easy to be certain about this material reality — it's all solid. But when you experience inner reality there's a sense in which it isn't. So one learns caution, tentativeness, not to be alone in this, to seek out peers. Maybe they seek you out — if chance it be. Ram Dass, several others I've worked with closely, are treading these boundaries and, even better, have trod them before us. Just as I now work with others as a teacher or guide, who were, to some degree, younger; there are one or two older in chronological terms.

I recently saw a speaker at a gathering. While somebody was speaking I closed my eyes and could see something else taking place. It was in a realm where bodies are not bodies, the physical is not physical — a timeless, spaceless place. I opened my eyes, and I saw this person with what, in my interpretation of this reality is, was some shadow walking behind them and it didn't feel comfortable.

So I have to work with that and say, "Is that an illusion? Is it a product of too much champagne the night before? Is it da, da, da?". But I have learned to trust those experiences that challenge the work I have to do on them. My spiritual practice is how I work with them

Do I go up to that person, as sometimes people of that mentality have done with me, and say, "There is a real shadow walking around behind you, watch what you're doing"? Because I don't know what the shadow is; whether it's real or not. But I know that I experienced it. And drifting between two worlds, and knowing some of the nature of the shadow, it doesn't feel comfortable.

I do feel that person is carrying something, or moving toward something that may put them in a place, perhaps, of physical ill health. So do I just ignore it, and let destiny take its course? Why does that reveal itself to me? Was it a revelation or delusion — the very fine line between imagination and revelation? All we are left with are our powers of discernment rooted in our experience, or faith, or surrender.

In this recent situation, it felt right to approach that person, simply because of the subject they were talking about. I sensed they must, in some way, be attuned to this sort of stuff. I was interested to see how that person would respond. I would come to them sensitively and say, "Look, just while you were speaking the other day, do you mind if I say something about what I was noticing? And it may sound a bit strange, but I'd just like you to interpret it with me".

I would approach it from what I would hope was a participative, non-diagnostic, non- controlling way. And see how the person responds to it. They may either say, "You're completely freaked out, and I don't want to hear you". Or, if they were the person they projected in their speech, they would be hungry to hear it, and want to work with it and see what teaching it had for them.

I do sometimes get a sense of being guided in this interaction, but I would hesitate to say where that guidance comes from. It is absolutely benign. There are tests that I apply when I am involved in something — either personally, or through a process I am going through or some experience I am having; or when I am working with somebody else. I am checking, "Is my ego in this? Is my desire to be clever and be able to tell somebody 'like it is' involved in this". I checked. No, it doesn't feel like it's there. Does this feel like it's coming from here the head, or the heart area? Does it feel loving? As a result of the experience, do I feel more, or do I feel less? Is there a sense of danger in it or not? Does it invite me to work with somebody in a loving and nurturing and supporting way? Or is it possibly threatening or frightening in some way?

Then you have to do the weighing, the checking, the balancing. In doing the weighing and checking and balancing, I am making reference to both worlds, in myself, yes; and the client, depending where they are — yes and no.

The information comes from the rational world and the non-rational world. The answers come from the rational world and the non-rational world. We have it all there available to us. I could stick with one, and stick with the other. I think those of us who get into this place of working with different states of reality probably have a greater challenge in the world. A more scary challenge, if you like, because you've got this extra stuff to work with. I can see why where I was ten years ago, as with so many people I work with now, many prefer ordinary reality. I refused to get out of this reality. It was safer, and full of certainties. I give drug X and a reasonably predictable response, Y, will occur. People needing certainty usually come from a place of fear in themselves because to move beyond that certainty is just too terrifying.

Where I am with this, is I think I negotiate, and I do not negotiate. I move with it, and have remained still within it. My spontaneous response to this question is that at some point I have to trust very deeply. Sometimes there is no contest to that trust. If somebody is saying, "I just had a vision, James. I know you have these things. And my vision is telling me to go and kill my children," I would have no hesitation in saying, "We need to look at that. We need to take a reality check here". Because that's one of the tests, to me. If the experience — be it visual, drugs, whatever — is asking you to harm yourself or others, then there is a gigantic question mark coming from it. At that point I'd say, "No. From my point of view, since you mentioned it, you're out of line. You've got some wires crossed, and we need to look at this".

People who I think get caught in that, have not had the advantage of the deeper work. They have not finished the work that's cleared out their stuff so they can avoid get easily attached to these certainties.

* * *

I've gone through these many times — I've received these guidance, these revelations; I've witnessed, I've experienced things on many different levels, venues, times. I can see the hooks. I make a habit of it, opportunities to be great, powerful, the centre of somebody's attention, whatever it is. All the things in my ego that are openings for me to get attached to these things.

I am thankful for this ongoing work that enables me to be illuminated, to see those things when they hook you, and to be able to unhook oneself from them. You can then be available without your agenda. At this point, I regularly get into places where there is no option but to say, "I'm surrendering here. And it is not my will, but Thine. Help me here. I don't know what I'm doing". It is usually in positions that are extreme — either for myself, because I'm deeply concerned about something, or disturbed about something, or when I'm with somebody else.

It's like a faith, a surrender, and a trusting, in God with whom I have a deep personal relationship. We chat like you and I chat now. I know that that would horrify some, and I know it could be classed as my projecting something onto some part of my ego or soul that I need to have a chat with. Doesn't feel like that. I have this regular confab with a humanist friend of mine — a devout humanist — if you pardon the pun. While I accept huge amounts of what she says about the experience of the super ego and the collective unconscious and all this type of thing, I end up saying, "Well, I can't have a conversation with a collective unconscious".

James

This is deep and personal and, from time-to-time when I feel in need of guidance, I go quiet. I learn to sit still and shut up. And listen. Sometimes it's a sort of inner dialogue. There are no words — I'm using dialogue but there are no words; just a symbolic interaction taking place, in which understanding comes through. Only occasionally have I responded to inner guidance that has said, "I want you to this". And then I think, "Oh, I'm unsure about this".

The doubt is a useful tool. I use doubt, and I use questioning to check things out. I'm making it sound like it some endless struggle or tussle, but by and large it isn't. It's fairly quick, spontaneous, fun.

The issue of discernment, is important. Yes, it may sound egotistical, but I'll say it because egotism is part of my spiritual practice: I don't think you can get it unless you've done the work. There ain't no short cuts, there are no bypasses, no quick leaps. While I think it is important to have the techniques and the approaches — like I've learned Energy Healing — without the personal work, in psychological terms it's working on the ego or the emotional work, or spiritual terms it's deepening one's connection with the Divine or "All That Is". I think all of them are needed to develop discernment. Everything in a holistic universe is enmeshed, all connected. Holism is about absolutely everything being connected with everything else. There is no separation — of anything.

And I don't think one can truly grasp that unless you've trodden non-ordinary reality.

James

Chapter Nine

MICHAEL

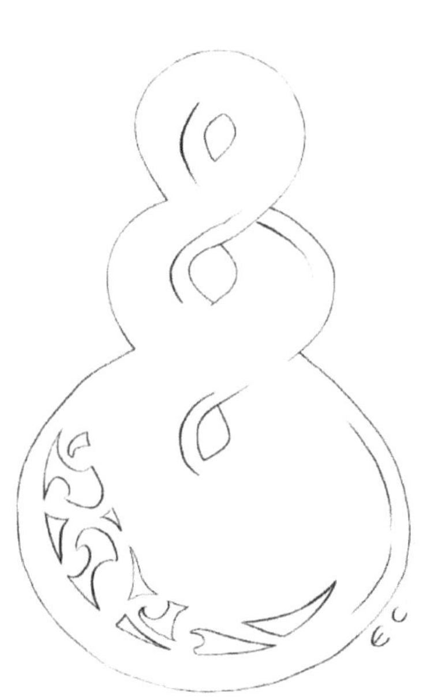

Michael

Michael and I had known each other for years without me being aware that he was a healer. We spoke on the back veranda of his home. I was fascinated by his poetic and articulate accounts of his journey as a healer, at his connections with Indigenous healers, and how he was integrating his spiritual healing experiences into his everyday life. I was also deeply moved by the healing journey around the deep wounds he sustained in his life.

I was lucky to be in a very good training school. I learned, from one of our tutors, a beautiful Maori woman, about the spiritual aspect of nursing. She spoke — openly and eloquently — about caring, and about the importance of touch, and healing. So, from day one that was just a given in the curriculum; not necessarily the established curriculum; her curriculum. I had a clear understanding of the spiritual aspect of nursing from the start.

I was young and don't think I'd thought a great deal about nursing before then. But I felt led to do what I was doing; some universal accident had got me there, though it wasn't something I'd had ambition or desire for. It came across my path — it just worked that way for me.

My first understanding about healing was about the importance of touch. I hadn't probably ever thought of it consciously, but I understood innately it was correct.

Until then, healing was something to do with care. The words "care" or "caring" were involved. I understood that. Subjectively, as a child, when I was cared for or unwell, I understood what that meant; not necessarily the lotions and the potions. It was being soothed, balanced in some way. That was my experience growing up. I hadn't ever challenged that.

There was a history of caring in my family, in my mother's family; I received a lot of extremely good nursing knowledge as I grew up. There were directors of nursing in nursing homes and convalescent homes. So, self care, as well as the ability to care for, was imparted in my childhood, quite naturally.

The women in my mother's family had an innate understanding of the principles of medicine, and the principles of the body. Lay knowledge, social knowledge, in a way, but quite grounded. In my first year of nursing, a lot of what I was taught to see as care and nursing was something I'd already learned. I understood how to care for those with measles and chicken pox, normal childhood illnesses, from conversations my aunties would have between them and my mother. From women who home nursed their children I learned the more social caring, sensible caring.

Michael

I worked within the framework for a large part of my nursing career; accepted that tenet quite easily. Where I came from, the spiritual aspect of nursing was promoted. Nursing was a vocation, rather than a job.

* * *

For a period of time my focus was on gaining skills, becoming an expert — you know, Benner's model.[82] I went through all the stages, and learned very fine somatic cues; why is this happening or that? I learned from books advanced learning of physiology, biochemistry, and so on. I worked in high-tech areas, so for a long time I needed to learn those things. As I became more senior in nursing, management and teamwork were a really a large focus for a long time.

I gave good care in nursing. I knew the power of touching was really important and that increased, rather than decreased, over the years. Still, I didn't consciously think about it, as a phenomenon, until one or two events occurred.

I remember that while working with ventilated patients, I'd have a really strong pull to put my hands on them. When I look back on it, it was more like Reiki. I would sit with head injury cases whom the doctors felt weren't going to wake up, and also pull them to consciousness when the drugs had been weaned and they were on ventilation. I would concentrate and interact with that being as I turned and washed them and physically cared for them. I had no expectation they would reply. And, I didn't necessarily accept the diagnosis. I also had no problems in stimulating consciousness in others, in many of those cases.

My spiritual belief is strong; it always was. I believed then that one soul was talking to another. I believe that spirit is attached — in quantum theory — in the space between atoms. So, spirit innervates the body. It's evident in the first breath of the baby. For example, caesarean-section babies who are completely asleep when you bring them forth out of the waters... when you prickle their nose, and you watch the neural prickle, when they first take that first "Ah" breath, and the little buds on the body all over the skin turn pink, and then the pink fuses. Then they start to move and they become collected. Certainly with that first breath, I've noticed more than once, what appears to be a cloud, a wetness around the baby, disappears. I thought at first it was just the shine of the lights on the baby, but rather, it was like a camera going into focus; you could see their outline a lot more clearly.

Michael

And certainly I've observed a lot of death over the years, and I have seen something leave the body. Not all the time, but once or twice definitely seen something leave the body. So I believe that the flesh is a willing participant in the connection between spirit which innervates, and body which reacts.

If one of the people in the Indigenous population was sick, I would relax and do healing touch around them, because the relatives expected that. They would look into my face, and say, "No, put your hands on them". They saw me as a healer, a little bit more than that. I was always given that place. And so if the curtains were pulled around the bedside, and there was an Indigenous family there, I would place my hands while they prayed and move energy. It was definitely energetic.

Certainly, stuff did happen for me which was hard. I had a lot of trouble with doctors. Perhaps it was part of healing or knowing, but I was able to diagnose very quickly. For example, when the unconscious came into A&E, I thought, like Benner described, it was minute somatic cues and excellence. Looking back on it, I realise it was a little bit more celestial than that. I would know that there was something wrong with their gut, or it was their head, or something else. Partly, a profile of somatic cues — I'd seen that phenomenon many times — but in mixed, multi-systems failure, I was still able to pick up the leading cause. Quickly. Now that insulted the medical fraternity; they got very threatened and challenged. They didn't know how I would know and would argue with me until the tests came back. (I would, as an advocate, demand certain blood tests). I just would want those tests to prove to what was correct, in the patient's best interests.

I became increasingly uncomfortable within the system. Not with people, not what I was doing, but within the system and, as a result, I restricted myself. What I was doing wasn't quite kosher, or wouldn't be regarded well by the system.

I was doing a fair bit of reading of esoterics — Taoist thought, Zen thought. Chinese medicine I really liked, and understood instinctually — and developed a broader understanding of homeostasis and medicine. I watched for years, and compared what I'd learned from Chinese medicine with what I was seeing before me in the wards. Over time — it proved itself again and again — I saw how the system or the method of Chinese medicine held true.

My abilities were eclectic — intuitiveness, with nursing knowledge. I became a nursing expert — an expert clinician and, around that point, I started doing more hands-on, or energetic work.

Michael

Coming to be a healer, and living as a healer, has changed me. I had a huge acceleration in my thirties, to the point where I disconnected from a twenty-year relationship. I was growing in awareness and understanding but certainly had to undergo my own healing journey. Very subjective, very difficult. I had three kids. I didn't have mentors, or a guide, or compass, or any comfort. Yet I had an intuitive understanding that it had to be that way.

So it was a very difficult time in my life. I reached a stage where I thought colour was draining out of my world. I was living in black and white, some could call it depression. I don't feel it was, it was more of a spiritual distress. I had started doing healing work with men's groups at men's festivals and gatherings. At that time it created a lot of trauma and anxiety in my relationship with my wife — there was fear and mistrust.

I found a dichotomy as I felt fine and high when I was doing this work but it would take me a couple of days to ground afterwards. If I'd been away for a two- or three-day gathering which had been growth orientated it was very nourishing for me. But it really caused direct problems in my relationship. As I said — fear and mistrust. I found that difficult to cope with.

I realised I had to dig into my own depths and go through my own healing journey, to move forward in life. I hadn't realised I needed to do as much inner work. I'd done work for everybody else as a nurse, and self ignored. Brought up three kids, self-ignored.

The men's gatherings can be 100 people at a time. When I step into the circle of men, something grows, accelerates inside me; I can breathe in and breathe out and something — calm — radiates, and men relax with that. Men who have had no experience before of "heart country" will relax. I have the ability to make people feel at ease, and I could accelerate or augment it, to get even 100 men at once to feel it. I would do some body process work and, as a result of putting them in a space, along with a bit of guided imagery, a lot of men would cathart. It might be dropping into their own grief, into their own stored or suppressed feelings, and then it could be a release. I was able to hold the space; allow that to occur, within some sort of boundary so it wasn't chaotic. So I would feel a great deal of peace, and joy, and knowing in that space.

I did have a sense of being assisted, indirectly, with this process. It also felt as if I was directly observed. The best way I can say it is I felt the weight of others around me; like the elders were with me. In the spiritual. I have always felt a strong spiritual presence in my life and been guided by it; kept

Michael

safe by it. Sometimes, you know, I've been warned about certain things. I've had a sense that if, for example, I'd gone down there, or moved over there, I would have been in quite a lot of danger.

The men's gatherings were heart space gatherings where my consciousness was heightened. Not altered, but heightened. When I came home, I felt very tender, very vulnerable. It was like a skin or two had been pulled off. So a bit raw, very open, and needing quietness and stillness. I felt quite light on my feet, didn't really want to eat that much and wasn't really feeling like I was in my body very much. Certainly had no feelings of sexuality, or, say, the usual base chakra appetites at all. I felt like a helium balloon slowly landing back on the ground, in myself, and it could take a good forty-eight hours to occur. Two or three other healers who worked in the same space have told me they experienced the same thing.

I always gave myself time, so I didn't have to go directly back to work, but the usual day-to- day life matters were still there, and some of them would be quite pressing. I was working in the esoteric world, but we live in the temporal world. I still had the demands of bills, children. It was a bit chaotic around that energy — pressing in quite quickly.

When I was in the more esoteric space and, for example, be on a bus or train, a plane and so on, I'd have people responding to me in a different way and, sometimes, people would cathart next to me. I got upset about that for a long time, but realised it was just spiritual energy.

One time, I was coming back from a gathering and waiting in a big city train station. I got talking to a Maori woman and her twin sons. And she told me that her husband was dying of liver failure. And he was on so much Doloxene and other pain killing pills, but not processing all that stuff. He was mad as a rabbit — pharmacologically insane. He'd been for a walk and as he came back he was throwing up into the rubbish bins. He really wasn't in good physical condition and, obviously, heavily drugged. He was also aggressive and frightening to his children but I could see, too, his verbose "out there" behaviour was shaming his wife. As she was there, he came and sat down. It was next to me. He calmed immediately.

And he told me I was an Indigenous healer, like a medicine man. I said that I did that sometimes, and told him a bit about the gathering that I'd been on. He talked for a while and then he walked with me to my train platform. To others he might have appeared a drunk insane man, but he'd got it. He got the message.

Michael

I spoke to him on that platform. "Go home and see the elders. And stop taking drugs, because all you are doing is running away from your own death." And he started to cry. When I speak with that sort of authority, I feel something different coming from me; I know I was giving him essential spiritual knowledge. He saw me onto the train, and did a tribal farewell to me on the side of the platform, as a mark of respect. He had promised he would go home, and stop taking so many drugs. He realised he had to face his death.

In the beginning I found these things upsetting — I didn't know where the energy came from and was a bit scared I might be a vessel for something I wasn't sure of. What was I being used by? I wanted some knowledge around that.

* * *

I had been brought up, or socialised, as a Christian. So I had a fear that I might be being used by inappropriate forces. That idea came and went for a while. But as the energy grew, and as people's reactions to what I was doing in healing circles became bigger, I realised that, in some way, I'd augmented it. I'd instigated it. At one festival, for example, a man shared in his heart space, got up, walked out and projectile-vomited black bile. It seemed like gallons came out of him. When he returned to the circle, he was pink. I saw that, quite simply, as a discharge of hatred and bitterness. So did all the men there. But I still wasn't sure where that energy came from, so I was a bit scared, at that time.

At one time, I was initiated by an Aboriginal man, in one of the men's gatherings. He was prominent nationally and had written a book. He had the knowledge, the unbroken-lineage knowledge of his people — one of the oldest Indigenous clans.

He knew he was dying and wanted to impart some of his knowledge. At the gathering, he spoke to me, almost continuously, and I couldn't quite hear him. It was like my subconscious was open, and I knew I should accept because I trusted this man — accept and take it in and the understanding would come out later.

Some Indigenous tribes will keep the children up at night and give them the knowledge while they are sleepy and their consciousness is dropping away. The children take in the knowledge, they can recall it later. I understood the principle of what he was doing, and I accepted it, because I understood that

Michael

process. What I didn't know was, as a result of that, he had accelerated something in my effect on people. I think I was shocked and surprised by that so, my distress was a personal reaction out of fear; I just didn't know where this was going to take me.

I also had a fear of being seen, in some way. I didn't want to be in a position of vulnerability, to be "stoned in the marketplace" so to speak. I didn't want to be thought of as different, or as having the ability to create that dynamic in people.

I was only developing, and really strongly accelerating. Though my knowledge of humanity was derived from nursing, the intuitiveness was in my family lineage. I understood something about being able to look into people. The nursing knowledge is a layer on that — the apprenticeship to the body over thirty years. It certainly grounded me more into the human condition. Then doing this other work, especially with the old Indigenous teacher, had accelerated it to another level; to one of energy transfer.

There is, too, my own healing journey. My opening and widening, which I think is developmental in the thirties anyway, was in process. I started to question a lot of things along the lines of, "Is this all there is? Is this my life? Is this where I'm going?" .Up 'til then I'd been quite happy to grow my children, increase my professional knowledge and standing. Quite happy. But suddenly I felt as if I'd been moved a few seats up the grandstand — I wasn't in the arena of my life, I was more looking at it. While I did appreciate that was part of growth and maturity, there was something else going on inside me. Within this, my desire to heal people other than in a nursing way, or the structured way I'd been taught, was increasing as well. I didn't know where that was going to lead me, but I felt compelled to do something about it.

As a result of the widening, I also felt my storage, the emotional history storage, starting to bubble and move in me. I had to deal with aspects of my childhood that needed healing.

And the fact I had always given myself away, and never, consciously, thought much about myself but, rather, about others. I had not nurtured or nourished myself enough. And there was a lot of grief around that.

I was waking up to the fact that I had, out of a loving sense, been wanting to help other people, so I'd become adapted to everybody else's needs. So much so, I didn't know who I was. Now, I knew I needed to know who I was.

Michael

I was also starting to get a few grey hairs on my head and, while this is more developmental, I realised I was only learning this stuff somewhat late. Why didn't I know this years ago?

So, I went to a counsellor — a men's health and wellbeing counsellor who I found really good. I did some rebirthing. I went to men's gatherings.

Yet, what was the inner process? Going to the counsellor was about emotional release. The first time I did emotional release work with him, I saw a myriad of overlaid blueprints of scenes of destruction — people dying; children dying in my arms; blood, guts that had come from the years I'd worked in emergency. While I had handled those experiences at one level, I'd never discharged the emotion of them. And so great grief came out of me around that. I was surprised at the number of memories that dominoed in that cathartic process. I was able to discharge my grief.

Also, counselling helped with my rage and pain around some of the difficulties I had as a male in nursing. The unfairness of my treatment, in the early days. It was good and I thought, "Well, job well done".

I realised, however, there were other aspects. I had never dealt with the toxic dynamics in my family. Nor had I dealt with my mother, a very destructive woman; it was time to deal with that. Two years earlier, I had isolated myself from her; resigned as her son and I didn't know exactly why. So I had to work through that.

There was a process I also had to face. An area opened within me about sexual abuse in childhood, that I hadn't been aware of. I'd carried it, but I wasn't aware of it. To find that, was shocking. I couldn't believe that I'd lived my life, in my body, and not been consciously aware of that. Yet, I'd helped so many other people through that phenomenon, and never ever related it to myself. Never integrated my own remembering/forgetting thing of abuse. It was an intense inner time for me.

I knew when I separated from my marriage, I needed sanctuary and time out. Emotionally, I felt I was dying and I needed to save myself. I didn't know anything else; not what that meant, or where it was going, but I needed it. I took it. To save myself.

I did that for six months. I did go back into my relationship after six months, but soon left, finally. It was a good decision, a healthy decision to make. I'd learned a lot more about myself.

Michael

I didn't really start one-to-one work till about five years ago. I think it's "physician, heal thyself!". And you've got to sample the wares. I couldn't find anybody with a key to accelerate that process for me. I felt like I had a machete and was hacking through the undergrowth creating the path and, though it seemed tough, I had some sense it was necessary. I really wanted a mentor — I wanted somebody to help me. If I could help other people, I wanted to find one of me somewhere. I couldn't.

I felt as if I had no choice but to engage in that process. The stronger the healing energy came up in me, the more sacrifice I had to make. For a period of time. I lost everything in my life — my family, all the wealth I had accumulated. Prior to that intense period, I'd lost the relationship so, it was a period of total loss, and detachment, really, from the physical aspects of life. I had to know that that part really wasn't enough. It was huge, and very traumatic.

Somehow, though, I had a great sense of calm inside, and obedience. I felt like I was peeled open and a strong search light was put on me, and all I could do was have humility and be obedient. All I could do was really go with it. Not struggle against that. It was profound, prolonged, and strong. And I felt broken, as a human being, but also, in a certain way, quite intact. I felt it was part of a process and I had to trust it.

It was deconstruction and reconstruction. But in a funny way, the reconstruction... no, deconstruction, was more archaeology. It was blow-torching off the unnecessary. The essential me was more me. The essential knowledge that I had was stronger. Not new, really. It was like remembering or rediscovering, rather than discovering. So I'd have to say probably more deconstruction. In that deconstruction, the scaffolding of my life — social and family and material — was taken away. This allowed me to expand rapidly. I fell off capitalism, and the expectations that the culture has about a capitalist middle-class wage- earning man. I fell off all that. I had freedom from the enculturation of all that. That accelerated my growth enormously. I really understood that life was the power, the important thing. The rest is an illusion.

It certainly accelerated me and gave me a fearlessness. I think fear is the contractor that we all have and it makes us close down if we keep defended.

And the deconstruction took away my fear — burnished it. What could I be scared of — I'd lost everything! I wasn't starving, the sun was coming out every day, I still had my bodily faculties, my mental faculties. My feelings

Michael

about all that were not joy or euphoria at all. But, at the same time, it didn't matter. I had a sense of the peace, which I'd always had somewhere inside me, growing.

As a result of that my work increased enormously. As did my ability to put hands on to help people cathart, read their emotional history. Now, when people come to me I can read their emotional history very quickly; often it's a matter of minutes. I scan them and tell them — through the body map I use, and my intuition — where they've been all their lives. They all go, "Yes!". It's 100 percent correct. I don't think I would have been able to do that, if I hadn't suffered myself, and felt what I felt. I would have had too much construction around me — too much filter to allow that process. So the increase in work was an affirmation, I guess, of the suffering I'd had. It wasn't "gathering" work now. It was one-to-one, and very powerful, very profound work. Often I saw a major transformation for those people.

The initiation I received from the Aboriginal man may have accelerated the process, but it didn't make it happen. That unfolding was already going on and meeting him was a part of that journey. I saw him as a beautiful being, surrounded by enormous metaphysical power. And I trusted him — his heart and soul. I guess he was sort of a role model. I realised you could live in spirit, if need be and it didn't have to be destructive. And here was this good, good man, whom I admired and respected. And he could move energy.

Not that he would have called himself a healer, because he wasn't, inherently. But he was a keeper of the law and the knowledge, and a bestower of those things. He could do that, that was this job. And he picked me as a healer. I never spoke to him about that, but he picked me, and drew me from the others; to give me knowledge.

There is in my story that of the wounded healer. I think all healers will tell you the initial part of their growth as a healer is to deal with their wounded healer. In the first phase the gifts come, and they are utilised, but they can be a little bit chaotic. You can get a bit carried along by the expectations and needs of others. I never officially opened my doors for practice — it happened. People started coming. I can't remember how, but it started. And I felt, once again, out of control of it; I was just responding. I'd worked for years in emergency work and if something happened, I did what was needed. In this journey it was the same thing. I didn't know there was a button, or switch I could control.

Michael

So it hadn't been until my thirties that I realised I had absolutely no boundaries. I'd never erected any for myself. Working in nursing didn't help; you don't have boundaries and neither do your patients when they are sick and dying or in need, or grief, or pain. The need allows the intimacy, and allows the boundaries to drop. Nursing is the only profession I know where you can put a drip in somebody's arm, or put a catheter up their bladder, and then ask what their name is (when they've finished choking). You can absolutely crash people's boundaries, and I've also been crashed all my life in emotional ways, without knowing it.

I think that declaring boundaries is an inherent part of healing as well. At first, I think you've got to experience "boundary-lessness" in order to allow incoming energy. I think you learn to control it later and it's true, from the ones I know and the readings I've done, that wounded healers have boundary issues as well.

I think if we had strong boundaries all our life we probably couldn't be good healers. I think the incoming energy is too filtered. When I talk to thehealers, especially the Indigenous model healers ,I hear a familiar story from most people who deal with hands on or energetic. I follow an Indigenous model of healing. In the beginning when the gifts pour in, and you get overloaded, or swamped or, even, caved in, you've then got to physically, consciously, erect boundaries.

When I feel swamped and caved in, it's about people demanding, needing, wanting. When I put a name and shape on the healing it felt contained. And I'd done healing for many years before that by talking to people. People might call it counselling, but it wasn't; there was a transfer of energy. I never advised them, but they would get something from talking with me.

It created difficulties within my relationship for a number of years. Yet, I couldn't not do that — I felt compelled, that I had to be obedient to that process, because I knew I could affect people in a very positive way. I think that probably took up a large amount of my time and, in some ways, my family did suffer.

When I started in practice, and had a start, a middle, and a finish, to a thing called "healing", it was a different story. Having said that, people would ring continually, and almost expect the response, "I'll come around now". It might be nine or ten o'clock at night. I started having people come from other countries and I would find their requests hard to refuse. I'd comply,

Michael

regardless of what that might do to my life at the time. "Oh, they're coming from such a distance, I'll have to see them".

I had to learn to say, "No, it's not really suitable for me now".

I think I did have issues around withdrawing myself from other people in a more energetic or emotional sense, around boundaries. I found it difficult to create boundaries, and I felt like that especially in the relationships I've had. I was changing some construction there. I do know that withdrawing, or really defining myself more clearly, hurt some people. I'd been so available to them, and suddenly I wasn't. My friends felt I had separated from them in some way. Definitely. It didn't affect my children, because I wasn't doing that with the kids. There is a "boundary-lessness" about children in some ways, in the growing years.

But certainly in my relationships with women as well, because I was going through issues of my own sexual abuse, it meant I really did learn to withdraw and give myself space. I found that very healing. I didn't have to comply with the wishes or needs of other people. I had to deal with my own needs. While I felt anxious about that, I had to see what that really was. It was irrational, but very unsocialised, and very eerie. I learned that I could say "no", and that I could shape and make this. And the better I was, the better it was going to be for other people, anyway.

The emergency imperative was quite trained into me — everything needs to be done in three minutes, and you can't say you want to have your tea, or go to the toilet or whatever. You deal with the discipline of having to do what's needed, immediately. I had to de-socialise from that. I needed to realise that sometimes a healing crisis isn't as urgent as somebody choking to death. No less important, but not quite as imperative. It was a difficult apprenticeship.

Social boundaries were not that difficult for me. It wasn't anyone ever making me feel powerless, or feeling powerless around them. But somehow if they needed something, I would feel invaded more by their needing than their demand. I could keep demand at a distance; I'm quite eloquent when it comes to defending myself. And I can push people energetically, I'll back them off, out of my space. But if I felt obliged or, in some way, compelled to help them — the victim calling — that was my invasion. That was just patterning from childhood. I've got on top of that now.

My belief, I think, around being invaded by the victim would be that I was responsible. For making them better. It was certainly reinforced in my

Michael

childhood, and in nursing. So, I had to really learn that I was not responsible for anybody else. And it took a while for it to feel okay. The more of the work I do with energetics, the clearer that sort of stuff becomes.

I really like clarity — the clearer I am, the clearer that I can be with other people, the easier it is for them to find clarity. I say to people, "If you know yourself, then you'll always know fifty percent of any social equation".

This is what I was talking about before — learning to know the human part of me. Who I am. But I've been working fairly consistently with energetic healing for five years. And a spin-off is that you to get some spiritual knowledge. And some clarity is part of that.

Spiritual knowledge, for me, I guess, is a sense of knowing; knowing that this thing — a thought you have, or the way you were perceiving a situation — is correct. In the healing environment, when I look into somebody and can tell them the emotional facts of their life, I feel much larger than I usually do. I feel quiet and still, and there is a lot of radiant love that comes out of me while I do it. And people receive that — I can see it by their reactions. And it removes their socialisation so quickly that they can go, "Yes, that's right. I forgot about that". They will react, and feel it because I promote a container of safety around it. It's more than counselling — it's telling them their life. It's done with conviction, because it's felt very much in my belly, and in my heart, and in my head. A very centred feeling.

That knowing is, I think, part of the old tribal knowledge. And has different flavours, too. When I deal with one particular Indigenous group I am, at one level, aware of the culture and their history, but I can speak with authority to this particular people about their issues.

I also speak with authority to other Indigenous people, and they receive it in the same light. There is the base village. The culture is the brightly coloured clothing that clothes the body of humanity or, in this case, the core of the village. So the authority comes from the human village that I feel spiritually linked to. And there is a lot of lineage and wisdom in that. So I can impart it, yet — while it comes through my mouth, sounds like my voice, and it doesn't feel like anybody else — the knowing is greater than me.

I'm not instructed — I'm not given words that I just spit out. They are inherent at the time. I know it, and I speak it and it comes with great love and clarity. I can do that one-to-one, or one-to-a hundred. They do hear that, they feel the groundedness and the solidness of that.

Michael

And they give way to that, in some way. They feel humility, they feel peace and can take it in. There is no ego there, no defence there. I can counsel people, and advise them, and it's my life knowledge, and my nursing knowledge (knowledge about human beings) which is a different layer of understanding.

When I touch people, sometimes I have a knowing about an event that happened on that part of their body. I'll give you an example. A client from another city came down, saying she couldn't understand why she couldn't initiate and go forward in life and wanted to do some work around that. We were doing some work, and she was in quite a deep relaxed state — I use music, frequency as well. She'd done one session with me, was quite comfortable in the second session, but was scrunching up her shoulder. And I put my hand on her shoulder, and grabbed it really hard to overawe the message that was coming out of that shoulder. I knew that a schoolteacher who had sexually abused her had grabbed her on the shoulder. I knew in that instant, and spoke it as I knew it. And I pulled that energy from her. She screamed and catharted, and I cradled her and her memories came open. Dominoed open. And she had not had conscious access to that since she was eleven. She had just blanked it out.

At these times I feel much bigger than ordinary old me. I'm a vessel, and there is sacredness working. And it's obedience. That's how the "ordinary old me" accommodates the great expansiveness of the experience of healing. That's what sacrifice is. Where you allow yourself...

I guess it's like the temporal world and the esoteric. Really, it's walking two worlds. So, I started to walk two worlds as a nurse, and do healing. You know, there was this temporal, socially constructed, organised thing called "nursing". And the other deeper spiritual stuff, and it was about aligning the two. The Indigenous at home taught me to walk two worlds. I learned that when I was young.

I think I was always aligning the two worlds. But I think the boundarylessness helped to integrate it. I've learnt more of that when I go away and do bush gatherings, it's very real, but you can't live in that. I would come back to bills, and crying children, and homework and my studies. I couldn't suspend the temporal world so I learned, to not exactly separate them but to give each shape and boundaries. Certainly I have a start and a middle and a finish to healing things that I do.

Michael

I was given this knowledge about opposites. You know, that it's "all of the above". First of all I took the knowledge on in a theoretical sense and had some illumination on how to view everything in my life. I had felt for a while that this healing journey included going off to a monastery. And leaving my children behind. Or being in a big garden, and having people come to me. I had to give over to that picture and lose my life as it was, in some way. It was either/or. Now, I realise how my constructed thought had given me the problem, rather than the energy itself.

It was a painful time, accompanied with loss, and the truth behind the saying, "The old must die before the new is born". My old died, let me tell you, it cracked! In all ways, in all directions.

It took about two years and, though it was a shock, I realised I wasn't dissembling; I was growing, expanding. So when I lost fear, I think, I integrated and I don't think I had a struggle after that. I just kept evolving — I got the formula right, if you like. I'd given up the idea of either/or — opposites, polarities. It was about blending all.

When you look into a kaleidoscope you see, really, only illusion. The kaleidoscope is all of the colours; all that you see. And I started to feel my life in that way. The total mandala, total matrix — with the rainbow in it. At any given time it was just about stirring that, and blending it. So, if I lifted a spoonful of that... and another of this... out of myself, it had all of the elements in it. I didn't have to have compartments, separations, in that way.

Since I've done that, I've learned that I can augment components of myself at any given time. Just like you can summon sadness or joy or fear or anger and, really, healing is part of that too, in some way. I am a human matrix, an interface with all the other things going on. And healing is one of those things.

It's not all that I am, it's not all that I do, but it is a vital part of my mandala. At any given time, if I want, I can put my hands on somebody without a preparation exercise before it. Although I do have ceremony around that, too. Certain cleansing stuff that I do before and after. Because I want to complete that. I don't want to share or mingle that energy, other people's energy with mine. I've learned, you know, I understand that sort of stuff.

The symbology, though I'm not very precious about it, is comforting, good for us. I understand the power of it, in a start, middle and finish sense; it gives things shapes and boundaries.

Michael

I think, through loss, pain, and personal suffering I got to blend. The rivers ran, you know, all the rivers ran. It all became one, rather than lots of different parts of me. And I think we learn a bit of that going through life anyway. I think when we're younger we have the social self, the family self, the work self.

We show different projections, different facets of ourselves everywhere. But I think we do integrate through life, hopefully, if we are successfully growing up, anyway. So healing was part of that process too. You know, it's part of that expansion. Because all creation expands. And so I'm expanding with it, and I see that, very much. That's a good thing.

I don't have struggles with any of that now. I view my working life, I guess, from the idea that there are always polarities, and we work with integrating the opposites. Somebody screamed at me at work a few months ago, and said, "I don't know what's wrong with you, you don't seem to get upset about anything!". And that, to me, is the fundamentalist view challenging an integrated esoteric one. That's the way I perceived it. I said, "Well, I don't have to get upset about this. There is no point". Part of that is suffering, too. You know, learning in comparison — relativity. Suffering widens your relativity. You can take more on. I think learning is about increasing capacity. So I think though the capacitor's suffering increases — the influx is greater, and therefore the outpouring can be greater.

I talked about the process of coming to be a healer. Living as a healer. I do identify myself as a healer now — I wouldn't have, once. It's quite a strange, chaotic life at times. If I had anyone staying with me for period of time, they'd see the different people that come and go, spontaneously, from this house and they'd laugh. There is a lot of mystical, and the metaphysical joke is alive in lots of ways. They are like a series of one-act plays. And that's not me being displaced from it, it's just what is attracted to my door. Sort of spontaneously.

So living as a healer is... I have lived alone for quite a period of time, and I needed to do that. My life pattern has changed. My understanding of human nature and human beings, adding the spiritual element, has changed. Certainly made me a lot fussier about my relationships. You know, like what I want to have near me in my life, because I know what I know as a healer is a completely different paradigm to what I first had. I've probably thrown away most of the paradigm. You know, the living happily ever after, the capitalist messages — everything slowly sliding away. So I'm learning to live

Michael

without labels. And it's part of the integration — I'm not either/or. Probably all of those things, which has given me greater freedom to be human. And the greater freedom I have to be human, the more I can help others in their transformation.

There is a layer of personal transformation that I can help with. There is a deeper layer of older knowledge that comes up in people when they are healing. Old knowings that I can also help with — earlier lineage, you know, where they've come from, energetically. Which is different to just their life. I also have learned to help people cleanse themselves from experiences, trauma — I can physically resonate them. So people who have been raped or abused, I can make them feel clean again. And that's really important. It's a gift, and I understand how it works now. One day I will impart that technique, because there is something about technique in it. You know, like I'm learning and growing still.

I know that I can't tattoo or pierce my body. Because I am a healer. I have to be as pure as creation made me. I just can't distort or change my body in any way. I just know I couldn't live with a tattoo on me. It wouldn't be right.

I couldn't pierce myself either. It wouldn't be right. It's not as creation made me. With the exception of cigarettes, which is an old pattern that I'm slowly eradicating. Because there's a physical addiction there, as well as probably psychological ones. I find I can't drink, that I have no interest in drinking very much. I don't want to smoke marijuana, I certainly don't want to poke other drugs into me. It's not necessary for me to do that. The natural is rising more in me. So when I need something, I'll go to the sea, or go to a high place, and I will get the energy I need from more natural things. More than those constructed by humans. It's definite changes like that.

I think my ability to unconditionally love has climbed to another level through the healing model; it's certainly well taught and well practised in nursing. You know, through healing I can be much more unconditional and not give of my bone marrow while I'm doing it — which I probably tended to do in nursing.

It's all a good thing — certainly has been a maturing, and a change. And nursing, and healing people in nursing, is somewhat responsible; whereas people that come to me — the "worried well" who come to me — are fully aware that I walk their pathway with them. I am not their pathway, I am not responsible for their pathway, or their soul journey. That has been a difference.

Michael

Chapter Ten

MOIRA

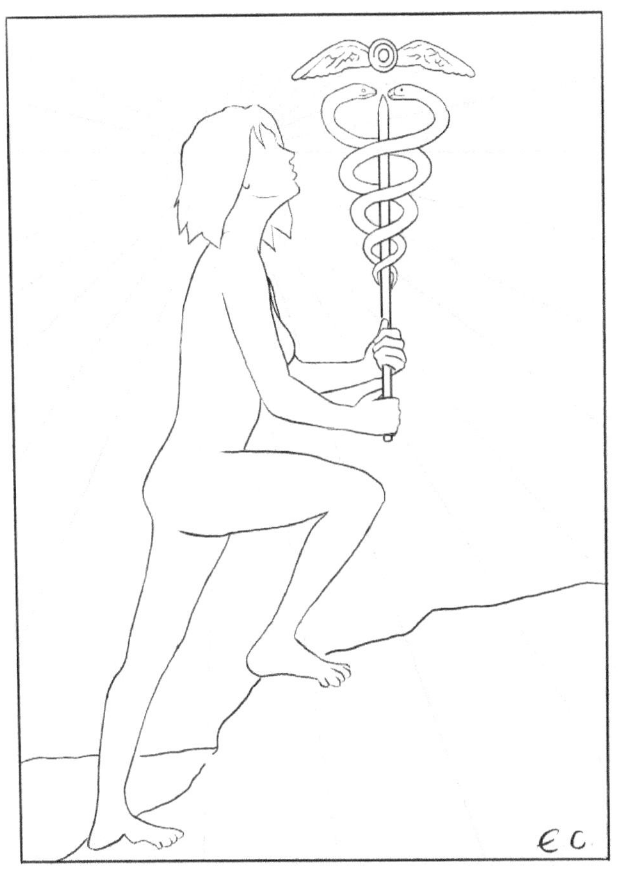

Moira

When I met with her, Moira was completing her RN training having previously worked as an enrolled nurse. We sat down together over cups of tea in her little unit. I was struck how Moira was ever-conscious that the theme of suffering in her life, rather than being a separate, debilitating and fragmenting element, was necessary to its wholeness, its integrity, and to its potentiation in a spiritual, meaning-full sense. She also spoke about her deep experience of being a healer, and the sometimes beautiful, sometimes difficult manifestations of spirit she encountered.

It's a lot of years ago, that I started on my journey. And I guess it started when I had close death in my family. I lost my brother a month before my daughter died, nearly three years old, so we had a lot of death. I had to deal with it, because I had another child to live for. And it was a really really hard time — it's hard to know how you get through a time like that. But, I remember having a vision. I saw my daughter, and she was with a lady who looked very much like my grandma — my mum's mum — though I'd never seen her.

I saw a lady with glasses, and when I described her to mum, later, it seems it was my grandmother. She was in a field of flowers, and my daughter was with her. And my daughter was very happy. And that was shown to me, to comfort me; I was heartbroken. Very alone; I'd shut myself off from everybody. I just wanted to see her again. And I guess I was asking, "Why?". And, without realising it, I asked the Universe, and I saw! I was awake. Wide awake.

I had had a premonition, probably six months before my daughter died, that one of my children was going to die. Of course, I didn't want to know about it. And I wasn't quite asleep — I was in that state where you just slowly go off. I just forgot about it.

I realised, after that, that I would have visions — they would come like a reel, a film, rolling, of how my life would be six months down the track. It's happened to me several times throughout my life, from then on. I never used to take much notice of it. Now, of course, I do and I get strong premonitions, feel a strong intuition. I'm a lot more attuned to it, mainly because I worked on my broken heart.

I did years and years of counselling — with different people. Some counsellors were into the spiritual side as well as practising normal counselling methods. They helped me get in touch with my pain, and it was crucial at the time.

Moira

I was already nursing, about probably ten years after I started to have counselling on a deep level. In getting in touch with my pain I realised I was healing, so I could heal other people in a similar state. That meant a lot to me. And I was working as a health aide with the district nursing service, where I lived. I did four years with them, two of which were in palliative care, on night shifts. A lot of people died during those night shifts. And for some reason I wasn't scared of it. I wasn't scared because I'd lost my own child. I knew she was in another place — another realm, somewhere and I thought, she's gone, wherever. But she didn't really die — the soul doesn't die. I know that for sure.

I was nursing one day, working with a lot of people in palliative care. I was laying them out, cleaning them — the whole bit. during my Enrolled Nursing training. One particular lady, an Italian woman, died and I saw her soul leave the body.

I wasn't scared. It gave me faith in knowing that people were there; could die and they were still there. And, so we went and got a rose from the garden and put it on her. It felt like the right thing to do at the time.

I used to take a lot of care, and talk to people, while I was laying them out. I think that was very important. Even though people would say, "Why are you talking to a dead body?", I would still do that. The person wasn't dead to me — the soul had just left, that's all. And there was a shell. So that was easy; I was speaking to their soul. It always seemed very comfortable for me to do that. And I still do. Even more so, now, I feel it's important that we do this with people. And I can't tell anybody on shift; they'll think you're crazy. So you just do it in your own way — even if it's thought forms. I feel that it's translated in thought form, anyway.

I say, "thought form" as in the thinking the words, and you speaking. Universe, I don't think, has to have words spoken, as such. It can be through touch, or through speaking in your mind — your higher consciousness, whatever you like to say.

I do see a distinct pathway through my life, looking back now. I find it very distinct though I didn't know then; didn't recognise that as being even a healer, until later. I just thought I was doing the things that come naturally. I did what I felt was right at the time. I didn't have any training in healing, until later on down the track.

Moira

My sister was a masseur, and got papers in that. We used to massage each other and one day I thought, "I'll go and do massage". So, I did massage, though I didn't actually sit the exams. I've done acupuncture, for nearly a year but it was hard to be doing full-time university and raise two children on my own. I'd left school at fourteen, so... I had no formative years. It's been a very difficult road.

When I decided I'd go and do a healing course I took a weekend workshop, and I did this thing called "Ki Force". I found it very interesting. At one stage, I felt like I was an electric light bulb. I guess that's the energy, someone else tapping into your energy. I felt like I was opened up to something else — I had more potential. I was a very unconfident person, so I wasn't sure what was happening any of the time. But I went to put my hands on somebody (we were going to heal each other) and he said, "Whoa, nearly knocked me over!" I didn't realise what had happened; I just thought, "Well, it's not me..."

What I learned from that was that it doesn't come from me. It doesn't come from anywhere but the Universe, and I get permission from the Universe if I need to heal somebody, or get the feeling that I should heal somebody. Or if somebody asked me to be healed, I will ask the Universe for permission. If when I get the answer that it's okay, I will do it. Other than that, I won't.

My hands might be on the person's body, they don't have to be unclothed. I found in nursing, it can be done while you're giving someone a shower, or whatever. If, say, the patient you're nursing is dying, it's good just to give them some nice gentle healing while you're rubbing their back, or whatever care you can.

I feel sometimes, when I ring the agency (it will be a spur of the moment thing) I'll meet someone on that shift that I can really help; it happens time and time again. Once you're there, and you meet your patients, there is quite often one that makes you think, "This is why I'm here tonight". Or "This is why I'm here today". It's really good!

One time in particular happened while I was doing my clinicals, in the second year of my degree. A young girl in my ward had had a nose operation. The packing was still in her nose and they couldn't get it out. I just happened to be at the nurses' station at the time, and the RN in charge said, "Oh, we can't get this packing out — she won't let us do it! She's having anxiety attacks.". I said, "Would you like me to try?". "Ooh, if you could," she said.

Moira

I went and sat with the girl, talked to her for a while and I asked her to breathe, and just be strong in her mind, knowing she is in control. I got her, more than anything, to not be anxious any more. And then I said, "Can I put my hands on you?". It didn't matter where, and she was under the blankets, so I could just rest my hands on her legs, or hold her hands, or whatever was appropriate, without being invasive. She said, "Yes".

She was such a tiny thing — and she was a mother. It turned out that her husband was a very dominating man, and she was going home just to clean up all their mess. She said she had anxiety attacks all the time.

I got her to breathe, and I could feel the healing. Then I said, "Do you mind if I help you get this packing out of your nose?". And she became very calm — it was interesting, how she calmed down so quickly. I knew that I could get her to do this, but she didn't know. No one else knew. So no one was with me in the room; it was okay. Then I said to her, "Well, how about if you do it yourself, and I'll just sit here?". I spoke to her, got her to breathe and talked her through it, as well. In the end, she was able to pull on them, with the forceps — with the breathing, and me soothing. I probably had my hands on her, as well — I was feeling some energy going into her — and she was able to pull them out.

* * *

I do see a progression around my experiences with healing. I don't think I have to go anywhere in particular to tap into it any more. I don't have to spend heaps of money on courses — though I never have, anyway. I like to hear about people's experiences — I read a lot. I ask for guidance from the Universe, and I call on my own guides. I tap into that. Over the years I've become confident in what I do. And it's okay that whatever I'm told through the Universe is right. I believe, and I trust, and I have faith.

I probably couldn't count the number of times that things have come up for me, over my time. It's been a very different life, anyway. If I would have, twenty years ago, sat back and seen myself now sitting here speaking about healing — I wouldn't have believed it. Or seen myself at university, doing my degree. I never felt I was capable. But I know, now, I am.

I've had times when I've packed up the car — my daughter, cat, everything I've owned; sold whatever I couldn't fit in the car and moved from one part of the country to another — because that was where I felt I had to live. This is at an intuitive behest — absolutely! I trust my intuition I'd say now ninety-

Moira

nine percent — or, well, 100 percent. And I never used to. I listen to myself now, I listen to my intuitiveness. I used to always listen to it as a woman but now I listen to it as being one with the Universe —just not being so separate.

I was helped a lot by a man who was our communications lecturer. He was bald, dressed differently to everybody else and was a psychiatric nurse. One day he pulled me aside, and said, "Moira, don't be afraid to be unique". I said, "Thank you," but I wondered how he saw that. "Do I stand out that much?", I thought. Anyway, he stood out too, and he wasn't afraid of it, so I think he saw it in me, felt it, and said it. That gave me confidence to be myself. In feeling confident, I feel I can trust my intuitiveness more, too. Each time I trust it, the stronger it becomes. You breed the strength of it. I guess, it's like fear breeding fear and it can accumulate — cause that chaos effect. I think that's what it does.

My intuition has taken me to some strange places, strange situations. When I don't trust my intuition, I can get into trouble. It can give me protection; help me sense people that I really don't ever want to be around.

I had a thing happen to me years ago and I know, now, it was because I was getting around with a certain type of people. I had dark forces come to me. It was very frightening. So I grabbed my child, who was there at the time, and ran out the door. I believe the woman I was friends with at the time, was tapped into the darker forces. Well, maybe it was just a way of warning me that there is dark out there; there's evil as well as good and I should beware. It's never happened again; I'm very careful who I associate with in that way now and I protect myself with the white light.

I think I have gone through a journey around protection. I've actually had times where I'd feel like things are a bit beyond me. Or there is another energy around that's not good, or whatever. So then I will send the white light around me, or whoever.

This sort of energy is very dark. I can intuit it more than see it. I don't see a lot; don't usually see spirits. But I sense things. I've seen flashes. I can even sometimes smell things. I've had times where basically the hairs on the back of my neck can fly up. It's like all my senses just come alive, I feel and I know there is danger around, or there is a situation that I shouldn't go into.

One year, just after Christmas, my daughter and I were driving long distance, and we broke down on the road for, I think it was, five hours. It was getting dark. I was in the car with the cat and my daughter — she was quite young then, not quite twelve. I remember believing that we were looked after, so strongly. I saw three eagles circling in the sky; I believe we were protected.

The highway was full of people going past. I didn't have a mobile, then. Someone stopped and asked if we were all right. They had a phone and used it to call road service for us.

Then, they left.

We waited and waited. No one was coming to help, but I just had to trust — I had to trust so strongly. And then a policeman went down the highway on his motorbike, and I just waved to him, as if to say, "Come over". He turned back down the highway and came up, and just said he would look out for us too, until we got the car going again. By the time we got the car fixed, it was right on dark. So it could have been a very frightening time, but I felt I was looked after. So it was okay even though we were out in the middle of nowhere.

I learned how important protection was quite early — from reading, and from hearing stories from others; people on the similar journeys, healing journeys. My sister, who was older than me, had actually told me a lot, because she went through it a long time before me. But I did go on and take my own path and journey.

I guess sometimes protection comes up when you go to a hospital. Hospitals have got some different energies floating around, because of the places they are — a lot of people dying, and a lot of sick people. So, I've learned you have to give yourself some protection. It might not be even when you go in, so much as when you leave after you come off a shift.

I've had times when I've been, wired up running around for hours on end, and I don't stop to really think about what happened. Who did I meet? You know, sort of, what patients were there? I guess, more so in psychiatric units than general.

The protection is not so much about disconnection, as it is about cleansing myself, my aura. Having a shower is a good way of doing it. Or, just shaking it off, depending on how strongly you feel, I guess and how it's affecting you. Sometimes, with what medications the patients are on, or what's happening to them or who they are, they may be in that state where other entities can slip in and get in with their soul (whatever you like to call it).

Moira

I think people could be taken over in that state and you get a lot of bad energy. It could be anybody, we don't know. They look all right as they lie in bed, dressed in their pyjamas, and their gowns, but we don't know where they come from, or what they've ever done in their life. I think, being intuitive and sensitive like some of us are, we sometimes pick up vibes and energies. I think it's important to protect yourself against those things.

I think just feeling it helps; recognising it's there, I can deal with it. I haven't had anything actually really go wrong, because I've been aware of it. I just sense it's a bad energy; feels very uncomfortable. I don't feel like I'm being invaded so much, because I can allow myself not to be. I can feel just like I've got to protect. So it's not directly inside, not around my personal aura space, but sort of out there. So, I don't let it in. For me it's cleansing — just to cleanse myself, like after you do when you've given a massage, or before a massage, with your own energy.

And that need for protection can happen with some staff, too. It's important for sensitive people to recognise that. You know when you meet somebody on the same path — you recognise that as well and, when you're in a hospital, or in nursing in general, it's refreshing. And in life in general, yes!

I don't think we would be healers if we weren't sensitive. Especially if you can put your hands on somebody and feel where their body is not well, or feel something that isn't quite right within them — whether it's in their aura, or in the shell of their body. I think we have to be sensitive to that, to recognise it.

I do see the process as a spiritual one; definitely a spiritual journey. I think it sets us up for the next realm we go to. But I also think it helps people who are not quite fortunate enough to be shown, or who've learned, in his life, what the possibilities are.

I think, with my experiences, it's been a very hard life. I've had a lot of inner pain. Sometimes physical pain, too. I believe we grow with pain — without it, we don't. I couldn't have got through what I got through in my life, if I didn't recognise that pain was growth.

And be able to rise above it, and become a better person for it. Become more compassionate, more empathetic, if you like.

Otherwise what's the purpose of me being here, too? If I can show somebody that it's this journey, or make them feel better if their body or mind is in a very sick situation, (I believe mind and body aren't separated)

Moira

then why not? if we can work on giving them some time out from any of that — why not? If I'm one person, giving even one person a year a bit of relief from some pain — why not? I can't prevent their pain from happening all the time, but I can at least help them through, somehow.

I've had people help me — and it works. The first counsellor I ever met who I liked was on a spiritual path as well, and I could see that she was integrating the two. I instantly felt at ease, and felt, "This is the one I need to meet". It's a very private thing. It's helping us get through what we need to at that time, with someone understanding who we are, without being classed as having something wrong with us.

It's good to show people that they are in control of their own emotions, and their own self, even by suggesting a breathing technique, or whatever it might be. If they give you permission to give a bit of healing, well, they will experience whatever — it might be just a feeling of comfort, or whatever. We've always laid our hands on people as nurses, so to be able to let them know that there is comfort there, that's a great healing process for them, as well. A hospital is a very lonely place for most people.

I would call a healer a "spiritual healer" rather than a "psychic healer", because I feel like "psychic" is spiritual. I prefer the word, spiritual but it's all combined and everybody's psychic, everybody's spiritual — they've just got to tap into it. I think that some people don't understand it, so they're scared of it for a start. Wouldn't it be nice if more people were not so afraid of it? At least in this day and age, we can discuss these things now. It's important.

Healing power is not from me. Even though people will say, "Oh, gee, you really fixed that", I'll say, "No I didn't — I'm the vessel. Universe is doing everything else". Or God, whoever you say is helping. It's not me — we're just the means of application. I think it's important people know that, too. Because otherwise it becomes a very egotistical thing, for some people to say, "I'm a healer", "I'm this", "I'm that". Really, we are just the vessels, and the means.

Still, I do definitely have a sense of guidance. That's why I ask for permission. I ask if there's anything that needs to be told to this person while I'm giving the healing, any messages they need to know? And that's where you've really got to trust, too, because it might seem so way out, or you might not have ever heard the word that's being given to you, or who knows? It could be that it's just meant to be for them and they will understand. You've got to

Moira

be really confident in giving a message — because it is not for you, it's for them.

I ask, "Is there anything this person needs to know, while I'm healing?". Then, I get it in thought form of, or I might get a picture, a vision of something. I'll translate it to that person the way I see it. Or what I have been told. If it means anything, they'll know. If not, well, it's okay too. But most times you'll find that you're right, and they can understand where it's coming from.

I do have a broader sense of guidance, as in everything I do in life. I've learned to listen to myself, and it keeps me protected, healthy and well. Even around times like the Christmas period — it's a real party time. So, if I tend to have too many drinks or something, my body will say, "Hey, hang on a minute! This is not good!". And I can listen, pull up, and say, "That's it! No more!" If I have a couple of cigarettes too many, it's, "No more, that's it! You can't keep doing it — your body will get really sick." My body has been very ill, and been given a disease, and that's a real kick up the backside.

* * *

I do relate my intuition to guidance. I think it's everything. I trust my intuition so much that it is my guidance. It tells me what's right, and what's wrong. I think it comes from the spirit world and all my guides, and whatever else's out there, but it's translated through me. I know our intuition becomes heightened as we evolve.

Something that comes up with healers, is coming to terms with how we are affected within ourselves by other people. I used to feel like my thoughts weren't me. I'd ask, "Where does that come from?" whether it was a horrible thought, or whatever (but, more when it was a horrible thought). I'd think, "Why am I thinking like that" and get uncomfortable. And it wasn't 'til one day I twigged that that's me picking up what the other person's thinking and feeling. From that day I felt more confident, knowing that it wasn't me. It was a big lesson for me.

Sometimes if I was sitting next to a guy, I'd start feeling sexual towards him. I didn't feel it really within myself, so was thinking, "What's going on here?". Then I recognised that it wasn't me; it was what they were thinking. It might be a girl or a guy, but was mainly around sexuality, and feeling. That meant a lot to me, because as a youngster I had been abused by my Grade Six teacher. I only talked about this a couple of years ago; realised I used to

Moira

blame myself, and felt so guilty. I was only a kid. I didn't get love in my home life. But, the abuse? It wasn't my fault — I was a kid. It shouldn't have happened. But up until I was about thirty, I blamed myself.

So, knowing where such feelings are coming from, and understanding they are not my own feelings, was a breakthrough. I think it's really important that people understand just how energies can be passed, and how strong intuition can be.

The way I came to recognise this was through one of my counsellors — a very spiritual person — who used to do guided imagery. Through working through my stuff, one day I had to really go into my own pain and the idea of how energies are passed. As I said earlier, I'd had my heart broken from losing my own child and my brother and my dad. And I avoided it for years twenty years, probably. But, when I actually went into it, it didn't kill me! That was really good. I could say, "I'm alive, and I went into that pain, and I healed my heart". It feels mended now — I feel whole again. I had always felt empty.

I think it was through that process that I realised what picking up other people's stuff could do — and how vulnerable I was. I was vulnerable because of my pain, and my hatred for myself, and my guilt, and all that. I think I was, also, really open. And I think it's important. We talk about protecting ourselves, and we also close ourselves down energetically so that we're not like an open wound, susceptible to people and entities coming in, whether it be a passed-over entity, or whatever. Being so open meant that I was just being vulnerable to people's different feelings; probably pain, probably everything. Anything that's not seen.

This is problematic.

This was probably a year-and-a-half, or two years ago, when that change happened through counselling. Prior to that time I was still vulnerable — I think I've lived most of my life like that and had times when I would adopt other people's pictures of reality, because I didn't discern they weren't mine. I'd chastise myself. "How can you be such a nasty person, thinking those things or feeling that?". And then, I would think, "But I don't. It's not me".

Now I know what I was doing — I was taking on other people's energies and thoughts.

I still slip back sometimes, but being aware, you can guard against it. When I made the shift I felt free. I felt... well, I didn't feel guilt, I didn't feel like a

Moira

"horrible person". My confidence went up. I started to become the whole person I should be, and everyone is entitled to be.

When I'm thinking other people's thoughts, it's not as if they are even aware of it, either. It can be just the energy they carry with them without even being aware of it. When I became aware, I would just not take it on board. That's the difference now. If it happens — taking something on which could almost bring on an anxiety attack — I can just cut it off straight away. I don't have to process any of it. It's not me, I don't have to wear it, and I don't have to carry it, and I can shut it off straight away.

My process is protection with the white light, or the gold light, or whatever. And I'll just give the feeling or thought or energy, gently back to that person — they own their own stuff and I don't have to.

I have a ritual for that. One that no one would even know I was doing, because it's all in thought form. You can protect yourself with white light, and just give the bad thought back. I think it's important. And sometimes you forget to do it, too. Then all of a sudden, you'll think, "Why am I taking this on? It's not me!". And you can be doing it while not recognising it's something you have to give back.

There's an emotional and a spiritual growth process around vulnerability and protection. An important question, though, is how can we be healers if we don't know how to protect ourselves, and protect the person we're healing as well?

For my own answers, I had to go back through my own life and stuff, and work through it. And face it. There's emotional hurts, as well as past happenings, and whatever happened.

My life. Worked through it, with a trained counsellor and it was a spiritual counsellor who helped me, because we could see that side of things as well. And throw it away — get rid of it for good. And push on. So I could become a clearer vessel, I guess. To receive whatever I was meant to. I think that's important.

The guided imagery I used to go through with my counsellor was really important. Because it gave me the responsibility to be in myself — no one put words in my mouth. It was all my own stuff — really exciting and interesting. I did seven years of it. It's been a long journey, but, by gee, it's worth it!

Moira

The first counsellor I met took me through, to my inner child, and worked with that. And my daughter who I lost, as well. I played with her — and I realised I could play with her any time I wanted to, if I wanted to call her. Things like that were really important. And you're there with them in the space that you go to, like a meditation. And that's good.

I think my attitude changed along with the process of getting things out; facing everything. Some people talk about being hypnotised and I think that can really work too. I felt I had to face my stuff, to become who I am now. To be able to be strong, and say, I can work with this stuff, and say, "I really know. From my own experience". That's important because I don't want to teach something to anyone else, or do something on anyone else, like healing, if it's not from my own experience. I can't read a book and do it. It doesn't seem right, seems false to me as it's only someone else's words.

I think the healing work I do becomes stronger, as I work through my own stuff. More situations come up where, out of the blue, you're driving on a Sunday afternoon, and something or someone — an animal, human being needs to be helped, or picked up. It might be just someone crying in the park, and I'll ask, "Is there something I can do to help you?". My daughter goes crazy at me when I do that. I picked up a drunken girl on the street in Melbourne one day and she was just so grateful — she and the guy with her. She was so sick, probably too much alcohol and just had poisoning. She was only young — sixteen or something. I was able to get her home safe. If I feel it's right, I will do it. If I know, and I get the feeling, the intuition, it's wrong, or it's going to be a danger for me — I won't be able to do it. If I feel the fear and the natural instincts happening, I won't get involved.

About my spirit guides? I used to say, "I've never met my spirit guides. How do you meet them?". My last counsellor said, "Just ask your higher consciousness if you are allowed to meet your guides". About six months ago, I was having time off uni. I was very stressed at the end of second year. I was very ill and my disease was giving me a really hard time. So, I decided to take six months off. I lived across from the beach, I could walk it any time and I was walking on the beach one day — I think I was upset and crying.

Things weren't working out — I was broke, and had no food. I was just walking down the beach, and I asked if there was a spirit guide, who I could meet, please tell me who it is. But I got better than that. I saw a large American Indian guy wearing buffalo horns. "I'm Buffalo Horn," he said. "How you doing?". And I just went, "Wow, okay. Hi!".

Moira

Now, when I tend to forget he's there, I get a little reminder, like, "I'm still there". I do think guides can come and go, too; I think we have different spirit guides, for different things. If I really need to know something, or if I'm really lonely or sad, or broke (as in no food, no petrol, no nothing) I can ask for guidance, for what I need from the Universe. "Universe" and "guides" go together for me — yeah, that's where they are. Usually you'll get an answer, if you listen closely enough and just be still. I'm more still now. Oh, I can get upset, but not half as much as I used to. I think they're a form of comfort, as well. Some would say that's all it is. But I know, in myself, and that's what's more important than anything; that you know, yourself, who they are and what they're there for.

None of this we can prove empirically. It comes from what people say about what they feel when they're channelling energies. Yes, it is a knowing. And knowing is very important.

I believe in God now, whereas once I never used to. That's another thing. I used to hate God, when I lost my daughter. I used to think there was never a God or why would he take her? But after a number of years, I realised that was just a reaction. And that I was given strength to get through it all. Everybody else asked me where I got it from. Where did I get it from?

At the funeral people said, "Where did you get your strength? You were the only strong one there. "I don't know". I said. But looking back, I knew — but I didn't want to admit it.

I know that I get strength from the Universe, and other places, when I really need it. And if you ask for anything, you will get it — if you really believe; it's about believing, and, more than anything, I think, trusting. Trusting in your own self, too. That you have been put here on this earth to accept whatever the Universe has to provide. It works! Yeah, it's pretty good.

When I got into the district nursing, when people were dying, I think that showed me a lot. I think that taught me to get through my own child dying, my own family. I wasn't afraid of death after that. I think by knowing what you know about your guides and yourself, it teaches you confidence, and knowing and feeling you're a part of the Universe, and life here and now. I feel so privileged to be here, and have this life. Whereas, once upon a time, I didn't feel I had a place in this life, because it was so painful and so hurtful.

Now, to be able to do my work as well as heal people (in another sense) is very rewarding. And to tap into both worlds, in a healing sense, with nursing

Moira

and hands-on healing, is wonderful. And spiritual healing? If we could convey this to people who were suicidal, or just felt they didn't belong on this planet earth, as we know it. Well, what work we could do! Just to give them some sense of... self.

I actually healed my own heart through guided imagery. This was after six years of healing and counselling. it was wonderful — it was the best moment in my life, in a sense of healing in my own heart; healing in my own life. My heart was so shattered that I didn't ever think it could be mended.

Moira

Chapter Eleven

RACHEL

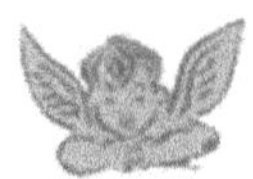

Rachel

Rachel and I met at a coffee shop near her workplace, a large metropolitan hospital. Although not an academic, she was already well known as a spiritual healer and visionary. I feel grateful and privileged how deeply she disclosed about her sacred journey, about the so- difficult challenges attending her opening as a healer, and her struggle to find balance between the spiritual and mundane worlds she was negotiating. I was particularly struck by the spiritual visitors and their guidance she described in our conversation, and by her openness around her personal struggles and how that related to her journey as an evolving nurse healer. She painted an intriguing picture of the evolved healer, one who came to "have her bones read".

I came to nursing because I wanted to help people — as lots of people do — and as my nursing evolved, I realised I was skilled at helping their physical existence but there was much more that needed helping.

I guess I was conscious at the time of my nursing training that there was something missing. Always something missing. As a young nurse, I'd sit in handovers, thinking, "There is something missing for this person". And while I didn't know how to articulate it, I knew there was an emotional, mental component to it. When I look back with today's insight, words, ability to articulate, to my training days, or days when I was on the ward, it was still my desire to work in that aspect; still an influence. But yet, care for the physical body.

So all through my training, I had times where I wanted to do more, but didn't know what to do. Wrestled with the idea that there was nothing to do — it was like, "Oh, that didn't seem right". And now, when I look back at those instances, it wasn't necessarily because it was not right, it's that I just didn't have the skills. Of course, sometimes it is right to do nothing. But there wasn't anybody, either as mentor, or teacher, who could guide me during those first years in training.

I always wanted to work with children. So, after I finished my graduation at an adult hospital, I went and became a children's nurse, and then became a midwife. It was at that midwives journey that things began to happen, both personally, and professionally.

Personally, I got married. I had been with my husband for about four years and when we got married, it was, "Oh, yeah, this was the right thing to do". But I had a lot of baggage that needed shedding once I came into a partnership. And maybe the baggage had blocked my ability to work more deeply with patients as a trainee nurse.

I think the baggage came up as I strived to become helpful in the emotional realms for patients — in understanding what it was, and giving some... In

Rachel

those days what I thought would be a great was a one-liner or a word or whatever, that would help people and would stop their struggle, and you know, life would be fine. You know, that Pollyanna, "take the pill and fix it".

I think when nurse healers begin the journey to becoming a full human being, we need to get rid of the baggage. For me that happened around the time I became a midwife.

Midwifery, if you have a look at the specialty, is about transitions and sitting with transitions. It's about moving through powerful stages. It was here, where things kicked off for me — being involved in such transitions, and questioning life and life's purpose.

I enrolled in a counselling course, thinking that's where I needed to go. I was there to get rid of my stuff. I hadn't realised — hadn't been still long enough to understand — that as a healer it's not the words you say that affect people, it's actually what's in your bones. And most people, when they are vulnerable, don't listen to your words, but they do read your bones. I still find that so evident in what I do now; that people don't care what you say, but they know who they can trust — it's that knowing. And I guess that that is what I call "reading your bones". People just know.

I didn't know my bones — I assumed that people would go, "Yes, what you said was right. Thank you very much". But I didn't realise that being was enough. That my baggage made my being so clouded that I thought that knowing it didn't really matter.

I had the sense that if I learned the right words, used the right tone of voice, then my being didn't really matter. What I know now is your being matters, and the words come later.

* * *

To clear my baggage would be all-encompassing — I guess I needed to look at my philosophy of life. That meant looking at my family of origin, and what I had gained, learned from them. And questioning those. In astrology people refer to such deep questioning of your life as your Saturn return. You question everything that you knew about the world and that's usually happening about the age of twenty-nine. I think I was younger when it started, probably about twenty-four. And all of a sudden I was an adult in this world, and I didn't really have a life philosophy — I lived for the moment — as you do, coming out of your teens. Yet there was something bigger, something bigger that I needed to do. Or something bigger I felt —

Rachel

something incomplete, something I was striving for. Yet I didn't know how to get there. And I didn't know what it was.

Part of the process was needing to redefine who I was now, as I had come out of my childhood. I was now an adult, and could make adult choices — even if they were all based on my family of origin, or about those friends and family, or experiences that I had gained through the eyes of a child. So what became a real focus was to clear the baggage and to get a sense of self, and to have a self-esteem that could then generate the journey onto other things. That was years of things like psychotherapy, things like journalling, things like drama — things that allowed me, encouraged me and helped me to express who I was.

I also chose things that helped me understand who I was. I saw astrologists, who would say, "Ah, now, looking at your chart, these are the aspects that I find… and this would mean that you would be this type of a person". I was getting a clearer picture of who I was — the complexities about myself. I mean, who we are as people; who you are in the past, in the present, and what influences you.

In the journey as a healer you have to do that work. It's hard work. It's emotionally, mentally and physically consuming. It takes a lot of energy and, unfortunately, I don't think there's a way out of it. It's usually work that you do alone, because it is of such a personal nature.

One of the difficulties I experienced during that time was, that as I wanted more and more to be that authentic person, or have my bones read by others, or feel that my being was enough, I became very, I guess, vulnerable about others. It was like shedding clothes, or the layers I had, and thinking that everybody knew everything about me. It wasn't only about other people feeling that they knew, but even more that it felt a lot out of control.

I thought the speed of my shedding happened very quickly. I was one day a normal human being who signed up for a counselling course and then the intensity grew rapidly. All of a sudden the teachers talked about having the ability to meditate and still the mind. "I may as well do that," I thought. And as I tried, I opened up that spiritual connectedness.

I think part of being an authentic human being is having a spirituality about you, but my spirituality came in the form of spiritual visitors. Beings who were as real to me as any other person sitting next to me.

Rachel

During this shedding, I also realised the marriage... I had gone into that pretty much like Cinderella thinking that marriage was, you know... this was how it was, and we would live happily ever after.

And circumstances in the world, high interest rates, and a mortgage — that was not what life was about. I didn't really have anybody who could give me concrete examples of how this was supposed to work. So my marriage was falling apart, as I was falling apart. I left my husband — we separated — and I went to live with some friends.

My first real spiritual experience was hilarious. Well, it's hilarious, now; it was terrible at the time. No, comforting at the time. I was sitting to meditate, and I didn't know what this meditation was. All I knew was that if you sat on this stool (a meditation stool) something might happen. I sat, thinking, "I wonder what'll happen," and then, with my eyes closed, yet as if they were open, straight in front of me was an angel. Dressed in the usual garb, you know, wings, opaque gown.

I thought "Right!" and I remember the conversation was something like this: "So you're my guardian angel?". "No, no," he said, "I'm not your guardian angel". "So, who are you?" "I'm Jim." "Jim? Oh, okay." And I thought, "Well, Jim's a reasonable name". I said, "What are you here for if you're not my guardian angel?". He said, "I'm here as a go-between for the moment". "Oh," I said. "So you think I'll get a guardian angel?" "Yeah, I'm sure one'll come along soon." "Oh, okay. Well then, how will you help me?" And he said, "Whenever you feel alone, or frightened, I will be there. All you need to do is call my name". "Oh, great! Okay, thanks Jim. See ya." It seemed like just a walk in the park.

Yet, afterwards, I thought, "Isn't that amazing! I have this angel called Jim! Wow!". But it was so matter-of-fact, so real that it became how life was. I would often call Jim when I felt lonely. I didn't really use Jim for a lot of clarity on things, back then.

When I meditate now, however, I use my connection with spirit to gain clarity and insight, and to also offer me other ways of operating.

So Jim was a being that became very comforting and, having realised that that happened, I saw that this energy healing had something to offer. I was going to see somebody for Reiki, and that would feel better. Then she would do something, to make my emotional being feel better; but also my physical being would feel better, which was like, "Wow!".

Rachel

At the same time I was still nursing, feeling more vulnerable, being impacted more, and being more aware from an energetic point of view; realising that the chest pain I had might not be physical but that it might be an emotional pain I was registering in my heart. Then my own health began to break down, and I began having allergies where my throat swelled up, or I would break out in hives for no known reason — just spontaneously, walking along the street.

One day I passed an alternative shop with a drawing in the window of somebody in the lotus position, with the chakras overlaid upon them. Around the chest area, was this emerald green and a label saying, "This governs the immune system," and it was my immune system that was breaking down. I went into the shop and asked about the picture. The shop assistant said it was a drawing of the chakras and went on to explain what chakras were.

Not that I had any idea what she was talking about. But I had always loved emerald green — and still do. Mmm, I thought, there was something to do with that.

What was happening was that as I was unloading baggage, my health was deteriorating; the spiritual experiences were coming; my emotional being was in crisis, because my relationship had broken down. It was like a total stripping back to my bones. And from that, then, I became more aware. It was like fasting — you become more pure as everything gets stripped away. Then I began to put on the layers, or strengthen the parts that I wanted to strengthen.

I decided that the spiritual "thing" was very important to me, and I began asking about that, and reading books about people having experiences like mine — seeing angels, those sorts of things. I found out that wasn't a common experience. So all of a sudden, not only was I bare, but I was also alone. But I still had Jim. Even if Jim was a spirit, I was never alone. It was more of an isolating experience than aloneness, because I was isolated from human beings.

As in anything that I do, I was trying to maintain the balance. In this instance, the balance was between a physical reality, and a spiritual existence. And I had swung — because I had, I guess, dropped so much of my load — I had swung into a very spiritual experience. So I was living in a physical world, having a spiritual experience.

Rachel

I had not ever known anybody to have done personal work. So dropping the baggage was a bit frightening. I had never had anybody in my life to demonstrate personal growth work — getting rid of the stuff that doesn't work for you, and picking up new stuff. Part of my isolation was that I didn't think people went through this; I had no idea that this was, can I say, a common occurrence for evolving human beings. I had no friends or family talking about it, so my only point of reference was things I read — and they were all from a spiritual nature. Some of the Bartholomew books all talked about this lovely heaven angelic realms. But I had nobody to model that for me.

I think that's the hard part; not knowing what is happening to you. So, I can relate to some of Caroline Myss's ideas of the dark night of the soul — where you actually think that you're going mad... Part of my madness was I'd never seen anybody go through this before; so it was quite a daunting time and a scary time.

I found out it was quite unusual to have those sudden experiences of angelic beings. I assumed that as people became more spiritual and more into energetic healing, that being confronted, or having the visuals, was normal. I assumed that everybody talked to spiritual beings, or had that ability. I'm coming to appreciate that everybody's ability is a different, and not many people start out with visual impressions.

I think the variations come from trust. I guess I am a little different to everybody, or to some people, in that I believe that everybody can see — I think that's just an ability you have. I think if you trust enough, you can, and I had nobody else to trust. My marriage had gone; my family of origin was dysfunctional; I wouldn't speak about this to anybody I was nursing with, because nobody else seemed to be having these experiences. There was nobody else. So the aloneness and the isolation were paramount. There was nothing else. So when somebody comes along called Jim, with wings and an opaque gown, my response was, "You'll do, if you want to be my friend!".

Now, my family of origin was brought up in the Catholic Church. So there was this... it may well be connected. Jim came in the image of an angel, because I guess part of my history would be to trust an angel. So it was like, "Ah, yes".

From the Jim experience, as my emotional being got more and more confronted by having to let go of more stuff, I also became more aware that there was more than just Jim out there in the world. The next evolutionary phase was to realise that everybody had angels, and that I was lucky enough

Rachel

to be able to talk to them. And I could use the information they gave me to understand a situation more. Originally I talked to them, literally, in words in dialogue. It's become more refined, to be accepting of feelings and ideas, and not needing so many words. Like a knowing, but more like a fast movie. Originally, I would talk to Jim like I'm talking to another person; now I still talk to my guidance, my higher self, like I'm talking to another person but I'm much more open to having ideas come into my head — I have no idea where they come from — and being open to that telepathic, almost, communication.

* * *

I should go back to what happened after the Jim thing. Being so alone, and having such a spiritual slant on the world, I started to become dysfunctional in the physical world. Going to work was hard; keeping to a routine was hard; my physical body was exhausted most of the time — and all of this, I'm sure, was because it was changing so rapidly. So keeping a full-time job was out of the question.

I cut back my hours and worked part-time, and spent a long time just, I guess, doing nothing. I spent time outside journaling, or just sitting, contemplating. It seems like a real life of luxury, now, but it did take that time, and I'm sure that's because my bones were changing — I mean, the level of change was so deep; that's how it had to be.

Many people didn't understand that — many people would think I was out of control, was obviously "losing the plot". Because I did require that time, and that nurturing. It felt like I just wanted to be cocooned from everything. Yet I still had ties to the physical world, I still had to earn some money to eat, to live, to do those sort of things, you know, which was a good thing, I guess. There was still an incomplete relationship with my partner, that neither of us could do anything about, other than to be separated.

So there were the ties, or links to the physical world, but the pull was so strong to the spiritual world; so strong, to just sit and chat to angels for hours on end, or to just have a meditation that could last half a day. Think of it like a seesaw. I was way down the spiritual end, and even sliding off the spiritual end, because it was so lovely. Nothing happened there; nothing unpleasant would concern me there.

I was slipping so far down into the spiritual realms that I could have easily taken my own life and gone to spirit. It was a fine line between leaving, and

Rachel

staying in a physical existence — because spirit seemed so much better. It was such a heightened experience — it made me feel good about who I was. It was friendly; it was all of those things. There were days, I remember, thinking, "If I could just kill myself, if I could just end it, I could be spirit and life would be fantastic, wouldn't it?". It was like they never had a problem — it was just this physical world that kept holding me.

Having to go and be a nurse in it made me think, "Why did the trauma that I was seeing around still have to happen?". I was way out of it! That's right, it was like that. I was in it, but I was out. Absolutely!

It made me ungrounded, made me have ideas that were fantastic. Absolutely fantastic! But, almost like a mental illness — so grandiose. I remember at one point, when I was sliding, we were having a party day at the hospital. Each ward had to decorate itself in order to change the environment — that sort of thing. I remember being so out of touch with the physical reality that my idea was to make it a day in fairyland and we had the most amazing party day. My idea was just so that we could, you know, get out of the reality; we had hundreds of metres of tulle everywhere; we had people dressed up as musicians. All that magic, all that out-of-the-physical reality. But it was absolutely so big, and so grandiose, that it had no reality to the physical world. It was a really good metaphor for how my life was — it was so "out there".

At that time I was also deciding I couldn't hurt animals by eating them, so I was a vegetarian. So there was nothing to ground me. I was having the most amazing time, in terms of being high — it was like being on drugs all the time. But I had lost my balance.

I was still in my two-year counselling diploma and the people there were very concerned. They detected the slide. Yet, everybody was very interested in the spiritual side — "Oh, who did you talk to today?" or "What are they saying now?". So the spiritual stuff was very addictive. The energy work was gorgeous — I had sensations through my body that just were such a high. It was so lovely! And then, to come back to earth was such a bummer!

And all this was being juggled with trying to work as a nurse.

What I know, at that time, was that being so almost out of your body, or so high — you became impacted by all the people that you met — all those people who were sick, all those people who were in emotional crisis. I was

Rachel

working with children with cancer at that time — you can't get much more emotional than that. So it really was a jarring time.

I would be emotionally and physically impacted. There was a time I went to see a child who had horrendous complications during induction surgery, and was in a vegetative state. Not the child's fault, just an accident that happened during an anaesthetic. He was young — about two. He was unconscious. Yet, being so spiritual, and having talked to spiritual beings and especially telepathically — I then had the skills to talk to this unconscious vegetative child. And I remember I went to him — it was nine o'clock at night — and we were tucking all the kids into bed.

I tucked him into bed and, as I was tucking in the sheets, I pulled out my hand with all this stuff on it and I thought, "Oh, my goodness, what is that?". I shook my hand, and watched black stuff fall on the carpet, and then disappear.

"What is that?" I thought and then tucked my hand back in, wondering if I was in a reality, or where I was. I took my hand out, and there was the black stuff again. I put it on the carpet, and it went. "Am I imagining this?" I thought. "Is this real? What is happening? God, this is scary!"

Then, I begin to feel sick, "I feel sick — this is terrible!" I thought. But my hand went back to his cot, and then onto his abdomen. "Oh my God!" I thought, and I pulled and more black stuff came out of his belly. What I know now is that was moving into visualising psychic or energetic stuff happening. I didn't know that at the time. I was frightened, I felt sick — but there was part of me that knew I had to keep doing this. Which I did.

All of a sudden the child looked awake to me. "What are you doing?" I said, and he said, "You're helping me". Then I said, "I don't know what to do". And he replied, "Keep pulling it off". And I kept pulling it off, thinking, "What is going on?". And somehow the conversation got into how angry the boy was, so angry at what had happened to him. That he had become crippled by a mistake.

I just remember saying to him, "I can't do this any more, I feel awful". And I had pains in my chest, and I put the cot side up, and went out of the ward, and vomited — because of the impact on me. I went back in afterwards, thinking, "I'm losing my mind!". And I said, "I don't know what to do for you". He said, "There is nothing to do for me — but for you, you must go and study light and energy". "Well, where..." I said, "I don't even know what it is,

Rachel

or what I should do. Like, where do you go for that?". "The back of the Wellbeing magazines has a list of places," he said. "Start there." It was like, "Okay". And that was the end of that. But I I remember, I had thought, at that moment, "I have slipped, I have slipped off. This is not real! What am I doing here?".

And that was the one experience — I had nobody around me who knew anything about that. I had nobody in the nursing fraternity who would even understand that. Then, after I'd come out, gone out to the room and gone back, somebody said to me, "You should go home — you look awful!". I said, "I feel shocking!". Which was the truth. "Oh," I said, "it must be the flu". Not talking about what happened.

And from there, I found somebody with whom to do a Reiki course. I realised Reiki wasn't enough for me — that I needed to be more conscious about what I was doing. So I went into a two-year energy work course, where I could learn the spiritual stuff. For the first three months, yep, I was out there really, you know, flying high, having a great time. More spirits came, more information — but I was still unbalanced in the physical; still impacted by energy, or energy things.

Once, I was sitting next to somebody on the bus and burst into tears, crying, thinking, and saying to myself, "I don't know why I'm crying, I don't know why I'm crying, I don't know why I'm crying". And the lady said, "Oh, have you had a bad day? I have, as well". It was like, "Right!". Got off the bus, and thought, "It wasn't my stuff — what was happening here?" It was her stuff. So it was like that, being so open...

As that evolved and I got more into the spiritual course, it was more energy, than spirit, but you were connected to your guidance, and your higher self. After about two months, I met my higher self in a meditation. I was just gorgeous. My higher self was somebody that I, as you do, recognised for a long time. By this stage Jim had gone, and then there were spiritual beings to help me through anything I needed to ask. So I had got into that transition now; they were my friends, but they were my teachers as well.

When I met my higher self, it was like having part of me back. And I remember thinking, "Wow! Now I've found the bit that was missing". I didn't know what that meant, other than it was the bit missing. One of the first things my higher self said was that to exist, and to do what was required of me, I would need to have my grounding work done and corrected.

Rachel

What he meant was I needed to come back into the physical world.

Then a new experience began. New in terms of the level of being that I worked with — I worked predominantly with him. He was also the teacher whom I would ask about spiritual things; about energy work. What I am seeing in this person? Is there a blockage here?

There? What does that relate to? He would be able to help me interpret that. But also he became more of a balance — more saying, "Well, you know, you're in the physical world, and there is a purpose for you being here in the physical world. You now need to work on that".

So that was the type of sliding. I went from becoming progressively more spiritual, I guess, throughout my life, or having a physical existence where I was hoping for something better — to sliding off the scale on a spiritual experience and now, being told by spirit that my purpose was to be back in the physical. Well, I didn't like that very much.

* * *

My life circumstances now ground me in the physical — and I wish I was more in the spiritual. It's forever going to be, I believe, that balance — that to be a nurse healer, you need to have the balance. So many evolving healers, and people that I thought were just so endearing and loving, and so spiritual — and they were so good — they were the people, like me, who were having these experiences, talking to the angels, and seeing stuff — they were tantalising. I could have sat with them, and talked with them for ever.

Now, I know that that is an addictive quality, to escape while you're here. I still don't like it! I don't like having to be so focused on the physical. Yet the work, the spiritual healer's work, gets done on the physical body, energetically. Like that's the problem that we all have. No matter whether we bring in issues from past lives, from dual realities — it impacts us in the physical.

So, a healer needs to be able to understand the physical reality in order to get their life organised. I guess my journey as a nurse healer has been about that swing. And today you find me focused on a physical reality, because I have two young children and dependent people keep you focused on the physical. And I'm incorporating a spiritual life into that.

Rachel

So it's almost like it's swung. Now when I think about the nurse healers I admire — they're the ones who are grappling with that spiritual experience in the physical. Not the physical experience in the spiritual world. It's like, it's that movement. That, I think, makes a mature healer.

Take the issue of money, which I think it's just a fascinating mirror, and probably where I've been doing lots of personal work. In my heightened spiritual experience, I couldn't have cared about work; I didn't care about eating; money was not a measure of anything. Because it didn't really matter.

But now I know it's important to have money, as an energy, in order to achieve the things I want to do. It has a priority now... because I was so spiritual, and, you know, thought I could walk on water, almost; I didn't need to have that reality. You know, I remember not eating for days — there was almost like a magical existence.

Whereas now, heavens above, I feel my physical reserves going down, and knowing that, I can't meditate if I haven't eaten. Like I can't stay focused during meditation — I drift off. And drifting off is okay, but you need to bring it back to the physical — you need to be able to get back in your body, and for your body to be reasonable to get back into after you meditate. I now watch nurse healers who are striving to maintain a balance between family, between job, between energetic work, healing work — and being authentic people. They're the people I admire, now.

It doesn't mean that I have lost the connection — in fact, the connection is much stronger. I have the ability now to actually ask, "How do I demonstrate this in my physical reality? How do I carry your light, or your presence, or your energy in my physical environment? And how does that then make

a difference?". And what I know is, before I could say, "Yes, you've got an energy block in your heart" or "around your liver" — whatever. Now being sitting next to that person — can help balance all that out. I don't have to do anything.

It's more than presence — because when I think of presence, I think about, I guess, somebody just being there. But it's actively being there. Sometimes presence can be a passive sort of thing. This is an active thing. An actual valuing of what my bones can show you, communicate with you. There is an exchange of something. That exchange then brings me to ask things of a spiritual nature, or of a more holistic nature, as a nurse healer.

Rachel

In the work I do, one of things I can talk about — I don't actually talk about angelic healings, or that sort of thing (and yet I know it goes on) — is that it's really important to demonstrate compassion and authenticity to others. Showing them you're a real person in the real world has a huge, huge impact on people.

One of questions we rarely ask our patients is, "How is this experience for you today?". And that's one of things, as a nurse healer, if I could say that was the question I'm curious to know about everybody I meet. It's the one thing that leads me into both a physical help and support; but also leads me into their emotional journey, and their mental journey, and their spiritual journey. It's a holistic nature of the nurse healer. That is in the now.

The other day, I was nursing a family and the child was out of the room. The mother and grandfather were there and I pulled up a chair, and said, "I've just come on. I'm Rachel, I'm looking after your child today, and you guys today. I have fifteen minutes, and thought I'd just have a chat about how life is for you today". They looked at each other, and I said, "Because I know, given everything what you've been through, that sometimes we forget to ask we just assume that everything is going along. And what I can tell you is, by looking at your notes I'm concerned about your child's weight. Therefore I want to know about nutrition, and things like that. I also know that you've been in and out of hospital for, you know, "X" number of weeks, and I wonder how that is impacting on the rest of things".

They both sat there and I thought, "Oh, dear" — you know when there is that silence. And grandfather said to me, "What's your name?". I said, "Rachel". And he said, "How long have you been in this specialty?". I said, "Oh, a really long time — probably about ten years." I've not seen you here before," he said and I said, "That's right," and gave him the reasons. "Is there a problem?". "I'm actually a GP," he said, "and I have never seen anybody come in and ask so precisely, and articulate the problems that they thought we were having, and that was so accurate".

I laughed at that, or smirked, thinking, that wasn't just me — that was my guidance working with me, looking at the charts, highlighting the things I needed to do. Also using my knowledge of the physical — the need for sleep, diet, that sort of thing. But also knowing struggles and bringing that all into a five-minute question. That family had been in and out of hospital for two years with the same child for the same problem. Nobody had ever asked, or sat down and said, "How is it for you?".

Rachel

So part of me gets carried away... part of me wants to say, "Well, the spiritual things are really good," but what I know, for that family, that had more impact. That responding to the physical and emotional needs was more healing than all the spiritual stuff.

It's that sliding, that... or balancing, I guess, that all nurse healers will go through. What now happens is that I have the ability to empathise, be aware of those on a sliding scale. And that's a good thing, because there will always be people somewhere on that linear model of to-ing and fro-ing in their existence. I guess I'm lucky that, having been almost to both extremes, I am able to detect when people are at the extremes, and offer some help. I think that's valuable, because anybody who is at an extreme is not of value. You know, you try and live in the physical.

* * *

How has the process changed me? I really like who I am now. I think that I'm a more authentic person. I feel more grounded — less airy-fairy; much more of a healer. I'm very comfortable with who I am now. Now, having all those spiritual experiences, and angels coming to talk, and being woken up in the night and asked to work on people energetically, and all that sort of thing, is wonderful. But you still have to get up and be in the physical environment. That still happens, but it's much more of it being a time for that to happen, as opposed to getting a high from being asked to do it.

I know the potential is there — it's like having all the potentials you could ever want at your fingertips — but knowing you don't have to use them. Somehow, it all balances out.

For me, that's a much more balanced point of view — less egocentric, more able to weather the storms. Formerly, when I come across a family that's extremely emotional, I would leave with chest pain, having taken on all that stuff. I now register, "Yep, that is happening — but it's a mirror for what they're going through". Even if I said something to them, to the effect of, "Hearing your story makes my heart hurt" (which is what I know to be my heart chakra overloaded or full or blocked) clears me. But also asks of that person, "Is that happening for you?"

I think people always read your bones — I think that we like to think they don't, but everybody does. And especially when you're in a vulnerable position as a patient, then it's like a primitive way of knowing who you can

Rachel

and who you can't trust in the system. And I think that as a nurse healer that's something that happens.

So from being very empowered, but in the spiritual, and having been through the aloneness, the unsupportedness — to now. What I have let go of is the need to be special. I think that's one of the themes — the need to be special. To be so special that the angels chose you to speak to them — that sort of specialness. Now, I know that it's not the specialness that counts that everybody has this ability. It's the trust that you place in yourself to carry the light, or do the work. And also, the ability to be content to be one of the crowd — not different.

I think, in all our lives (and when I think about my family of origin, all the baggage I had to get rid of) one of the things that happens along the way, is somehow our specialness gets lost. And it gets lost because your family doesn't honour it, or whatever. So what you crave is that specialness. The spiritual experiences give you the specialness, and then they say, "Go back and be like everybody else". And I can say, "No! No! No!". I think the journey is to find that ability to be special to yourself — but also special because you value what you do — and then your spirit friends agree.

I hate the word "ego", because one of the directives when you're developing your spiritual existence is, "Let go of the ego". I never believed I did it. I believe they did it, and that was fantastic. So I didn't have an ego — I had a lack of ego. When I look at nurses who I think are healers, because of what I see in their bones, or what I feel in their presence — I wonder if all of them have a difficulty with their ego, in that they don't have a good self esteem. They don't value what they do.

I've got that reality now. One of the things I used to assume, when I was on this spiritual high, was that I would not be challenged by the limits of my physical existence any more — as if illness and stuff would go out of the window. That was wrong — it's absolutely there! And one of the journeys in coming this way is to accept that there will still be things that occur to you — not for you to heal, but for you to sit with, and live with and be happy with.

So at the moment, my allergies and everything that caused me to be thrown into the spiritual have now re-emerged. They came back eight months after my first child's birth and again, eight months after the birth of my second child. My challenge is to understand that that's just the memory in my body and that's okay. Even when energetically I can't cure it; even when I have to

Rachel

take medication from the physical world to make me able to live in the physical existence and if I didn't take medication, I would die.

I continue to be challenged on my agreeing to stay in the physical world. One of things I discovered going through my heightened spiritual journey and then trying to get back into a physical life, was that I had set up a number of situations through what I call my "etheric blueprints", that would have me die. Yet, as I've cleared them and thought, "Right, great, I will stay, I will do the work, I will until I believe I'm no longer needed," it comes back to challenge me. So, at the birth of my first child, we had a lovely labour and delivery.

But after that birth, I haemorrhaged dramatically! I had done a twelve-hour labour with no pain relief — so that for me was a great ego thing. I'd used "the boys" (spirit) for guidance, and I knew, I'd been warned, that there would be problems. I had not asked any further about that, other than, "Would I be all right?". "Yes, I would be all right." "Would the baby be all right?" "Yes, the baby would be all right." Okay. I could live with that — I didn't actually want to know what was going to happen.

So all through the labour and delivery they'd check the baby's heartbeat. I'd wait and hear, "No, it was all right". "Oh, yes," I thought. I had this baby in my arms, and I was crying and it was just the loveliest time. Fifteen minutes after that, I remember my higher guidance said to me, "Things will start getting hectic now". "What does that mean? " I thought.

The midwife said, "Rachel, just hop up on the bed, because I need to get this placenta out". I said, "Something is not right here" and she said, "How do you know?". I said, "It's the knowing". She said, "I'll get a doctor". "Yep," I said. "Get a doctor". I had begun to haemorrhage very badly and that was a really difficult time. I remember being run down to theatre; they were running.

I remember saying to my higher guidance, "Get me out of my body! I cannot stand the pain". My uterus was filling with litres of blood, and pushing my kidneys out of the way — so the physical pain was horrendous. "Get me out of my body!" I said. And he was saying, "Stay in the pain". "Get me out!" "Stay in the pain." "Get me out!" "Stay in the pain." I'm thinking, "What is going on here? This is not good!" I remember some part of me saying, "I have just given birth to a baby who needs me. I am not going to die! It is not my choice". Then I had a "thud" in my abdomen and that was about it.

Rachel

I had a spinal anaesthetic, I had a retained placenta. I remember hearing things like, "She's lost so much blood, oh my goodness". I continued saying, "It is not my choice — I have a beautiful baby waiting for me. I will not go now". I was being rechallenged about my desire to be in the physical environment, like, I'm not finished.

My second child's birth was better — and yet my allergies came back again. Now this is three years of solid work on them, and they are back here again! "So," now I ask, "what past life, what present life, what dual reality, what... what have I not done?". In meditation the other day, and I got, "What if it was just to be with it?". But I don't know. What would that be challenging?

Part of the journey as a nurse healer is, I think, being active. Also, sometimes it's about being passive and accepting is what is supposed to happen, despite all the skills you have. Maybe it's just acceptance and I think that then goes into acceptance of the self — and your self esteem. As your self esteem becomes more solid, no longer do you have the accentuated spiritual, energetic experiences — but no longer do you need them. You know you can have them; I know that I could have an amazing spiritual experience, or energetic experience, if I truly needed it. I don't need it. I know it's there. It's like knowing you can have all the lollies in the lolly shop, because you've got the key. But you don't need them — why would you need them? Some days you do, but the majority of times, no. It's enough to know you have the keys, knowing you're the keeper of the ability to do that.

I think spirit is there when you need it — it's when it's needed, I guess. It is also when they need you, now. Whereas, before, right in the beginning, when I talk about Jim — I'd call. "Jim! I'm lonely". And poor old Jim, whoever he was, would come along, in spirit. Now, I don't have a need; I know they're there. It's that complete knowing, that you can be their hands. I know that they're there, they know that I'm there. That's the change.

In the last three years I hadn't stopped to think how had my spirituality changed, other than there are some days that I miss the highs, and think, "Oh, God, that would be good". Then I realise, "No, that wasn't a good time. That wasn't a good time". Now I would say that I was in the physical, because having two young children — they don't care about what you do energetically. They want things like food, shelter, cuddles — it's a physical existence.

Rachel

Now I find myself having slid, on the continuum, past the middle — into the physical. My youngest is now nine months old, and I'm coming back into that spiritual middle. And that would be how life is continually, I would think.

* * *

A final reflection. I guess that I thought about the aloneness, and the isolation and I felt how much that was a necessary part of the journey. Part of me wants people never to feel alone, and never to feel like there's nobody there, in the physical world. I think that humanity is about being in connection with others and while I want to say, "I don't want that, I don't want others on the journey to feel that," I know it was so necessary.

I couldn't shed the illusions of who I was, with everybody — it had to be a personal, intense journey. That was one of the things I had wanted to change, and still struggle with having to do; yet, knowing that the aloneness was so important.

The unsupportedness... Now we have more writers who write about it — people like Caroline Myss who, you know, write about the journey of the healers and this stuff about the wounded healer journeys. I think that's really important to know about — know that there are others who've done it that way. I guess I'd like to see somebody write an autobiography about it, so that people can think, "Well, that really did happen! That was a journey!". So that people know that while you may not have somebody to walk that way with you, there are others who have been down that path, and survived. Having gone on the path, you can have a realistic outcome; an outcome that is attainable.

I still have to shop at Woolworths, I still have to feed children, change dirty nappies — do practical things. Yet, it's now much more in line with who I am — as opposed to having that heightened spiritual experience, where I forgot to pay bills, I forget to eat, I didn't really want to do the shopping. At that time, who cared about taxes and those sorts of things?

Now I'm part of the world that I chose to be born into — doing an integrated version of a healer.

I wonder if this is what a matured healer looks like. Or is this a point that a healer gets to, after all the acute stuff goes. Is this the level of maturity as a healer? Or something about that process. All the while knowing, that I can also say, "This is a mature healer? Get serious! I've got years of work to do!".

It's that juggle — that juggle between the two.

Rachel

Chapter Twelve

ROSE

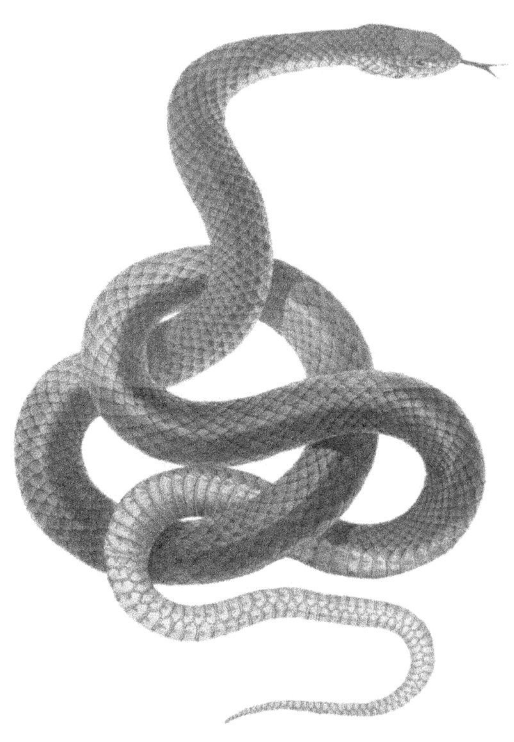

Rose

Rose gave me the vertebra of a snake when we met, and introduced me to the protecting and healing spirits of the land where she lived — the huge fig tree, the animal spirits and the people at her lake. She spoke of the many woundings of her life, and the strength and insight she drew from the healing of these wounds. She disclosed her isolation and deep connections, and spoke of the blessings and challenges of being a healer.

I guess the first big thing that happened to me was the death of my mother, when I was four. It was a major thing. She also was clairvoyant, as was her mother, so there was probably a big spiritual attachment with her for a start.

From that point on, talking about her was forbidden; it was very upsetting for my father, apparently, and I was forbidden to mention anything about her. I had this feeling as I passed through life, that there was a great big hole, something huge missing. I suppose a lot of things happened through that; I felt very different from other kids at school, and I was told by the other kids that I was different. My father was a brilliant journalist and writer. He was also alcoholic; a good deal of stuff arose from that.

When I was eight, he married again and my stepmother was very cold and he was very flamboyant but unavailable to me. I learned very early to keep my mouth shut and keep invisible. That was my role at that time, you know, keep your place and be suppressed.

I spent a good deal of my childhood alone, because I felt different from other kids and didn't make friends very easily. The friends I did make always seemed to leave; there was this sense of, I suppose, rejection. I developed a fairly rich inner life, from quite an early stage. I was always finding lame animals and bringing them home, looking after them. I was always doing a little nurse number.

So I was always nursing animals and, in retrospect, I think I took on waifs and strays in people as well — I had friends who were older than my parents, and a lot of them were real loners themselves. I had some good solid friendships with them. Maybe they weren't so old — maybe I was so young I thought they were old.

So I got through school and then we moved out of the city, because my father was ill, and alcoholic. We moved to the country, "doing a geographical" I guess, for him. It was an isolated place, and that suited me because I didn't have to be intimate with anybody. I still kept in the background because of dad's volatility — it was better to keep out of the way. He was never physically abusive, but he was constantly verbally

Rose

abusive. I would hear his car coming home, and think, "Oh, he's going to be drunk, and I can't stand it," and I'd disappear into my room.

I was quite isolated in that way, I guess, and had developed strong relationships with animals. I was able to get animals to do things I wanted them to do. When I look back on it now, some of these things were unusual. I could get cattle and horses to do what I wanted, by looking at them or being with them. If they were distressed in any way, I could walk up to them and put my hand on them. These might be wild cattle that hadn't been seen for years and they'd just be like small, calm dogs. At the time I didn't think there was anything peculiar about it. It was just the way it was.

I went to the big city, and started my nursing training. Almost immediately I started having feelings about what might happen to the patients; that something would happen that was pretty awful, or they'd bleed, or their blood pressure would drop.

When I voiced those concerns, I was in trouble and was sent to matron. People would say "You're not here to talk with the patients, nurse". "Well," I'd think, "What am I here for? It can't be just bed pans". So, there was always the notion that, yes, there was something a bit deeper in, apart from being a nurse on the staff. I suppressed a lot of that.

I then met my first husband — a doctor — and he was very cold. We were young, so it was hot. But he was very unemotional, cold. When I talked about my experiences with patients, he would tell me I was mad, just crazy. We had met in the psychiatric block of our training, and we had a bit of fun with that — both busy diagnosing each other, I suppose, and he was doing all sorts of things to me. Abreaction and stuff to make me cry. Well, it was pretty sick.

It was, though, the first time in my life I'd been in love. Part of it was amazing and eye opening. Because I was in love with him I trusted him with my innermost feelings. I would tell him about all these psychic, I suppose, experiences I'd had. The things I'd seen on the wards, and that happened to me when patients died. I would often be aware of the soul of the person leaving the body.

One old lady, who had been unconscious or partially conscious some of the time, for about a week, was of particular note. Whenever I'd come into the room when we were giving her two-hourly mouth care and turns, her breathing would change. To all intents and purposes she was unconscious had a certain breathing at that time, it wasn't Cheyne-Stokes, but it was stertorous, laboured breathing. When I came in and put my hands on her arm, her breathing would change and she'd become very quiet.

The last day of her life — I was on night duty, and she died. That last night, when I went into her room — gives me the shivers to remember it — she was lying flat on her side. But I could see her form above her body. I realise that's probably what it was. But it was as if there was another level of her above her body. I had never witnessed that before. And when we were laying her out, I could feel, as we were washing her body that whenever I'd move my hands and my arms over her "shell", I felt another energy above it.

It was like putting my hands in one of those blowers in toilets where you dry your hands. The wind wasn't as hard as that, but there was this other energy and it gradually moved up. The next time I came into the room, it was gone. So, I suppose that was seeing her aura, and seeing her detachment from the physical body.

I didn't think of that as being out of the ordinary at the time; not even thinking, "Oh wow! I've never seen this before!" It felt a fairly normal occurrence.

Looking back over the years, I was used to strange phenomena. Well, they might have been strange to others. Like that stuff with the animals; like knowing sometimes what an animal was thinking, and being with people and knowing.

Even when I was a kid, I could be with a group of adults and know what the dynamics were, and what was going down with them, and what they were thinking. I suppose I thought it was normal. I could accept it straight away.

I remember a few people who came into casualty who I realise, in retrospect, were psychotic. Pending somebody jabbing them with Largactil or whatever we were giving them at the time, I always was able to walk in and calm the person down. People who were tied down but had been very distressed.

It only seemed unusual when people started pointing that sort of stuff out. People would say, "Oh, send nurse Goode in, because he's really ratty, and she can handle ratty people". I assumed it was something I could do, but didn't see it as special. As I got older that idea probably made my ego swell a bit, but it didn't then. I was naive, and very unsophisticated, and had very low self-esteem. I wasn't willing to accept there was anything special going on, perhaps. It was very much part of my everyday experience of the world.

The main thing I remember feeling, and still do in similar situations, is no fear. I remember one man in the accident unit, bundled in by a couple of ambulance men, and a couple of cops. They left him and took off.

It was left to my girlfriend and I to handle him. He had a Gillette blade in his hand and he was slashing himself. Chop, chop, chop. He wasn't cutting deep, but he was absolutely covered in blood because he'd made all these superficial wounds. And the huge cops and ambulance men shot through! They didn't want to know.

I said to the other nurse, "Right, let's get him". Now he was a huge guy — massive, but very fat. Big, you know, and we're little ladies. But we advanced on him. I grabbed his arm, and I had a pair of artery forceps in my hand. I grabbed his wrist, with one hand, and grabbed the blade with my forceps and ripped it out of his hand. We wrestled him to the ground, and I felt no sense of fear at all, and I was lying on top of this man and then he went, "Ah, phew". He totally relaxed.

I had an absence of fear, and overwhelming compassion for the person; they were suffering badly. I still feel that, when somebody's having a bad time, I have a very intense feeling. It's not sympathy, and it's not deeply emotional; I feel a bit detached, but I do feel something moving through though it's not coming from me in total. Some of it's coming from me, but a lot is from — I would like to think — external, divine realms and moving through. Every person is aware of that, whether they consciously know it's happening or not. It's powerful that they feel it. In its presence they, whew, have a bit of a more relaxed state. I did feel ego about that from time to time. Now I realise that it's got nothing to do with me. I feel like I'm a vehicle for that.

After I finished nursing training and graduated, I went to New Guinea. There, I learned a lot about spiritual healing. I would see people who'd had the bone pointed, or a spell cast on them. They'd be brought into hospital and be on drips and drugs and everything, and they'd still die. I could see the power of spirit in that.

At the time, I was still married to this doctor, and he was quite violent. I was very much involved in using pethidine and alcohol myself. His response to my drug-taking was violence; beating me up. I was told consistently by him that

I was mad. Often beaten if I had too much to drink. I was raped frequently by him. There was a good deal of violence, and a good deal of drinking. A lot of self-violence, really. I was addicted to pethidine and alcohol, Valium, barbiturates... everything!

We came back to Australia, and I was working in the accident unit. I loved accident unit nursing. Now, I realise I needed the adrenalin to get the cortisol up in my blood, and that's probably another link to my having rheumatoid arthritis. Though I'm getting rid of it, actually. I don't buy into the fact that I've got it any more; there are a whole lot of biochemical things happening in this.

Consequently, my level of psychic ability fell away. It was being suppressed by the drugs, and by my life situation as well. At about thirty, I suppose, I decided to leave my husband and I lived alone. I went to AA, and stopped drinking. About six months after I'd done that, I met my second husband; he introduced me to marijuana. For years, I thought how wonderful it was that I didn't have any addiction. But I smoked dope every day!

I suppose the dope relaxed me tremendously, but it closed me off to reality, really. And here was I thinking I'd met this guy who allowed me to talk about my experiences with my first husband, and so forth, but it was a world of illusion, actually.

We were living in a small community, and a lot of people there were coming to me for clinical stuff. I had a suture set and did a lot of suturing (a lot of them refused to go into the hospital). I said, "Okay, all care and no responsibility — I'll do what I can". I had an auriscope, and people brought their kids to me with ear infections. That was when the ego started up a bit — not a lot, but I used to feel very proud of myself. Maybe it wasn't even ego, but a bit more self-esteem, or feeling pleased with myself. Husband number two had built me up and encouraged me. He'd told me to go for what I wanted and I was getting right up there. Also, I hadn't had a drink.

I started to realise, however, that all was not well in that relationship either. As soon as I'd been built up to a certain level, this guy chopped me down. I was under total control, and realised that here again I was with another authoritarian man, and my self-esteem dropped, and my ego went away, and everything went away. Then I had my son, who's now sixteen, and that was extremely difficult for me. I didn't want to have a child, I didn't feel I would be a very good mother and it was very difficult to go through that.

Rose

Around that time, I started having a lot of experiences, and one in particular. I was doing a lot of hands-on healing and learning a lot from other people too. I did some Buddhist meditation retreats, which were quite wonderful, and I was easing off smoking dope because of that.

I had a few healing events, and I started making a healing crème which was doing incredible things. My husband had cut his index finger, cut it to the bone, and he refused to have sutures. He said, at the time, "If this is not okay by tomorrow, I'll go to the hospital and they can stitch me up". It certainly did need sutures but I put this healing crème on it that night and bound it up. In the morning, not only was it healed up, but there was no mark at all.

And we went, "Oh, wow this is pretty amazing stuff!".

One day I was at the market and somebody called me. "Quick, quick!" they said. "Hannah is up here, and she's in terrible pain". I found this girl. She was sitting against the wheel of a car, she was green, and sweating like mad, and was having colic of some sort, probably from her gall bladder or pancreas. But she was in severe pain. She was a pretty heavy drinker — it could have been pancreatitis, or gall bladder, or whatever. I was kneeling by her side, and could see her situation. I said, "We're going to have to take you in to the hospital. This is quite serious. I'll send somebody to get a car, and I'll come in with you". I despatched somebody to get a car. Then she had another spasm, very colicky, and she was writhing. Her eyes went back into her head — it was very dramatic.

I put my hands on her shoulders, and I was leaning forward with my forehead touching hers. And I felt this huge wave of something move through me. It felt the same as when you feel intense love for your partner, or your child or something — a massive wave ran through me. I felt that, and I said, "Oh God, Hannah, I really wish I could help you!". And as I sat back on my haunches, she went pink, and sat up. "I feel great now!", she said.

I've never seen a patient do that. You know, it just doesn't happen when they've had that degree of pain. There is always that degree of shock with it. I was dumbfounded. And she got up. I said, "Well, go and have some water". She got up, toddled off, and went about her business.

That night, I said to Fred, "God, that was amazing about Hannah, I can't believe that!" And he said, "Don't you know you are a healer? Don't you know that when you touch people, they get well?". I hadn't thought about it. I guess I assumed that it was natural. I had, at the time, looked up to a few healers in the district; thought they were marvellous wondered how they did what they did. Then, I was doing the same thing, but hadn't thought very much about it at all. Maybe it wasn't part of my self-concept. I could agonise over that, but there's no point.

After I eventually separated from husband number two and came to live where I am now all sorts of things started to open up. I met a lot of people who were clairvoyant, and lots of people reading tarot cards and that sort of stuff. I became aware of a whole other life that was open to me. I stopped smoking dope (though I did start drinking again).

I had some hypnotherapy and learned quite a lot about myself through it. I didn't just have hypnotherapy from this woman, a whole lot of other helpful things happened. She laughed, delightedly, when I said I didn't think I was psychic; that I either thought everybody experienced the same thing, or I suppressed it so well, that I hadn't been able to deal with the realness of it.

I run a spiritual development group — new people are sometimes petrified that they're mad. They're not — they're very open, and they need to learn how to get a handle on it. I never experience that. I never felt fear. I was often told I was mad, but didn't ever feel that the experiences I was having meant I was mad. I'd accepted them as part of me.

I got to a point when I was starting to think a bit more clearly about myself, and who I was, and what I was doing. Though, because of the horrendous things that had happened to me, I was quite amazed I was still alive. I was into Louise Hay at that time, and I found a lot of sense and support in it.

My four-year old son introduced me to a man down the road, who became husband number three. (I'm sounding like Elizabeth Taylor. He's the last, he's the last!) It turned out that Peter was also clairvoyant, and a medium and he encouraged that in me. Then I did Reiki, and once I began, I was right into it. I found it wonderful. The Reiki master — a fantastic guy — has been a real mentor to me.

I was into my practice, doing Reiki 1 and seeing a lot of people. And then when I was doing Reiki, I would start to talk to the client, but by the end of the session I would think, "Did I make that up?". It was like I'd opened my mouth and, though it was my voice coming out and I'd talk non-stop, I didn't feel any of it was from my head. It was from somewhere else, but I wasn't

Rose

sure. And I'd think, "Oh God, what if I've told them the wrong thing? Am I bullshitting, am I making it up?".

I went ahead and did Reiki 2, and it amplified. I asked my Reiki master about this. "Am I making this up?". He said, "No, no, no! You're channelling! Didn't you realise you're doing that?". Well, I hadn't realised. Yet, as it became a conscious thing, it got more and more powerful.

Though I'd been practising for a while I was still drinking heavily. I would only ever drink at night when everybody else had gone to bed, because I didn't want anybody to see, but I was consuming huge amounts. I'd wake up in the morning feeling crummy, and think, "Oh no, I can't stand this!".

Then a couple of years ago, a few things all happened at the same time. I harboured a lot of anger toward my son's father, and one day a friend said, "I think that you're misdirecting your anger. It's about time you dealt with this. Stop blaming Fred, and deal with your own stuff". I felt very ashamed, and totally blown out that this friend of mine, who's got an anxiety neurosis, would find the guts to say to me, "I think you need to do some work on this". And here I'd been thinking I was doing well.

I went to an anger workshop called "Getting to the heart of anger". It was very confronting. If I'd known what it was going to be like I wouldn't have gone. We did this dynamic meditation, jumping up and down and screaming, and so forth. I'd always been very inward with my anger, and never screamed or shouted at people; I've always been very quiet. I was, in the meantime, though, beating myself up, but not actually doing it at people. Though I must have done a bit to this girlfriend, because she picked it up. In a way, it was a very intensive day. It opened me up incredibly, and made me realise that there was a lot down in there and I had to stop covering it up. It was a big journey from then on.

About the same time, I was introduced to the path of Tao and received my Tao initiation — another huge awakening and I've been cultivating that ever since. It's been a couple of years. Then I went back to AA for a year, and I haven't had a drink for a couple of years now. I haven't had any drugs. I haven't had anything. For the past two years, I've been totally clean.

I've been following this spiritual path, been cleaner and much more available to receive the celestial gifts and blessings. The more I receive that, and the more I cultivate that path of Tao, the more clients are coming, and the more people I'm helping, and the more benefit I'm having for the community in

Rose

general. These experiences, I suppose — I know — have made me much more compassionate.

Having menopause and the onset of rheumatoid at the same time was huge. I met a fellow doing Buddhist meditation practice once a week and I was doing that with him. He was in partnership with the woman who ran the anger workshop; it was he who felt, after hearing a few of my stories, that I had PTSD.

As a counsellor, he practises EMDR, and I had about three sessions with him. In the first I dealt with the loss of my mother; I was able to visualise the entire experience. Then there was an issue of an abortion I'd had without anaesthetic. I went through that; I went through a rape, and I went through an issue between my son's father and my son and myself, which had been extremely distressing for each of us.

After those three sessions of EMDR was, I think, when I began the major change of dropping my addictions. Now I feel there is still a long way to go, but I feel a lot of those spaces have been filled up. The clots in my brain that were there from those past experiences have been moved. My brain is able to fill up with good stuff. I think experiencing that technique was the most major thing that's ever happened to me. I have since sent a lot of people to that counsellor and they've experienced good results.

I have found that now that I've got a handle on what's coming in and moving through in my psychic development, it's also fostered my own personal power. I think I'm in my power at the moment. Yet, I feel like I'm scratching the surface; I'm at the tip of the iceberg and what's underneath is going to be monumental. Not for me, but whoever I'd come to contact with — it's going to flow out to them.

Having dealt with the emotional traumas and blockages — that means I'm freer in the spiritual sense and in the healing sense. Like there's a sort of an opening now. It's like seeing the light, but being in the light as well. Yes, I do feel on the brink of something great, of greatness. I don't mean that in any egocentric way at all. It's more a spiritual knowledge, I suppose.

When people say, "Oh, you must be drained" I never am — a lot of the stuff that I'm providing is coming through not arising from myself. Some of it is, obviously — but a lot is coming through from other realms, or other energies. I'm getting healed while I'm passing that on to somebody else. I'm not being untouched — it's not coming through and doing nothing for me.

Rose

All the experiences I've had — you know, all the ghastly things, losing mother, being raped, bashed, being addicted — that's been my whole life. And now I'm fifty-four, and it wasn't until I was fifty-two or something when all those things started to slide away — not slide away, but be dealt with. I don't regret any of them. I don't even think, "Oh wouldn't it be nice if that hadn't happened". I feel grateful, and I feel in a sense that I'm quite privileged to have been through those things, because they served to make me a better person, or a greater person, or more capable of serving other people. Because of my intellectual knowledge from those things, and from being able to look back on them too, and see what was happening around them, too.

Not "me me me", but the dynamics of the people who were involved. From the benefit of being a lot clearer, being able to see what was motivating them, what was happening for them at that time and not blame anybody. I used to blame everybody! You know, "Oh, why has this happened to me? What have I ever done to deserve this?". I think, karmically, that I did it all to myself, I mean everything we are, we've done.

I feel I am able to move into my wisdom as a healer, because of the experiences I've had in the past. I'm sure there are lots of factors, but that's part of it.

Now, I'm not a totally spiritual being. The other parts — the emotional, the mental and the physical that have experienced whatever — were brought to bear on what and who I am now. I feel that if I'm going to be out there as a healer, put my name in the classifieds, or promotional material, then I've got to be as good and as clean as I can get. It doesn't mean I have to be a perfect being, because I'm not.

I want to remain my human person who might drink too much coffee, or say, "Fuck" or be rude to somebody; you know, all those things that are normal.

I can't live like a nun and give all those things up because then I'm not balanced. I still have to be balanced to be effective as a healer.

But the things that I can clean up that will probably serve my clients, I have to. That's a little promise to myself. If people come to me — for, well, I don't like the word "advice", but that sort of thing — about a holistic approach and we look at what they're eating and how they're moving their body, and their work situation, their relationships and any of that, then I'm a hypocrite

Rose

to be telling other people what they can be doing if I'm not operating as well as I can in those areas.

I also know I always have to operate from the truth. If I see something clairvoyantly about somebody, or I pick it up in some way, I have to tell them. I can't think, "Oh gee, it might hurt them if I say this". How they choose to receive it is not my business — it's only my business to give it as I see fit. I used to not speak because I (a) didn't want to hurt people, and (b) didn't want to be rejected by them. Thinking, "They might not like me if I say this".

So, when I'm doing a healing and things come through, I always preface what I say with, "I don't interpret what I'm giving you — I simply give what I get". That's what I do. And most people receive it well.

From a long way back, I remember certain people who I haven't liked have come to me for healing. Yet, when they've left, after a healing, I love them. That doesn't change. I don't go back to my old dislike of them. I might have been judgmental of their behaviour, or something and that disappears. During the healing session, my intention is for healing, for them. My personal beliefs about that person or how they conduct themselves, have no place in what I'm doing. When I'm working with them I see their — not necessarily their openness, because sometimes they're not very open, but their — fragility. That always touches a chord in me. People are vulnerable and fragile.

* * *

I don't think I hate anybody now, but if I did hate somebody, full on, which I have done in the past, I would love them if they came to me in a vulnerable state. I don't know how that happens. It's a force much greater than me.

After they go, I am able to relate to them in a loving way. Maybe I should line up all the people I don't like, and give them a healing, and then we'd both receive something nice. It's very moving, too — sometimes as they're going, I'm overwhelmed by... ah... it's incredibly uplifting. It makes me feel like I'm in the company of angels. I probably am.

The angels have come. I did see an angel a couple of weeks ago, when a woman came for a reading. As we were finishing I was aware of a being behind me, and I turned around quickly. The woman said, "Oh, they can't get past you, can they?". I said, "Did you see that?". "Yes, I saw it," she said. She saw the being move past the window. It was a very beautiful thing to

Rose

happen. I can feel presences, but I don't always see them. But I do see them around people if I'm doing a reading.

I don't ever feel overwhelmed by the degrees of intensity or the largeness of what I'm working with. I wait until whoever is coming, arrives, and I'm starting to work the moment they walk in the door. I now always protect myself. Before I learned to protect myself, I used to get drained. Now, my feeling after a session is mostly joy.

About three or four years ago, there was lot of stuff happening at the same time — the anger workshop, the Tao — and I started going to a mediumship development circle. A group of us met once a week, learning techniques of protection, of opening the chakras; all of that. After some months of having learned various techniques of protection, I felt confident about that. I was talking about not having done a conscious protection with one of my Tao forerunners, and she's a great healer. She's sixty-four or so, and she's been doing it all her life. She said, "Oh protection! Heavenly Mother protects us all the time, anyway. No problem!". And I thought, "Well, that's right. It can be in the mind, it's only a thought away. Well, yes, okay. I'm protected". And I am! I also feel protected within this whole property. I think every person who's ever come into the property has said, "Oh, this feels great! It's wonderful here".

There's the fig tree, it's got a lot of amazing energy. I can't walk past that tree without feeling it. Even people who are very unawakened will walk past the tree and remark what a beautiful tree it is. It gives off an energy blast.

There are a couple of spirit people hang out in the garden here — George and Frank. And I've got a main guardian — a Tibetan monk — who hangs out around the ponds and he's very protective. There are a lot of animal spirits here, because we're wildlife carers. I've had many many animals over the years die here, and some I've had to euthanase myself. And I feel those strongly.

A couple of those have come through other people in our circle. One frogmouth hangs out all the time; we have a kestrel — a stuffed kestrel — who was sitting on a shelf over in Peter's house and a friend said, "That kestrel over in Peter's house wants to come over here. It wonders why you haven't brought it over here". I feel that hawk's presence strongly.

In the past, I felt very unprotected around one man, who'd rented the other house on the property; I was petrified the whole time. Had everything

Rose

locked; when I heard his car coming, I'd start shaking. Normally, I don't feel like that but he was very aggressive. I went to a girlfriend who did a session of hypnotherapy. She said, "You've lost your power. That guy's taken it".

One day I was walking down the street in town, and I could feel my whole body starting to open out. I felt like I was growing, like I was twelve-feet tall. I felt an incredible sense of freedom, and later I found out that was the day he'd left the area. There had been a lot of psychic attack from him, and no matter what I did, I didn't seem to be able to free myself of it.

I was not able to protect myself fully against that psychic attack. But that's pretty unusual. Sometimes people I have been with have had a bit of stuff stuck to them — nasty stuff. And I've cleansed them and felt myself very detached from it. You know, no way is that thing going to get me. Though, I haven't done any clearing of houses, or anything like that. I'm not drawn to it, at all, and other people do it. I don't want to spread myself too far — I want to be with what I'm capable of at the moment, and then as other things come, I'll deal with them when they come. You know, small steps.

When I was a child, I was very much a loner. I liked that. I'd go off with my dog, or whatever, and be alone and didn't ever feel I needed to be with other kids. I had a fierce reading and writing habit. I suppose that was my first addiction! I got rid of a good deal of my angst through writing.

Anyway, I never did like crowds. Maybe that's part of the psychic experience, one instinctively keeps away from people to a degree. I do remember, I liked New Guinea because it was very isolated. I always felt much more comfortable either by myself or with a couple of people. If I'm out somewhere, I'm not entirely present, and I wish I were at home, or somewhere by myself.

When the issue of doing readings at markets came up, I remember saying to my friend, Jane, "Well, I'll be so open there". I feel only psychically open if I do that specifically. It's a technique of opening and closing, and I have techniques of protection. But I still don't feel comfortable with that.

There have been times, before I started doing mediumship development, when I was walking through a crowd, and somebody might be behind me; and I started feeling "Whoa, whoa". The energy that I get from that person is almost tangible and if it's a negative energy I've got to move away. I can be with people, and feel a huge sense of irritation, impatience, like I've got to be away; and that energy will be coming from a specific person.

Rose

So, it's not the "largeness" dynamic, it's more an individual thing. But in a crowd, I stand to be affected by a lot of people. The only way I could deal with that in the past is if I've been pissed or stoned (that doesn't apply now), or if I absent myself to a certain degree, where part of me is held in a little box somewhere. The body's moving around and doing the body things. But the other stuff isn't touching me. It's dissociation and detachment; that gave me protection.

I'm sure most people could say, "Ooh, I don't like that person's energy", but I've got to move away from them. It's good in its way, because I can be more discriminating. It's not healthy for me to be around some people.

I decided that I would do readings at the markets. When I was doing them, there wasn't anything else happening around me; I was focused on the other person. I could hear the guy in the stall next door talking about his plants, or a friend walking past yelling "Hi, Rose!" or whatever, but nothing existed apart from me and the person. I felt protected that way.

One woman, I was reading for, I felt pretty edgy about. She was very angry when she came in. I did a cleansing for her, and calmed her down before we did the reading. I said to her, "You're really hot at the moment, we need to cool you down, because I can't read for you when you're in this state". And she laughed a bit and said, "Okay, cool me down".

I gave her a guided visualisation of getting in a pool under a waterfall, and it worked well. And it turned out she's a psychotherapist in Holland, and was already pretty clued in.

I was sitting (I read with my eyes closed in the main, because I see things, but I open them up and eyeball the person) with my eyes closed. Her husband had brought her a drink, because she was not only internally hot, she was physically hot as well. I had my eyes closed but I observed her throwing this cup of water at somebody. The next moment, my leg was soaked, and the cup that she had in her hand got splashed and soaked my leg. She was horrified, and I roared with laughter because I'd seen this happening. When I told her, she was horrified. She said, "I didn't throw it at you, I didn't throw it at you". I said, "No, I know you didn't throw it at me. I was visualising you throwing a cup, and that's what happened". It was quite amazing. Things like that do happen.

Rose

So, I feel now that as I'll be doing readings as markets I'm going to come across difficulties. But it won't be because I'm doing readings, it will be because that's... that's life.

Rose

Chapter Thirteen

RUTH

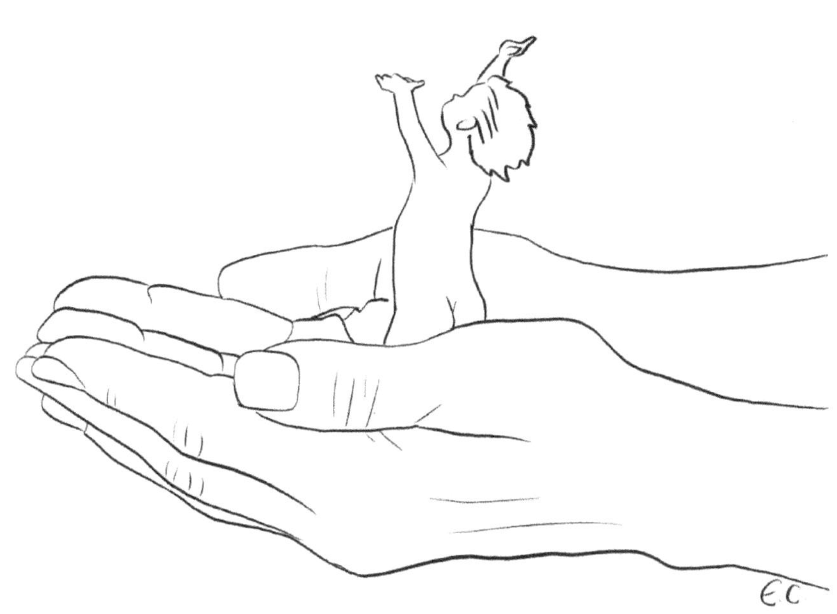

Ruth

Ruth, like some of the others I spoke with was quite famous as a healer, particularly in her nursing work with older people. She also gave healings to people at her home. She gave out a direct sense of heart and devotion and deep humility, and as we spoke her healing power was manifest but in no way intimidating. Ruth revealed how she lived in a wondrous world of spirit, and spoke of her deep woundings and her isolation through her life, and how her connection with spirit nurtured and protected her. I had the privilege to spend time with her a number of times through the years. I feel that the world is a lesser place for her passing last year, although she spoke often of welcoming a full return to the spirit realms, into the embrace of her beloved spiritual master.

My journey started off with a very abused childhood. Though, when I had nothing in my life, spirit was always there. As a child, I was moved from pillar to post, and ended up with the nuns; it was they who created my position of student nurse. They gave me a uniform and, that, as such, was my identity. Before that, I didn't have an identity. I was fifteen; that was how my identity started.

Somehow, whenever I had real trauma — like big, big stuff — spirit was always there. I could see them, or I could feel them holding me. That was from three months onwards. When I was three months old — that was the first trauma — my mother smothered me with a pillow until I was dead.

She rolled me in a grey blanket, and left me in a cellar. I know the place exactly. And I distinctly remember being in my light body, looking at her walking away; very aware that I was not in my physical body. I remember that what she'd done wasn't what hurt me, but the fact that she walked away without ever looking back. It was a bigger hurt in a way. It grabbed me deeper than even what happened. Then my Dad happened to come home. And I was revived by him. Still, I died. I went through this process.

When I was dead I was in a beautiful space; that's where I saw Jesus for the first time. Jesus touched my third eye, when I was in my light body, and that's when I came back. That's the moment my Dad revived me. From then on, I knew I'd been somewhere else, and come back. I always had this knowing, and the feeling, and the security of spirit.

Some years later, I worried that I was making up this whole story. But there was confirmation from my oldest sister. She recalled that I got lost as a three-month-old. Found rolled in a grey blanket in a cellar of that district; exactly the things I remembered.

Jesus has come to me three times. There was very bad abuse — sexual abuse — when I was eleven. At that time, I thought, "Okay, this time I will die". I didn't die. I went to the church that night, because in my mind, nothing

Ruth

bad ever happened in a church. Nobody got abused, in a church — well, that was my experience and so I went there. And Jesus came again.

And then later in my life, after I split up with my husband, I wanted to finish my life. I was in a very good peaceful calm space for three days, and I went to see my doctor, a person I'd worked with, and said to him, "I'm going to kill myself, and I feel very good about it". "No," he said, "I don't think that's a good idea, because spiritually you'll just have to come back and do it again". And I said, "I know, but it feels so right. It's just feels so right to do it".

Anyway, that night, Jesus came again.

Three times. I feel very blessed, and I'm very grateful.

When Jesus came the third time, I changed. I didn't have that need any more. I didn't feel like killing myself any more. He just looked in my eyes. He was right there, looking in my eyes, and everything changed inside of me. I was wide awake at the time. I saw him in the physical sense. Three times. I could have touched him. He seemed very substantial.

Sometimes during healings I give, a master can come and I can touch them. That's what it feels like. That's how close, how solid the energy is. So, I've always had a strong spirit connection.

I go back now to when the nuns gave me this position. It was great because, like I said, I identified — I became something. But, anyway, it was a very strict upbringing with the nuns. So, I went and did my training. I have been a nurse since I was fifteen and I love it. I loved it. Absolutely loved it.

Until I was eleven, my connection with spirit caused me to be isolated. I would sit for hours in a church or, if I was in an institution, in a chapel. But I wasn't touching other people. I wasn't there. Now, I've got five sisters and one brother, and all they ever say to me is, "We can't remember you, can't remember the times you were home".

I was partly in the world, and partly — mostly — not in the world. It was my choice, I think. My way of coping. I felt very safe and very good. I remember deciding, as an eight-year-old, that I would never let anybody in my heart again; would never communicate on a deep level with another human being again. That was my choice.

I grew up with this knowing and this experience of two worlds, I made no accommodation to it. No adaptation. It didn't come up to tell other people about it. Who would listen? There was nobody who would ever say, "What

Ruth

do you feel?". Or, "Are you all right?". No one wanted to share what was happening for me.

That's why I say I survive because of spirit. I'd go to school, and sit there. I had no friends; didn't belong, in a way. It wasn't like I couldn't communicate. But it was lonely. Still, I wasn't getting physically hurt or emotionally hurt and I didn't really worry what else went on.

Spirit replaces your parents. For me it did, anyway. There's always been more than one energy or picture or being, each was different. Mainly, there was Jesus. Buddha, Maitraea — Maitraea was very strong. Even after I was married, if things got bad, then Maitraea would come and hold me; as I presume a mother holds her child. As I held my own children.

In recent years, Sai Baba is with me. This all feels like being held, a nurturing, like everything is all right. Like it doesn't matter; as if I'm being told, "Look, there is this as well". It's hard to put into words, because it's mainly a feeling thing.

It is like I had two lives, in a way. And I do believe I was given another chance to learn whatever it is I've come here to learn. God only knows what that is. But, yes, it's like being in two places. There is always this other one, always. I might be in one world, talking, but there's always this other spirit world, where I can be me. Where I don't have to play a part and there's nothing to do. In that place, there's total acceptance, no such thing as good or bad. There is just acceptance. Where our souls meet.

You know when it's cold and you form small particles of air when you breathe out? It feels like I'm one of these particles, with the ascended masters and on the other side, my mum on that side, my dad on that side, and all of this is still moving around. It's like this cloud of air, and each individual particle can't... There is always movement. But nothing to do. Just an "is-ness". And it's nice to have that. It's a gift. I think it's a blessing, myself. It's pulled me through many things.

I do make light of my wounds, but I've worked through a lot of stuff. Accepted it. I now know that the work I do now is the positive side of all that has happened to me. Every time something traumatic happens to somebody, I understand that we have a choice — the choice that it's all just an experience. We can choose to make it a negative or a positive experience, and any experience we all have brings us closer to our soul. That, I feel, is why we're here.

Ruth

So, as I can, I drop more stuff, and serve — I wouldn't say better, but serve more honestly, with a greater compassion, with a bit more softness in my heart. Every experience has served its purpose — my whole life's purpose is for me to get those understandings and I feel very blessed. Because of that abuse, then compassion, softening of the heart, understanding people; all that has come from those experiences. They brought me much closer to my soul — and there is nowhere that anybody's soul is not.

So maybe that's why I can make light of my wounds — because they have served me well.

* * *

I don't experience the shadow — not with myself, no. But I do work with people who have those sides. I know they have them, and I just know I can get rid of them. In whatever way, I'm being guided.

What's involved depends what they are. There are ones we create ourselves in our thought form — actually create an entity. The same thought over and over creates an entity. Then there is the one in astral, where people might play the ouija board, or get drugged or drunk out of their skull, and as such the aura becomes opened, and an entity comes in and says, "Hello. I'll have you now, for a while". They try to get your light.

Then, there are ones from outer space, and I feel, I see those — like beings from a different planet. The energy comes through a funnel; often it's to do with people who have been on hard drugs where, after a while, they get cut off from their higher selves. That's when these beings move in. They find a being that's on their level.

Now it's my understanding, that everything in the universe constantly changes. Nothing stays the same. I believe that Earth is one of the very few planets where we have been given the chance to experience unconditional love. Often, it happens through also experiencing pain and suffering. So, the being is only coming to get to that light state. They come from a place where it's not possible to do that. They connect with a matching vibration here, and take its light. I believe a lot of schizophrenics, a lot of people in psychiatric wards, are being possessed (though that's not a nice word) by one of those astral beings. And really, everybody's intent is to get to the light.

However, these beings are trespassing. My method is to send them away in whatever way I get guided to. They all go to the centre of the sun, where they disintegrate, and where they can start again. Even if a person dies while

Ruth

being possessed by one of them, even then, eventually that person would come back around. Though spirit has told me, I have forgotten how many Earth years it takes for that to happen, but it is how it works. This cloud's constantly moving.

I asked spirit one time, "How come I can do this?", and was told, "It's because you've had that experience". I believe in reincarnation and, I was told that in one of my lives, I was possessed like that. So, in my being is this knowing. When I see somebody, or work on somebody, I know, "Okay, that's what happened to you," and I can ask, "What do I do, God?". Because of that, I know that vibration, and I can pick it up.

* * *

Now, in my life, I did what a lot of people do — I married my mother. Well, I recreated the pattern. Like, "Love me, or eat a bit more shit! You still don't love me — eat a bit more shit!". Shit sandwiches for years. (Until I realised you can have ham on it if you like.) And then my family migrated here. We came with two little kids. For about the first eight years, I didn'twork.

I started working at an institution when the kids went to high school. My qualifications as a registered nurse didn't count, so I had to enrol in a nurse course. At the institution, a beautiful old building, absolutely full of spirits, I learned about the mind. It is a gorgeous place and yet, a lot of people died there in agony. So straight away, as I started there, I was connected. That's the world I know. I could help them move on to the light. And I loved it!

I ended up in the old-fashioned long wards, some of which had seventy-six in them, men and women; seventy-six very advanced dementia sufferers in a locked-up ward. I loved it. I felt I belonged somewhere for the first time in my life, really. It was a type of nursing I was very good at.

I started there but soon I became aware that these people who have this mental agony, mental disease do know love. Their souls know love. Because of my childhood experiences and living with spirits, it's very easy for me to go past the personality; that part beyond personality, is the one I know best.

You could ask me, "What does that part look like?". And I'd tell you that it looks different with everybody. Sometimes it's a colour, sometimes it's just a light. Sometimes a feeling. Sometimes there's no word for it. It's different with everybody. But I know I can touch it. I've touched it especially with people who are mentally ill.

Ruth

What was happening at the institution was that, because I was having these soul connections, they would feel very close to me. And I, for the first time in my life, experienced love from another human being. Through their mental illness, they didn't have any inhibitions. All of a sudden, here was God in the physical, loving me. And I was able to serve.

I felt good because I was serving them — I knew I could make them happy; could make them sing. Because I accepted them for what they were. But, as I tell you this, there are tears in my eyes, because I had to give this work up.

I used to touch the patients, and the bones in the bottom of my arms used to hurt. While I could feel the hurt in my bones, they would say, "Ruth, I have no pain. While you touch me, I have no pain. At first, I thought, "Oh, yes, accidental". But, it happened so many times, even with the staff, that I had to acknowledge it. If it happened that somebody went off their face, I would hold them. Instead of three people having to sit on them and give them an injection, I could just hold them, and they would calm down. I could feel the pain, but I could also feel an electrical current, you might say — coming through.

When we moved to this area, it was like a last-ditch attempt to make my marriage work; I had to leave that job that I loved.

* * *

When I wasn't working, and I wasn't using my hands on people there was like a build-up of air. I was breaking a lot of stuff. I would push through, thinking I had to push, but — bang! One day, my husband went to see a chiropractor and happened to tell him about this. The chiropractor said, "She should go and do Reiki". So, I went and did Reiki — the very first, and the very last, alternative thing I've ever learned. I learned how to do Reiki. And I was put in alignment (whatever that means).

Some time later, I went to a local barbecue, where someone mentioned they smoked pot every month for their menstrual pain. "Look," I said, "I've just done this thing, come and see me". And she came, and I put her on the kitchen table.

What happened blew me out! While she was there and I had my hands on her as I was taught, I could see my hands — but they were inside her, doing stuff! And, of course, my training came in very handy, because you always pretend everything's right in front of the patients. I'm was reassuring her. "Okay, everything's right, blah blah blah". As soon as she went I rang up a

Ruth

friend of mine, also clairvoyant, and said, "You will not believe what happened to me!". (Now, it worked. She never had problems with menstrual pain again.) I told him what had happened and he said, "Ruth, you think this is weird? This is nothing compared to what you're going to be doing!".

Well, I went to work at the local hospital. It seemed like I was pushed; like there was way I could not have done that job. Every time I was on A&E duty, a particular doctor, Alan, was on. We were always put together. And if things happened in A&E, I would just do what my heart said — I couldn't not do what my heart said. For example, rather than getting oxygen, or sutures ready, or whatever, I would do whatever I was feeling to do with my hands. Alan said, once, "It's amazing working with you — I see the change with people". Later, when Alan started his holistic surgery practice, he asked me to work in there.

Soon after I began working again, my husband and I split up. I went away and worked in an institution in an Aboriginal settlement, with elders, from whom I learned a lot. I worked in another institution, also with Aboriginal people and they got to know my hands. If somebody was sick, rather than get the Ventolin, or whatever, they grabbed my hands, and made me put them on the sick person. These people know energies. So, once again, I was supported.

While I was away in the Northern Territory, my husband John was found dead. So, I came back here — I had given our property all to him, but he never changed the papers. And so, God gave it all back to me!

After this, I used to say, "Thank you" to John, but spirit said that wasn't quite right. They said, "No, don't thank him — he'd done enough damage, and it was time he left. He had enough opportunities". This was an amazing learning to understand that spirit will say, "Enough is enough", and then take a person. Until that time, it didn't fit what I was conditioned to think about spirit. However, I've learned since.

After I came back from the Northern Territory, I was given a job at a nursing home and was, again, in a dementia ward. The nursing home was run by nuns and, within the first month of my working there, thirty-three people died. The matron approached me one day, in front of all the other staff, and said, "Ruth, my mother-in-law is on the other side, in the general hospital. She's at the end. Would you mind, before you go home, going there and putting your hands on her and saying whatever you said to all the other ones who went so peacefully".

Ruth

I do exactly the same thing wherever I've worked. I don't look for support or for it to be charted. I don't have to worry about that. Because everybody can do what I do. Everybody. When you know what is, it automatically happens.

I don't do it — love does it. Love does it, not me. When you make a cup of coffee, it's the water that makes the coffee — not you. You pour the water into the coffee percolator — that combination is what makes coffee. That's how I feel about the healing I do. It's not me who does it; it's the energy coming through that does it. Of course, I acknowledge that it comes through me. However, anybody can do it. Anybody who has a connection can do it.

Is having a connection the key thing? I think it's that, and the trust. I have to say things to people when they come sometimes — but before I meet them I wouldn't have a flipping clue what it might be!

For example, one Sunday a woman came, and I said, "One of the rings you're wearing is your mother's ring. She's not here any more. If you let me hold it, I can give you some messages from your mother". I was thinking, "Holy cow, you'd better get this right!". Now it is always right, but I have to surrender to being thought a complete idiot. Yet, if it wasn't right, what's the worst that could happen? That I become an idiot. Well, that's nothing! We all are, in a way.

Maybe I did some big painful transformative things when I was very young, that other healers usually do as adults. I'm doing it again now. Because, twelve months after I began working again, after my husband died, my heart stopped. Now I've got a pacemaker and it has a tremendous amount of problems. It means I can't do my work any more. And, because my whole identity is tied up with my work, as a nurse and, more so than as a healer, I felt it was God saying to me "Okay, next step. What are you? Are you the nurse, who does this?

You've done that now for nearly forty years. It's long enough, now".

* * *

I have to let go of my identity, again, with more understanding than when I was young, when it was given to me. But, it's all I know. And so, I'm shedding tears again because this is a very painful time for me. I feel like a snowflake; I don't know which way I'm going to be blown. I know I'm going to land softly. I certainly don't mind dying. But, obviously, I knocked on His door twice, last year, and He didn't want me to enter. So, here I am — there must

Ruth

be something else I'm still to experience. And now I'm looking to get a bit closer to my higher self and work it. I have to drop a lot of stuff to get there.

So, where this will take me, I don't know. But it's another experience, and every experience brings me closer to my soul. And I yearn to go there. That's where I want to be.

There is this difference between my experience of spirit, and my experience of my soul, because it's my journey. Spirit comes — that's been my experience — so spirit will come during a healing. Whoever — I'll know them, and I will do whatever; or nothing, if that's the case. My journey is to pull in my higher self, so I can get strength from it, and get understandings, and get completion. It's like, I haven't learnt yet from my experience — like to have my higher self with me all the time — awareness of it. It's there with me all the time, but....

So, there's a letting go. That's happening now. And I do believe that's why God gave me this problem with my heart. So I can have that experience. I will experience it to the best of my ability — to the full. Yes, I am learning other things again, about spirit, I suppose. My own, this time.

There has been this situation with my late husband. Like I said before, the pattern that I had with my mother, is the pattern that I had with my ex. Before I married him, I knew that he was, in his earthly being, not a nice person, a very wounded being. For some unknown reason, I thought that because of my ability to go beyond the personality, it would work out. I see people's potential, so I would fall in love with his potential.

But in the meantime, it was like Jekyll and Hyde, and my light, what I am, drove him mad. Let's say you have a vibration that goes mmmmm [deep sound], and another vibration that has a different sound. Theirs goes hoooooo [higher sound], Well, neither is better than the other, it's just an experience in this life — and then the hoooooo will drive the mmmmm absolutely crazy.

With us, it was the same pattern. "What I can't handle, I will hurt — in any way possible". Yet, I always saw his soul. So, for thirty years, that's what I took. Until God finally put a stop to it. Every time it got really bad, I always thought if I loved a bit longer, and a bit stronger, and a bit harder, or "ate a bit more shit," it would get better — he would love me. Sad to say, it doesn't work.

Ruth

However, the positive side of this situation is that I would never have been able to love without expectation if I did not have all those years of experience. Because now, I don't do it for people to love me any more — I can just love now. That was his gift.

At some point, it got nasty. It was after we separated, and he lived on the same property in another dwelling. There had been many experiences of his using black magic against me; many times where Sai actually protected me in the physical from getting badly hurt. When my ex would see a wall of light around me, he'd say, "If I could get through that, I'd kill you!". But wouldn't dare to come close. At that time, though, the black magic got really powerful.

Something I didn't find out until after I came back was that there is a ley line that goes through the house, through the property, and he tapped into it. He was a very powerful man in the negative. And would stand in front of me, and yell, "I'm your teacher in the negative!". He was. Somebody has to do that job — that was his part to play, and it was my part to learn from it, to play that part. It took me a long time to learn that non-violence starts with yourself. So, if you let yourself be abused, you're not living non-violence. If you never hurt another thing in your life, but you allow yourself to be hurt, then you're not living non-violence. Anyway, he used the energy of the ley line. But spirit looked after me. I ended up with the Aboriginal elders, always, in the middle of their circle. They did smoking ceremonies with me. They gave me healings, corroborees for a certain purpose. I was always protected.

Though I've got a very strong connection with that place where I live, and the land about, I left the place. He programmed the energy of the ley line for bad, for me. It was earth energy — Indigenous people know about it. And spirit has always been there for me. Always protected me, been near me.

* * *

Some two years before I left that place, the last fully initiated elder in the area had died. But while she was still alive, we connected on a spirit level, and she taught me many things, in the physical. Still now, she teaches me in spirit. And when I do clearings that have to do with Aboriginals, she will guide me; there is other spirit like that, as well as the masters.

So, and it's only through spirit being there, and having the right people visit me, that we healed the ley line so I wasn't being drained constantly. I only

Ruth

found out what my ex had done after he died, as I was being drained all the time; the energy leak was still there programmed like that. I know this is "way out" stuff.

After my ex died, he couldn't get to the light. I knew that but, at first I couldn't get the light to him — that's how dark it all was. Then I did a pow-wow with a very powerful friend of mine, and we got him into the light. He came and said, "I've no... thing".

What I'm saying is, if you, as a healer, a spiritual healer especially, are around people who are of lower vibration, you don't have to do anything to those people, but the mere fact of what you are, and the spiritual connection that you have, can drive them deeper into their darkness. This is what happened with my husband while we were together.

In the physical he did some very bad things. Consciously. Dark things. And I, once again, in my ignorance, once again pushed him into the light, after his death. Well, it wasn't his experience yet to go into the light and so, in a way, it's interference, with his soul journey.

Well, it resolved, because of my spiritual guidance. It was as if God came and showed me, and said "Okay. And now you can use this to have another spiritual awakening". But, to get that, I have to let him go. I'm still doing that and I find it very difficult. I love him. But I will let him go. Because I want to get to my higher self, and I'm absolutely chuffed to have another spiritual awakening. Because ultimately, that's what I'd like.

I can't describe this spiritual awakening, because I really don't know yet. I truly don't know yet. It will have to do with me acknowledging me, and my spirit, and what I am. And that will be a tough journey, I think. Much easier to just let spirit come in and do it, you know.

Am I ready for a tough journey? I think am, and really? It's only me that makes it tough!

Ruth

Chapter Fourteen

MY STORY

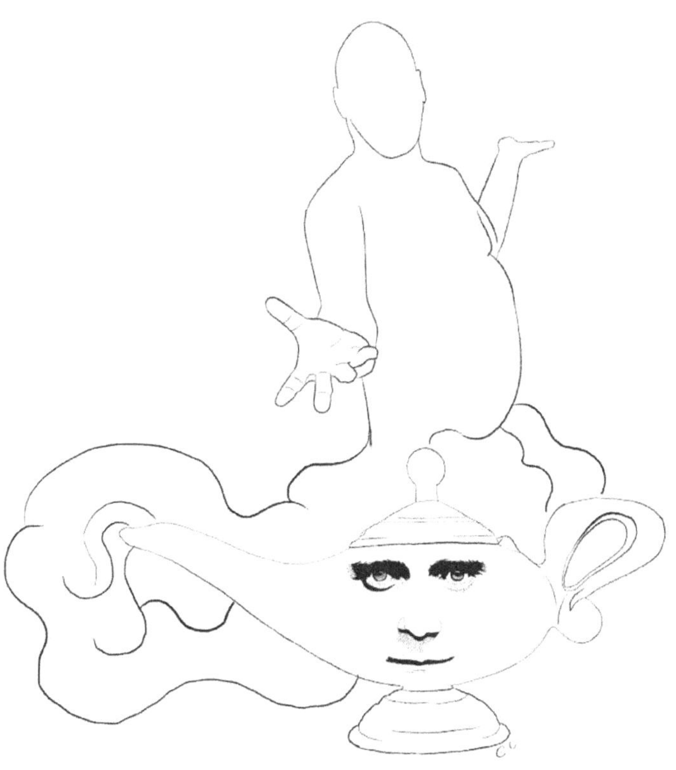

My experience of being a healer engulfed me in my late thirties, in ways that were astounding, and for which I felt totally unprepared. But as I reflect on it, precipitous as it was, it seems to have been connected to a spiritual journey I can trace back to my childhood. if I ponder certain occurrences in healing and therapy sessions I received over the years, this experience of being a healer seems to be connected to a mythic flow of experience running through many past lives.

I grew up in a quite strict Catholic situation. Religion was extremely important for my parents and pretty much all their family. I went to Catholic schools all through my education. As a child, it was very important for me, too. I was an altar boy, a very serious young person.

My mother was particularly intense in her religiousness. I recall her taking me to a church to pray, and she told me to focus so very hard in prayer, to fiercely put my whole mind in the endeavour. I did not really understand this approach to spiritual practice but, knowing no other, went along with it. My parents also passed on to me a very big focus on being truthful; this was central to my makeup. I would not be able to tell a lie.

There was no sense of anyone in my world being a healer, growing up.

Around my eleventh year my family moved to a new suburb and I went to a new school where I was bullied mercilessly. Taking pity on me, the nuns sent me to the next-door church at lunchtimes to serve as an altar boy. There were always funeral services — I was now in a suburb with an aging population — so it was a morbid experience, obviously, but on another level I have a sense that I was a psychopomp somehow, or at least being prepared for that, to shepherd the dead to the afterworlds.

My mother was diagnosed with paranoid schizophrenia when I was about fifteen, and my siblings and I were all lined up and told there was a good chance at least one of us would develop schizophrenia. Still traumatised from being bullied years earlier, I lived a very intense fantasy life at the time, and considered myself a candidate for madness. From that point, I fiercely repressed my fantasies, bent on transforming myself to be safe from madness. In a way that was the genesis of my quest for self-knowledge in this lifetime.

I was very disappointed with Catholic religion as it did not meet my craving for spiritual meaning, or speak to the deep angst I was experiencing as a sixteen-year-old. Much to my parents' disgust I stopped being a practising Catholic. There was a huge hole in my life after I left Catholicism; as a teenager I felt so isolated, empty, bereft, and was also very vulnerable to the ravening depression my mother was experiencing.

My Story

As a teenager and young man, I was very interested in touch; I was a "touchy" person, almost as a reaction to the stiff way that people tended to relate with each other at that time. Also, being a very alienated young person, it was one way I felt I could connect, for I was naturally affectionate. I liked to massage people. I recall being on a bus trip around Europe the year after leaving school, sitting in the sun somewhere in Greece, giving my fellow travellers massages in exchange for pistachio nuts.

The following year I travelled in Indonesia, where touch was very much more a normal way of relating. After that I learned more about massage and in my early twenties tried to set up a private practice. My interest in this led to a curiosity about massaging people's auras, but people I practised on found that unsatisfying, they wanted to be touched.

I turned twenty in the city of Solo in Central Java. There I learned meditation in a local spiritual organisation (or "kebatinan") called Sumarah. As I recall, Sumarah means "Thy will be done". The practice was identified as "samadhi meditation" (contemplation in Christian traditions). I was exposed to a plethora of ideas about spirituality, especially in the Eastern traditions — Buddhism, Taoism and Sufism. I witnessed daily the charismatic powers which attend mystic spiritual practice, such as telepathy, clairvoyance, and healing. I learned how they were treated in the Sumarah society as a sort of "epiphenomena" of the spiritual journey, to be respected when they visited but not seen as being of central significance; known to be, usually, quite transient.

I had a lot of confusing experiences in learning meditation, particularly rapid wild movements and strange speaking in tongues, which would inevitably emerge as soon as I relaxed into the experience of surrender. All my teachers could tell me was that it was something some young people experienced, to do with the kundalini, and that I needed to be wary of it lest I become possessed. That was unnerving, and led to me thinking there might be something fundamentally wrong with me. I did, to an extent, come to associate this with the release of repressed trauma from earlier in my life, a mechanism of self-healing from meditation.

The other big thing that happened while I was learning meditation was a kind of awakening. I was profoundly touched by the transcendent message of the Buddhist text The Diamond Sutra, which I read from the library at the centre where I studied meditation. Its truth struck me like a brick and the world never looked the same after I'd read it. But I couldn't comfortably live in that realisation. When I would enter into it, powerful and confronting physical experiences were unleashed. Also, in the background — even the foreground — was my fear of going mad.

I became very interested in processing my painful and traumatic childhood experiences. I read widely on spirituality and therapy. Arthur Janov's Primal Therapy appealed as it focused on powerful emotional expressions, releases, which was another aspect of the automatic movements and sounds that I experienced when I surrendered to meditation.

I would find a place where (I hoped) no one could hear me, surrender into meditation, and howl and howl into a pillow. While it provided relief, I didn't experience much life change from this self-therapy; to be fair to Janov, however, I did this without seeing a therapist.

Years later, I learned co-counselling and felt safe with its eschewing of the powerful therapist role, and was comfortable with its focus on emotional release as the mechanism for healing.

Although feeling thwarted about not being able to sit in deep still meditation, I remained interested in spirituality; I just didn't have a home or a practice in this. Until my late thirties, I was not interested in any theistic spiritual perspectives; even less in Shamanism, which I considered — if I ever thought about it — as delusional or a trendy showing off. I was focused on absolute transcendence, in the Buddhist perspective.

In my mid-twenties, I moved to the North Coast of NSW and studied nursing. After two years in general nursing, I studied mental health nursing. I have not ever openly practised as a nurse healer in clinical settings, although a decade later, when studying for my Honours and PhD degrees, and teaching in academia, I did identify as a healer and, for a time, worked under my assumed spiritual name.

Around age thirty-seven, I went through a lot of change, particularly in my emotional life. I left the relationship with the mother of my children — an enormous decision, but very important to my personal and spiritual development.

Some time after this separation, I attended some meetings with the spiritual teacher Barry Long, and at the last one had a powerful spiritual/energetic experience, like I was a rocket taking off. A few days after, I had a dream of Barry Long, and not long after I began to undergo odd and powerful changes.

My Story

The first was a sense of being very uncomfortable around other people and their distress; I ceased to function in my job as a nurse in an acute psychiatric unit. I could not be in social contact with other people; I lost the mechanisms, such as reading novels, to distract myself from myself.

For two or three months, I sat and smoked cigarettes, I went for long walks, not much else. I was full of something like anxiety, as if all the things I had repressed and stored in my body now seized my mind, while my body became unusually fluid and limber. I knew from the friend who'd introduced me to Barry Long that this experience was something others who followed his teaching and sat in his presence had experienced. Barry called it "awakening in the spirit", or "dying to the self" — something like that. I held a dream of enlightenment at the end of this.

As it went on and on, this time was hellish, and the methods that Barry taught to hold and integrate these experiences did little else but make me feel my whole being was exploding. I thought of suicide but had a clear idea it would not mean the end, nor bring relief. So, I persisted and was courageous with it. There were no helpful practices, but I knew it was a transitional time and on the other side was, potentially, some important change.

However, it seemed unending and I was a little haunted by my friend's stories of those who failed to negotiate this falling into madness. I had grown up with a fear of succumbing to madness — my mother was wracked with nasty paranoid delusions; I'd worked in psychiatric units as a nurse. These images were lurking in the shadows of my experience.

I had some supportive friends though they felt unable to help much. My housemate was concerned. Another friend said he thought I was depressed, which was unhelpful. I was determined to not pathologise what I was undergoing.

I was sleeping poorly, although I remained very energised. I recalled the powerful and strange experiences I had learning samadhi meditation in Java, my body flailing around, and talking in strange languages, and how that was explained as a kundalini thing. Still, I suspected that if I could not just be still and have the deep still meditations others experienced, there was something flawed in me.

One morning I woke up with the words in my mind, "They're experimenting on you". I had never heard voices before; it was very disturbing. Things were going very awry, this awful period was going on so long, not resolving. So, I phoned a friend at the inpatient unit and asked her to bring me some Melleril (a sedating antipsychotic). My housemate insisted I not take it, and asked if, before I took it, I'd see a friend of hers who was a healer and was about to arrive to stay for a while.

Heka, arrived at our home that day and we met in the kitchen. She looked at me and said, "I see your chakras have blown. I can help you with that". I was stunned by her words and, initially, withdrew. Then I came back and demanded she help me immediately. Heka told me to wait while she prepared. I sat on the lounge, she went to the other end of the house, set up her massage table in a small room and began to make strange high-pitched sounds.

Down the other end of the house, my whole being was jumping at these sounds.

The session was like nothing I had experienced, she walked around the table making sounds (toning), she put her finger in my ear, she spoke/channelled my spirit guides. I howled with relief of the pent-up fear which had been held inside me. I spontaneously voiced — as I did in subsequent sessions — advice to myself. "I must give up my cherished desire for enlightenment!" I said. I had no idea where those words came from.

There were sessions at least daily, where I would somehow know what needed to happen — I'd raise myself up from the table the moment Heka was about to lay her hands on my upper back, for example. There were messages from my spirit guides. I was opening up to a new way of experiencing, there was the awakening in me of an inner guidance, where I would receive answers to questions I'd put to my inner self. Heka taught me words of power to invoke my spirit guides. We'd say these together. I experienced a deepening and expanding of consciousness, spontaneous movements and sounds and the beginnings of healing.

Heka was, from the start, taken aback by the intensity of what was happening to me. Even more, by how she was almost involuntarily united with me in this. There was a juxtaposition in our energy fields where together we felt at home and strong; but apart, we both felt somehow deflated and vulnerable. This was unique in her experience and, initially, very disturbing. For Heka, energetically healing was all about obediently following the impulses of Spirit, and at this time she felt impelled to be connected with me. She was very uncomfortable with this, but as we grew to love each other it became more like a normal experience.

Heka was eleven years older than me. She was, when I met her, wild and skinny, outrageous and elusive. Full of authority and wisdom and spiritual power, Heka was also very much a human woman. She was hugely broken and wounded in every way, so much more than I could imagine one person being. Heka spent her life on the fringes of society, and had lived with millionaires, gangsters and psychopaths, as well as spiritual masters and healers. I loved how she was different, completely eccentric, which was such a relief from the constant pressure I have felt to be normal and fit in and look good. She trusted her inner guidance and spirit guides utterly; she had a constant dialogue, and checked in with her guides on almost any subject. She was both holy and irreverent, and obedient to the dictates of Spirit. I don't think Heka thought of herself as a shaman, rather a spiritual healer and yogi.

After the first couple of days, we slept together, platonically, in the tent she'd set up in the backyard. Then we spent two weeks in a cabin in a camping ground behind Mt Warning.

There weren't other people around at the time. On our first day there, in the forest by a stream, I sat and found myself toning for some time; the sounds were forced from me, intense and high pitched, visceral. Suddenly I felt as if a cork popped and from then I was different.

I was a healer. I knew what to do to bring healing to people. I only needed to ask inside and follow my impulses within the healing consciousness. Just do what I was guided to do. I would make sounds, sometimes directed into the part that was injured, I would look in a certain way and my eyes would heal, I would move my head and an energy from my third eye would bring healing. I would move around, speak in a language I did not know, speak deeply and powerfully or make toning sounds of different pitches. There was an occasion when giving healing to Heka, when I found myself bent over onto my head, with a gorgeous flow of energy pouring out into her from all down my spine.

Now the movements and sounds which I had repressed since learning meditation in Indonesia in my twentieth year, somehow were filled with meaning and love and the power to heal. Before this, they'd seemed uncontrolled and incoherent, even threatening to my sanity.

My Story

I had no idea before this that I would be a healer, it was not how I imagined myself to be or experience. I did know that healing was one of the charismatic powers that people following the mystic practices such as samadhi meditation could experience. When I was learning Sufi- type meditation in Java as a young man, I encountered people with clairvoyant or clairaudient powers, and the power to heal. In another mystic organisation in the same city there were people seeking these powers to do things like making a nearby volcano erupt, people learning Kundalini yoga who sat in caves and rivers to gather these powers. The Sumarah group I was learning with had no focus on that.

So, I knew healing power as a charismatic power from that earlier time in my life, from other people, but was astonished years later to find myself being unexpectedly visited by such.

* * *

I felt I had to follow all the impulses of spirit, and found myself engaged in so many astonishing and mysteriously meaningful actions. I'd do something whose meaning would only later become clear. Once, I was standing up and started turning around, I was spinning and spinning, almost as if I couldn't stop.

Afterwards I saw visions — dolphins streaming from Heka's heart — and the healing power grew much stronger.

On another occasion, I was giving a healing to Heka, and I suddenly was guided to stride away from our cabin into the forest. I was myself, and also somehow a powerful tribal shaman, looking around me for something, sensing and seeking. I walked into a clearing and did an intricate and symmetrical dance throughout the clearing, moving and rhythmically singing a deep-toned song. As I danced and sang, I could see an immense high tower of interwoven vine-like strands of light energy coming up from the middle of the clearing and reaching way into the sky. I knew the dance was making that tower. I came across a patch of lantana vine, and found myself trying to dance through it, but unable to. When Heka came to where I was, she found me distressed, in tears, because I could not follow my inner promptings to complete the work of the dance.

Most of the healing and other energy work I did was with Heka, who had been very abused and traumatised throughout her life. I somehow knew, completely and deeply, how to bring healing to her; to channel healing for the traumas she had experienced in her life.

There was a time in our healing journey when Heka was breaking oaths and curses and spells from earlier in her life, and from earlier lifetimes. This was very intense and potentially overwhelming, and I was helping, as a healer or shaman or witch doctor in that part. Other things happened, I broke curses, unravelled spells (for want of a better word); on one occasion a man began to manifest in the room, and the power came up within me to ward him off. Heka was saying out loud words to break the ties with this man, who had a lot of power.

I had/have the knowledge within me to do that work. Such powerful and mysterious work that even now I'm reluctant to write about, it is so far away from consensus understandings and maybe has a claim to be unspoken. Yet, it leaves me with deep knowledge about the unseen agencies and powers of life, how our incarnations are shaped by our own and others' intent which, when focused, has such force. I learned I know the power of words, how words spoken with clarity and intent command the world.

* * *

I have just written about the power of word. Of words spoken with awareness, intent and power. My shaman came with invocation, with me saying the words, taught to me by Heka, to invite my guides and helpers to come within me, to guide my actions and if needed bring healing or other agency to situations of need. Oaths, curses, spells and other acts of power to bind, change and influence, are invoked with word, spoken aloud from a very particular state of consciousness. Inviting and invoking the unseen gods, spirits and powers.

I found I know that part of the hidden worlds, and I have the knowledge and power within me to break those binds and ward away the acts of power of others. I know the words, within me, to exorcise and clear the energies and spirits who have come unbidden and unwelcome to influence others, myself too. I feel and understand how some energies are benevolent, even divine, in nature, and some are unhealthy. I can taste the unclean energies that attach to myself and others. All this came awake within me, by the act of invocation and following faithfully the gait of these spirits and powers. Embodying them, channelling them and allowing them to work through me.

My Story

This was all so shocking to me, never in my most bizarre fantasies would I have pictured myself having these kinds of experiences. Indeed, I'd always been dismissive of others who professed to have them. My fantasies of spiritual awakening were of deep serenity — pretty much just smiling and not doing much, living love and wisdom. The figures acting through me at this time were often powerful and beast-like, uncompromising and unpredictable, and directed me to act in ways that looked bizarre, were bizarre from lots of perspectives, and that had no explanation in the accepted norms of my culture.

It was all a massive challenge to my identity, particularly my fear of madness and my desire to be inconspicuous and blend in. So, while all that was arising was beautiful and joyous, it was, also, appalling and threatening. Of course, going through this with someone who was familiar with it and able to guide me, was enormously helpful. I also changed my name to 'Sananda' and the energy of that name was very stabilising; I've always had a good expansive feeling when others call me by that name.

Alongside this joyous light work, there were many challenges as I was precipitated into the unseen worlds. Not all is of a loving and benign nature. There was much that was difficult, enervating and even threatening. The beings working through me were, mostly, there to heal but, at times, attached to me were other entities or thought forms, which were less conscious and, usually, confused, hurt and lost.

As my awareness was now open to the unseen, I had to learn to protect myself. I had to learn to remove the other entities, which often meant assisting them. Sometimes, there were energies in things, such as clothes and bedding, which I found very unpleasant.

Physical and emotional illness, drug use, all had energies I would potentially be affected by. I would often be exhausted, bombarded by these things and even after energetic clearing work — would be flat and stunned. People's projections, for example, their thoughts directed towards me, could carry entities with them. Sometimes the emotional and energetic intent of others were unpleasant or threatening and, usually, beneath others' awareness, even completely unconscious.

This experience was not limited by proximity. I felt, for months, a physical sense of a knife in my back, which I knew came from someone far away who was unhappy with me and speaking about me in negative terms.

Despite all the negative consequences I was, from the outset, very excited with what was happening, being a healer. I was also so relieved to have come to the other side of that difficult period leading up to meeting Heka, that I wasn't at all discerning about discussing the experiences with others. I was naïve. It led to accusations that I was insane. Given my background, that was very distressing. I knew I was not experiencing psychosis. It was important to me to keep that distinction (although I feel less so now as a Process Worker).

I was always clear about at least two levels of reality going on, and that I could choose which level I experienced. There were powerful reasons to engage in the deeper states as there was much joy and adventure in those; also, to follow the prompting of inner guidance felt safe and true to myself. Further, my recent experience of more everyday reality had been so grim and painful, thus I had a strong incentive to experience what was deep and sacred and connected to the spirits.

Eventually, the healing gift largely left me and, at the end of a year together, Heka left too. The deeper lovely spiritual experiences became less a part of my life, but the more difficult aspects remained.

I knew from my studies of esoteric spirituality that the charismatic powers such as healing, clairvoyance, clairaudience, speaking in tongues, etc., are often a temporary part of the adept's experience. Nonetheless I felt bereft at the loss of this wonderful part of my experience.

What has become more and more clear over the years is that my inner psychic/spiritual nature is shamanic. Just beneath my everyday demeanour, I have constant tendencies to move, make sound, experience proprioceptively, negotiate with spirits in ways that shamans do. I may not always be in touch with the inner knowing of the shaman, but it is part of my makeup in ways that are intrinsic, essential in my nature.

Finding Process Work has been helpful in many ways, but particularly in that I have not felt pathologised in these experiences. Also, I have had the opportunity through therapy to find accommodation between these different parts of myself — the ordinary me who is quite timid and sensitive and inclined to be self-critical, and the shamanic me who is big and wild and often uncaring about its impact on the me in CR. This dynamic I would say is my *life myth*.

Section Three

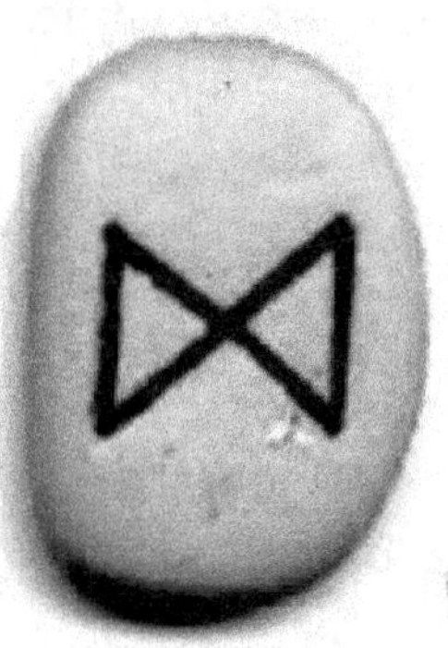

DAGAZ — Breakthrough

Drawing Dagaz marks a major shift or breakthrough in the process of self-change, a complete transformation in attitude — a 180-degree turn. For some, the transition is so radical that they no longer live the ordinary life in the ordinary way.
Because the timing is right, the outcome is assured, although not, from the present vantage point, predictable.[83]

Transmutation

Introduction

What can we make of these stories of nurse healers set out in the previous chapters? In many ways, it might be sufficient to read them and take in the detailed and panoramic picture of this important and little–reported part of human experience they depict. They may well stand on their own as memoirs of sojourns in frightening and beautiful worlds, and accounts of personal wounding, courage and healing.

Nonetheless, I feel it is a very worthwhile enterprise to pull it all together, as it were, to try to capture and present the essence of what these bold adventurers of spirit have given us, in a way that's relatively easy to take in. This takes the form of themes, which in the following chapters I've illustrated with quotes from my collaborators, as well as quotes from the literature of healers, shamans and others.

On studying these stories, I have found six themes which seem to express, essentially, their shared reality, their common ground as healers. These themes, or essences, are: 1. Belonging and connecting; 2. Opening to spirit; 3. Summoning; 4. Wounding and healing journey; 5. Living as a healer, and 6. Walking two worlds. The sixth, 'Walking two worlds', speaks to the deep process the nurse healers were involved with in bringing home the experience of being a healer and living both in ordinary reality and in the spiritual realities of the spiritual adventurer. For easy reference, these themes are set out below:

<table>
<tr><td>Overall themes (Essences)</td></tr>
<tr><td>1. Belonging and connecting</td></tr>
<tr><td>2. Opening to spirit</td></tr>
<tr><td>3. Summoning</td></tr>
<tr><td>4. Wounding and healing journey</td></tr>
<tr><td>5. Living as a healer</td></tr>
<tr><td>6. Walking two worlds</td></tr>
</table>

Chapter Fifteen
BELONGING & CONNECTING

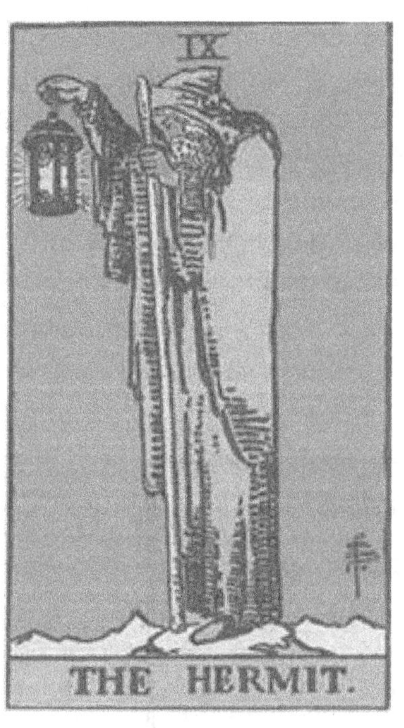

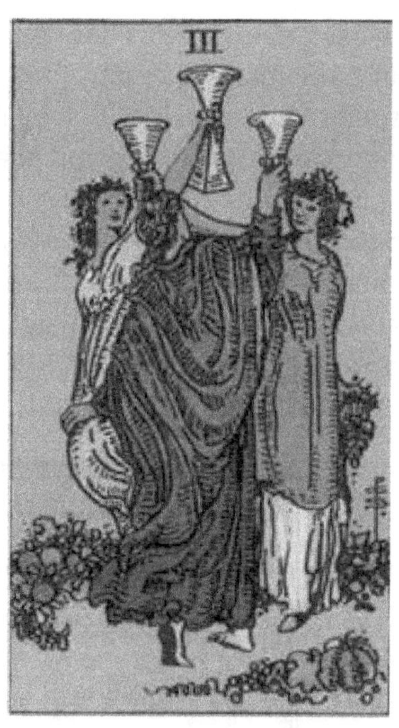

Belonging and connecting

Connection is about the journey around feeling a sense of belonging, and connection with other people, and with spirit, undergone by most of the nurse healers I spoke with.

Fundamental to pretty much anyone's journey through life is connection, so I want to set this theme out at the beginning. A number of the nurse healers experienced a strong sense of isolation from others earlier in life, and this seems to have provoked exploration of the inner worlds and a growth towards the experience of deep connection.

Isolation

> *I certainly felt different. I certainly felt as though there wasn't a place for me, in the world as it was. — Emma*

Several the co-creators of this work articulated the experience of not feeling they belong, feeling different and feeling isolated. They recalled that in childhood, and often well into adulthood, they felt alone, and not able, or sometimes even interested, to just play with the other children of their own age. They reported being thrown onto their own resources and into their own company.

Whilst this was a painful experience in the way most described it, it was also often a time of personal exploration on the inner levels, having contact with spiritual beings, and/or of deep connection with nature.

It was apparent that the experience of not belonging and feeling different and alone oriented a number of the healers to life in a way that encouraged a deeper exploration of self and spirit which is at the heart of the experience of the healer, as Rose's words indicate:

> *So, I developed a fairly rich inner life, from quite an early stage. I was always finding lame animals and bringing them home, and, you know, looking after them.*

Ruth spoke powerfully about the aloneness of her earlier life, connected to no other people, and how her experience of spiritual realms was almost her only reality:

> *Growing up with this knowing, and this experience of two worlds, I made no accommodation to it. No adaptation. It didn't come up in me to tell other people about it. Who would listen? Nobody there. There was nobody in my life who would ever say, "What do*

*you feel?" or who would ever say, "Are you all right?". No. So it
was not a question. There was nothing else in my life.*

It may be significant that some of the collaborators who did not report this
experience of aloneness and isolation in childhood (notably Gabrielle, James,
Michael and Rachel), experienced dramatic personal disruption (discussed
below) when, in adulthood, they entered deeply into the experience of the
healer. It might be that for the isolated young people, coming to terms with
the self and connecting with spirit facilitated a quite natural transition, in
adult life, to deeper experiencing on the non-ordinary realms of the healer.

Some of the participants discussed their coming to accommodation with this
sense of isolation in adult life — for instance, Rose spoke of her enjoyment
of her own company, and Emma spoke of the meaning of her power animal
the wolf for her — being a loner and running with the pack. Reflecting on
the healing of that sense of isolation from others, Emma stated:

*I think I do have a strong sense of belonging within my healing
community. Within the human place, I have a very strong sense
of belonging, and in the esoteric — in the spirit place, I have a
strong sense of belonging. So, all of these things have come
together.*

Accounts in the literature of the experience of nurse and other healers also
point to the centrality of the journey around belonging and connecting for
healers and shamans throughout the world. For instance, Barbara Brennan
spoke of a childhood of much aloneness with nature, largely separate from
other people whilst in deep communion with nature. Speaking personally, it
was certainly my painful experience from late childhood onwards that I felt
different and separate from ordinary society, feeling like I didn't belong. And
in some ways that experience persists to this day.

Another example comes from the personal account of the shaman Elizabeth
Cogburn, who reported a childhood experience of isolation from her peers,
and intense connection with the spirit world:[84]

*In many ways, I was very isolated as a child. School was a
nightmare. My peers seemed to be afraid of me and scornful of
me, and it was as if I was too much, too strong, too active, too
intense, too excited; my eyes frightened people. However, I never
felt alone, because of the myriad of unseen people who came to
play with me. And also animals. I was given to understand about
my parents that I was somehow different, and somehow special.
Everything in my young life corroborated that. I never fit into the
patterns of ordinary life.*

Rachel recalled how, in her early twenties she underwent a deep spiritual transformation as an emerging nurse healer. She reported how during this time she felt very isolated from other people, yet not alone as she had the comforting presence of spiritual visitors who communicated with her. She reflected on the importance to her journey and evolvement of going through this period:

> *I guess that I thought about the aloneness, and the isolation and I felt how much that was a necessary part of the journey. Part of me wants people never to feel alone, and never to feel like there's nobody there, in the physical world — because I think that humanity is about being in connection with others. And while I want to say, "I don't want that, I don't want others on the journey to feel that," I know it was so necessary.*
>
> *I couldn't shed the illusions of who I was, with everybody — it had to be a personal, intense journey. And that was one of the things I had wanted to change, and still struggle with having to do; but yet knowing that that aloneness was so important.*

Connection

The sense of not belonging, differentness, isolation and aloneness appears to be a lot about not feeling connected with other people — for whatever reason. The other side of this issue is the deep connecting with others which becomes possible as people come to terms with their inner terrain and process their sense of isolation, and other emotional issues. Some of the nurse healers I spoke with reported being able to relate more effectively as a result. For example, James reported a transformation in his relationships when he began to open to spirit.

> *it transformed my relationships. It was what love really was. People said I was becoming more available; more present with them. They noticed I was less caught up in my stuff, which meant I was more available to be for them, which conversely over the years one of the pay-offs has been.*

Heloise, who had not reported feeling lonely and isolated earlier in her life, described the importance of connection, which she discussed of in terms of relationship — enacted in her nursing practice; this is clearly at the heart of her experience as a healer:

Relationship is a big thing for me. I don't think that you can impact, or help, or be there with anyone else to facilitate any process, if there's no relationship.

Opening spiritually, and being sensitive to the energetic and deeper, more mysterious aspects of connection, lies at the centre of the experience of the healer, whose spiritual practice is enacted in connection to others in the healing encounter.

James talked of the sense of being at one and co-experiencing in the healing encounter, describing it as being together in the "pool of consciousness".

So here is the consciousness thing... we're both in the "pool" together. That's what's happening. I don't think it's telepathy, and I don't think it's projection...

Angelique spoke at some depth on the energetics of connection, and she brought to the fore aspects of experiencing which are usually not conscious. For instance, she told how she had observed that simply being in the company of other people affected even her dreams. She reflected:

... your mind and your energy works at a different way as when you have a dinner party with, let's say, people who are designing clothes, or dress designers. Your energy, your inner vision, your dreams move in a different way.

It's not just people like me who experience like this. I think, to different degrees, it is a human thing. I think, none of us are islands. I feel that to a degree, perhaps not to the same intensity all the time, we all are exposed to each other, and are influenced by each other.

I think that that is one of the most important things to discover for yourself to what degree are you influenced by someone else's mind, or by a group energy.

Being impacted by the presence of others, energetically, is an aspect of the experience of the sensitive healer which Angelique discussed at depth in my conversation with her. This connecting on the energetic level, and experiencing the impact of another's presence in a powerful way, is clearly an important aspect of the journey of most of the nurse healers I spoke with, and was reported also by Heloise, Emma, Rose, Moira, Michael and Rachel.

It certainly played a big part in my own experience. In healing sessions, the sense of connection — union — with the other was profound. Also, for years I became very open and vulnerable to how those around me were feeling and thinking, and would often take on the energies associated with their distress. This matter, as one related to boundaries and balance, is also discussed below.

There are some accounts in the nursing literature of nurses' experience in healing encounters which describe quite extraordinary — even transcendent experiences. Powerfully illustrating the deep nature of connecting with others experienced by healers, Stephen Wright wrote about a session with a client who'd suffered a stroke and had Alzheimer's disease, where he entered a union which challenged his ability to conceptualise the event. He wrote:[85]

> *Using my hands was barely necessary, my intuition if that's what it was, was in overdrive already. I kept having to pull back and centre myself, the impressions were so strong. His body felt utterly unbalanced — a deep hollowness of the lower half, searing pain along the right side especially. I felt drawn into him, into his experience... I just kept "hearing" this is what it's like for me. To be inside this body. I was close to tears and struggling to stay centred. The pain was awesome, I had never experienced TT like this before, so intimately, so powerfully, so rapidly.*

> *I was almost overwhelmed by a sense of what it was like to be Harry. I was being Harry. This was beyond being with him, beyond empathy or compassion or "presencing". There was no he and I. This was a kind of union. That place of mystery that I've heard about in healing work, where all the boundaries fall away and there is no difference between wounded and healer. We were both in the same place — and there was no we, no both, just being in the same place. It came and went, this feeling. At one moment there was just an immersion in oneness, at the next, a re-separation when I was flooded with imagery and impressions of what it was like to be Harry, to be holding that body. This was the place of knowing. I was rocked by the pain and the intensity of the impressions. I looked at him at one point and said, "Oh, Harry, how do you go on with this, what a tough one, what on earth are you doing inside that one...?" Suffering. A state of continuous suffering.*

> *I felt like I was reporting back. Like somehow I was being informed of that which he could not speak. And I looked at him and thought, "You know". At some level, he was not suffering himself. HimSelf. He was just watching all this. Experiencing it. Knowing it. Being in it. Yet in some way apart from it — witness and participant in one.*

Chapter Sixteen

OPENING TO SPIRIT

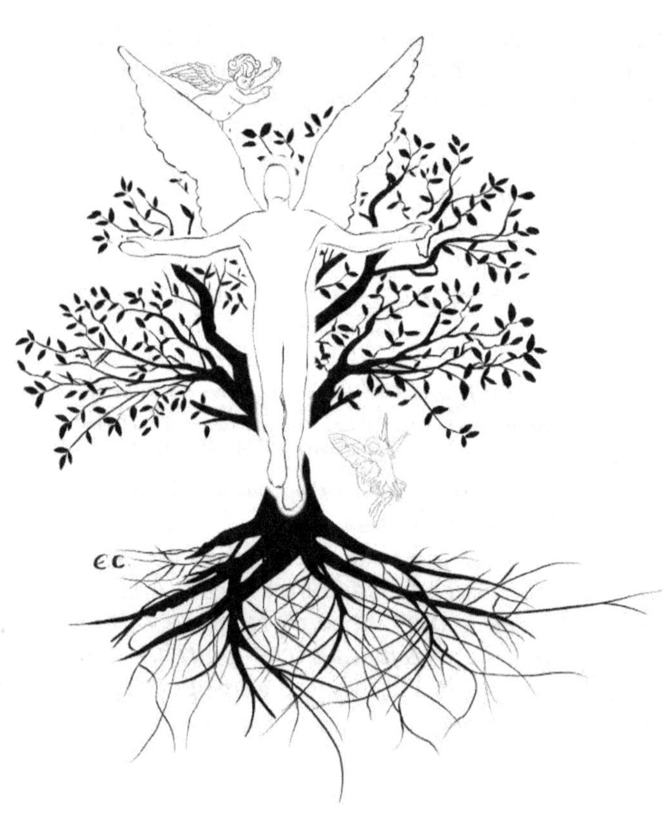

Opening to Spirit

A core theme in the lived experience of the nurse healers I spoke with, regarding their deeper, transformative journeys, was that of opening to spirit. Whereas a number of the nurse healers spoke of the role of spiritual beliefs in their lives, this theme speaks of the direct spiritual experience, little mediated by belief.

This theme was articulated in different ways by the collaborators, each reporting a highly personal experience of, and evolution into, that domain. Some, such as James, Rachel and Ruth, spoke of a dramatic introduction to the spirit realms. This is how Rachel expressed the first time she sat down to meditate:

> *And I sat there, thinking, "I wonder what'll happen," and then, with my eyes closed, yet as if they were open, straight in front of me was an angel. Dressed in the usual garb, you know, wings, opaque gown.*

Unfolding and deepening

Some, like Emma or Heloise, described a gentle unfolding, and a gradual deepening, as when Emma recalled:

> *Regarding my coming to know the spirit place, I think that my experience was very much more of a coming into it — a growing into it.*

Others, such as Gabrielle, described a lifelong process which sometimes was painful and terrifying, and at other times was graced with the gifts of spirit.

Whereas — as noted above under Belonging and connecting — several the nurse healers (Angelique, Chris, Emma, Gabrielle, Rose and Ruth) reported an experiencing of spiritual domains or phenomena from an early age, they nearly all spoke of a deepening over time in their connection with spirit, or their ability to experience different realms of existence, or develop an adeptness in that domain.

Some spoke of their experience of spirit, at the time we spoke, as a clear and consistent experience of spiritual realms (Angelique, Chris, Emma, James, Ruth, Rachel). My sense from others' words was of episodes of deeper experience, often at seminal times such as deep crisis, death, or powerful healing sessions. Almost all spoke of being permanently changed in this opening to, and deepening and evolving in, spirit, as suggested powerfully by

James saying how he felt like he was bent like an iron bar. This I explore further below under the theme 'Summoning'.

Distinct points of intensification or deepening of the process of opening to spirit were identified by some of my collaborators, for example on dealing effectively with trauma following therapy (Rachel, Michael, Rose, Moira) (also discussed below under 'Wounding and healing journey') or after undergoing an initiatory experience like learning a healing modality, or undertaking a shamanic journey (Moira, Emma, Gabrielle, James). Rachel made a clear connection between her emotional work — dropping her "emotional baggage" — and entering and evolving in spiritual realms; and her meeting the angel, described above, came while she was in a counselling course.

Some spoke of the deepening of spiritual experience as a gift of support from spirit, or God, at extraordinarily painful times (Angelique, Ruth, Gabrielle, Moira). A remarkable instance of this is in Ruth's account of dying as an infant, and meeting Jesus:

> *When I was dead I was in a beautiful space; that's where I saw Jesus for the first time. Jesus touched my third eye, when I was in my light body, and that's when I came back. That's the moment my Dad revived me. From then on, I knew I'd been somewhere else, and come back. I always had this knowing, and the feeling, and the security of spirit.*

My own experience was of a yearning for deeper experience throughout my life, followed by a precipitation into other worlds of experience, which I found utterly beautiful and yet at the same time bewildering and terrifying. This came out of a time when I experienced an intense "dark night of the soul" and my shaman healer teacher and fellow traveller arrived just when I felt I must give up.

Transforming

It was clear from the accounts of the nurse healers that the spiritual journeying was not something like putting on a knapsack and hiking through the bush — there was a transformative engagement where the person changed fundamentally as the experience unfolded. This is particularly evident in the accounts of James, Michael, Rose, Gabrielle, Emma and Rachel.

This is less evident for others, as in the case of Chris, whose being part of a spiritual heritage from birth meant that she was, from the beginning, deeply embedded in that experience. It was part of the familial world of her upbringing. Chris described her particular challenge to change as being more that of learning to operate in "normal" society. She said:

> *Challenging things don't really arise, for me, on the unseen levels. It's quite a simple thing. I have more struggles doing things socially correctly, you know for me that's been a bigger challenge. To not blow it socially. In my twenties and thirties, that was like a dilemma.*

Others who had had this very early experience of spirit, such as Ruth, Rose, Angelique, and Emma, also described a less dramatic process of inner change through adult life, but more challenges in living in the ordinary world.

The case of Ruth is remarkable in this context. For her, since infancy, her experience of spirit was all that sustained her, such was the awful nature of her early life, where she was unwanted and abused. This experience reveals the spiritual experience to be a gift and a blessing — a truth very strongly borne out in her story as it unfolded. It speaks to me of the ultimately illusory nature of "achieving" spiritual mastery, or evolving ourselves spiritually — all we can really do is obstruct the workings of spirit, and maybe not even that. When the time comes for spirit to manifest, then we are taken, and reminded that we were only ever dreaming we were separate.

In her book *Living the Therapeutic Touch*, Dolores Krieger, in describing healing practice as a type of yoga, spoke of the opening to spirit, the transpersonal implications and opportunities for personal transformation from learning and practicing a healing modality:[86]

> *Like yoga, the study of healing requires self-discipline, it demands a conscious commitment, and it entails a ready willingness to strive towards an understanding of the self-to- self interface, in this case the interface between healer and healee. As such, it is an experience at the transpersonal level, a state that harbours possibilities of awareness of the more profound reaches of human consciousness where enhanced perceptions may radically alter one's sense of reality*

Visionary experience

This theme — Opening to spirit — is of deep self-discovery and exploration, of encountering the unknown and the unexpected, the beautiful and the challenging. Intrinsic to the opening to spirit for my collaborators were visionary experiences gifted to them. In important ways, the opening to spirit is very much a visionary process — such is the significance of this experience in the lived experiences of the nurse healers I spoke with, as they discussed them with me.

All the co-creators of this work had wonderful accounts of their visionary experiences. They were not, however, all necessarily visual experiences, such as when Heloise recalled a healing session she received:

> *I had this experience of being so big — that I was bigger than the veranda, that my feet were over on the headland — I was monstrously huge! I was so expanded, I had a feeling of knowing everything — not a knowing of knowing it, but a feeling.*

What is evident in the above story from Heloise, an in the accounts of all the nurse healers I spoke with, and mine also, was the intense personal significance of these experiences — visionary experiences they relayed to me all related to, or were in themselves, significant and deeply resonant life events. Another example is from Moira, who found the appearance to her of a healing guide was very affirming and reassuring at a low point in her life:

> *I was upset about something. Things weren't working out — I was broke, and had no money, no food, no nothing. And I was just walking down the beach, and I asked could I meet him? If there was a spirit guide that I could meet, please just tell me who it is, or whatever? But I got better than that ... I saw this big American Indian guy — 'Buffalo Horns'. And he said, "I'm Buffalo Horn. How you doing?" And I just went, "Wow, okay. Hi!"*

Ruth's account of meeting Jesus during a near death experience, quoted above, was another strong instance of the significance of the visionary experience.

Every one of the collaborators spoke of contact with spiritual entities. A striking example (mentioned above) was the case of Rachel's spiritual visitors, such as the angel who manifested to her the first time she sat down to meditate. And from her account, experiencing spiritual beings was a consistent experience from that point onward in her life.

For Rachel, the spiritual visitors played a central part in her opening to spirit, and the beings she encountered were important in giving her support and guidance. Other nurse healers I spoke with reported the importance of the support and guidance of spiritual entities or deities in their opening to spirit (Ruth, Gabrielle, Emma, Heloise, Moira, and Rose). For instance, Ruth said:

And even after I was married, if things got so bad, then [the ascended master in spirit] Maitraea would come, and hold me, as I held my own children.

Gabrielle reported the angel of death, and Jesus, coming to reassure her just before her father died:

And the angel said to me, "Only those who need to be afraid of me, are afraid". And Christ was there, just standing in the distance.

Sometimes the awareness of spiritual beings was incidental, as when Emma as a child was aware of the presence of fairies, who showed no interest in her. She described her experiences with fairies, which to Emma were part of the spirit of nature:

I remember as a child I used to spend a lot of time with fairies. Now I don't know that I saw the fairies, physically saw the fairies, but I knew they were there. And they weren't very responsive to this kid that used to sit in the tree, and I really got the impression then that they weren't really responsive to humans in general.

Other encounters were of a less serious kind, such as when Angelique described playing with spirits as a child:

when it was hot and everybody was sleeping, I would be on the veranda and I would see these spirits that would play with me. And they would rooch back and forward across the veranda, and they would peek around the corner. And that's the way we were playing — hide and seek.

Discussed below under Encountering the shadow some of my collaborators also spoke of inimical entities they encountered.

Related to the above was an experience, for some nurse healers I spoke with, of being deeply involved with the spirit of nature. This is especially evident in the accounts of Emma and Rose, and is also significant in the stories of James, Gabrielle, Chris, Ruth and Heloise.

Here is a strong association with the Indigenous shamanic experience, with which some of the nurse healers I spoke with strongly identified (James, Emma, Rose, Moira, Ruth). Some spoke of "power animals" (Emma and Gabrielle) with which they were associated, and which clearly brought insight and understanding in their connecting with the wisdom in that association.

When we spoke together, Emma brought me a long peacock's feather, and Moira gave me the vertebra of a snake. These symbolised, I feel, the spiritual wisdom of nature, and their sense of the importance of bringing forth the deeper experiences of the journeys of healers.

Rose spoke of her relationship with the nature and other spirits at around her home, where we had our conversation:

> There's the fig tree. The fig tree's got a lot of energy. I mean, that's amazing energy. I can't walk past that tree without feeling that energy, … And you get this energy blast at you. So, when you've got that there, that's pretty strong. There are a couple of spirit people living here — George and Frank. They just hang out in the garden and I've got a guardian — my main guide is a monk, a Tibetan monk, and he hangs out around the ponds, so he's very protective. And there are a lot of animal spirits here, because we're wildlife carers. And I've had many many animals over the years die here, and some I've had to euthanase myself. And I feel those strongly.

It seems appropriate to conclude this subsection with the very sober attitude to the visionary experience voiced by James. Whilst in his conversation with me he recounted some astounding visionary experiences, both in healing and with the shadow. James did express caution about the significance of the visionary experience, particularly when offering healing to others. He said:

> My hit on that is that I am witnessing something that has filtered through my mind, which struggles to put a rational explanation on things. Therefore, if I experience something, like a light around somebody, or the presence of an angel, I am cautious with it. Because I am wondering how far that has been culturally embedded in me. That my culture knows about angels, I see this thing, and therefore it is an angel. Rather than, what one is experiencing in the healing space is somehow the rational mind in an effort to struggle and put an understanding on it — find a label for it.
>
> And so, for me, there is a wariness of what I rather judgmentally call a new age fluffiness, about angels and energy fields and spirits and all this stuff.
>
> And I know some people are gifted with a sense of certainty about something. I understand that, and share it. It happens with me many times, and I just hold that in the context of healing. But what I have learned to do, and I don't know whether I'm right or wrong, I really don't know, but what feels right to do is to keep my trap shut. And not start saying to patients, "This is it, this is what I see, this is what you've got, this is etcetera. Yes, I know this, I know this". Rather than, very gently, if it is discussed at all, is very, very tentative, very gentle.

Opening to Spirit

Tools, practices and guides for transformation

Several my collaborators spoke of tools and practices which assisted in their opening to spirit, as in the above example of Rachel sitting down to meditate, and meeting the angel. Others, such as Moira, Angelique, Emma, James, Gabrielle, Heloise and Rose also spoke of meditating as a practice they found helpful.

Other tools for transformation mentioned by the nurse healers participating in this research were walking the labyrinth (Gabrielle and James), shamanic journeys (Emma, James, Gabrielle), journaling (Rachel), participating in spiritually focused gatherings (Rose, Angelique, Michael), dreaming (Angelique) and having a spiritual companion (Gabrielle, James).

Perhaps of most significance to a majority of the co-creators of this work in their opening to spirit was the learning of healing modalities and other esoteric practices (Angelique, Emma, James, Moira, Gabrielle, Rose, Rachel, Ruth, Heloise), among which were TT, Healing Touch (HT), Reiki, Sufi practices, Trance Postures and Ki Force. This by no means exhausts the tools employed by the collaborators in this work in their opening and deepening into the spiritual realms, but gives a flavour of the range of tools that the nurse healers I spoke with found to be supportive of their inner journeys.

Of fundamental significance for most of my collaborators in their opening to spirit was the role played by spiritual teachers and role models (James, Chris, Gabrielle, Heloise, Rachel, Emma, Michael, Ruth). These individuals were vitally important in guiding the nurse healers in this quite uncharted terrain of the spirit. Chris spoke of the role of her grandmother, and the quiet yet powerful way she guided her:

> *She guided me, silently, really, most of the time.*

James spoke about the significant relationship he shared with his spiritual teacher:

> *always it's like, with him, he either tells me off... but recently he is mellow, he's soft, it's just like a gentle sun bathing when I'm with him now. A tremendous sense of what might loosely be described as energy, passing, or being brought down by one being for the other — what in Hinduism is known as "shaktipat".*

The significance of the spiritual guide becomes very obvious in the light of the bewilderment of the individual who does not have a guide for these deep passages of the opening to spirit, as Michael conveyed powerfully:

I certainly had to undergo my own healing journey. Very subjective, very difficult. I didn't have any mentors, any guide, any compass, or any comfort.

Information from spirit

Several of the nurse healers I spoke with discussed spiritual guidance, which is the receiving of information from a spiritual source. Experience and interpretation of guidance varied from individual to individual. Some described receiving information from specific spiritual beings (Rachel, Moira, Ruth, Emma). Michael, by contrast, recognised that guidance did not arise in his everyday consciousness, but did not identify a source of guidance outside of himself. Angelique also described a general sense of knowing, as of information arising in consciousness. Emma and Rachel and Rose articulated an evolution in guidance over time. For instance, Emma,

described an evolution from a general intuitive sense conveying quite vague information ("radar" or "antennas"), to a receiving of specific information from identifiable spiritual sources. She told how she had confidence in the guidance she received:

there isn't a scepticism, there isn't a lack of belief. And I think it's because I've been very kindly treated by the spirit world, in that it's been a gradual process.

Rachel disclosed how guidance had evolved for her, in terms of her communications with her spirit guides:

Originally, I talked to them literally in words — in dialogue. And then it's become more refined, to be accepting of feelings and ideas, and not needing so many words. Like a knowing, but more like a fast movie. … I still talk to my guidance, my Higher Self, like I'm talking to another person — but I'm much more open to having ideas come into my head that I had no idea where they came from.

Emma, who gave me a very clear account of the development of her inner guidance, told how she could determine the difference between spiritual guidance and the ordinary contents of her mind:

like my daughter would ask me a question, and the words would come out of my mouth. So I wouldn't think. Then, I'm feeling very peaceful, relaxed, and at ease. … if I was in that thinking space, my body changes. My body … gets a little bit tighter, because I need a tight body for my mind to work.

Chris reported being firmly cautioned by her grandmother, her spiritual guide, to not disclose her visionary experiences, unless specifically asked:

I was having all these visions as an eleven-, twelve-year-old — I was seeing things, both in the past and things in the future …And I remember my grandmother saying to me (staunch Irish woman) she'd say I mustn't say anything unless somebody came to me and asked me. That was amazingly helpful, because I'd see things and then they would happen. And then I'd be like, "Whoa, oh dear, what am I going to do?".

Whereas James and Chris expressed caution about passing on information they received from spirit to others, Rose and Ruth saw it as important to pass on what they were given for those who came to them for healing. Rose said:

I have to tell them. I can't think, "Oh gee, it might hurt them if I say this". Well, how they choose to receive it is not my business — it's only my business to give it as I see fit.

I end this section on messages from spirit with a quote from James, who gave a lovely textured account of his personal processing with inner guidance:

So, it's like a faith, and a surrender, and trusting, in God with whom I have a deep personal relationship. We chat like you and I chat now. And I know that that would horrify some, and I know that that could be classed as my projecting something onto some part of my ego or soul that I need to have a chat with. Doesn't feel like that.

And I have this regular confab with a humanist friend of mine a devout humanist — if you will pardon the pun. And whilst I accept huge amounts of what she says about the experience she says about the super ego and the collective unconscious and all this kind of thing, I end up saying "well, I can't have a conversation with a collective unconscious".

This is deep and personal, and from time to time, when I feel in need of guidance, I go quiet and still within myself. And I learn to sit still and shut up. And listen. And sometimes it takes the form of an inner dialogue. There's no words — I'm using "dialogue" — there's no words. There is just a symbolic interaction taking place, in which understanding comes through. And only occasionally have I responded to inner guidance that has said, "I want you to this". And then I think, "Oh, I'm unsure about this".

So, the doubt is a useful tool to have. I use doubt, I use questioning to check it out. I'm making it sound like it some endless struggle or tussle, but by and large it isn't, actually. It's fairly quick, spontaneous, fun...

Blessings of spirit

My collaborators spoke of the blessings of opening to spirit. For instance, a number spoke of the beauty of being in the experience of spiritual reality, or in the company of beautiful beings. Emma spoke powerfully of feeling blessed by the gift of spiritual experience:

> *being blessed enough to have that awareness of the spirit world. To have that knowing support of spirit in the work, in the things that I'm doing. To be able to connect with people on that etheric level.*

Emma also spoke of being blessed by the expanded sense of knowing in spiritual consciousness, that for her it was empowering and comforting. Most participants spoke of the blessings inherent in being healer, which I discuss later under 'Living as a healer'.

Ruth expressed the almost bittersweet gift of spirit as she described her experience of this other world she lived in:

> *Like, you know when it is cold, and you breathe out, and you have these little particles of air — that's sort of what it feels like. You know, like I'm one of these particles, and the ascended masters and on the other side, my mum on that side, my dad on that side, and all of this is still moving around. It's like this cloud of air, and each individual particle. And there is still movement, all the time. But there is nothing to do, there is just an "is-ness". And it's nice to have that. It's a gift. I think it's a blessing, myself. It's pulled me through many things.*

Insights

One of the great pleasures for me in the conversations I had with these nurse healers, and in transcribing and reflecting upon those talks, was the spiritual insights they expressed.

Whereas the path of the healer is by its very nature one which requires spiritual insight, there were some lovely examples which stood out.

Perhaps the insights which most impacted me expressed concerned the nature of reality, and on self in that. James reflected on the central understanding funding his transformation into someone living a life of the spirit:

> *absolutely everything [is] connected with everything else. Everything, everything is connected. There is no separation — of anything. And I don't think one can truly grasp that unless you've trodden non-ordinary reality.*

Another insight, concerning the nature of greatness expressed in the beauty and delicateness of a flower, was expressed by Angelique, who recounted an anecdote about a flower — a poppy. This simple story, how she told it, struck me as holding a deep insight into the meaning of essence, and greatness.

> *I was walking along a canal — along the water somewhere, and there was a poppy, in a green field. And I stopped, and I looked at it — and it was so exquisitely beautiful!*
>
> *... That is an example of. to be what you are — I think a flower represents that, to me, in a way. If you lose the sense of who you are, have a look at a flower — a flower that is beautiful, and cannot be other than what it is; and it has its own fragrance, its own qualities. And so I admire, and it's like the whole universe is in this poppy. I walk away, and I see another girl coming behind me, and she sees, "Oh, poppy!", and snatch! She takes it along, and then she puts it in her hair. And goes like, "Ouch!". But it's appreciating the small thing, that is so large! And this is simply an example, but it is also in the relationship, in a gesture, or in a look, or in the way you listen, or in the way you communicate.*

Rose's insight on the blessing of suffering, mentioned below, under Wounding and healing journey, also struck me. The simple and humble way that Ruth embodied her spiritual understanding impressed me greatly — no grand concepts, just living in the grateful knowing of being embraced by God. Heloise reporting a sense of, "I think God's happy with me", regarding her healing work. All the nurse healers I spoke with expressed spiritual insights which touched me.

Encountering the shadow

Not all of the reports by the nurse healers of encountering spiritual or non-ordinary realities were of the lovely and supportive kind. For instance, Heloise reported encountering the spirit of a deceased Aboriginal man, which terrified her at the time, although she did not believe it held ill will towards her.

Angelique, who worked at times with dying people as a mental health nurse in her patients' homes, spoke of the presence of spirits around dying people which might bring a very uncomfortable feeling to the environment. She also spoke of challenging energetics around death. Working with those who are dying, for Angelique, exemplified and brought to the fore a number the challenges facing a nurse healer, who is working on both physical and energetic levels, dealing with health issues both seen and unseen. The following quote from her story brings forth issues such as dealing with uncomfortable feelings; being challenged to act authentically, with personal integrity; the need for protection; mental, emotional and psychic strain; and working in an environment that denies reality of nurse's perceptions and insights:

> That takes a lot from a nurse — to be so close to a person who is dying, because there are a lot of energies from the unseen realms the person is processing. And working in an environment that does not appreciate the knowledge, or even the sensitivity to this, is very difficult.
>
> I'm talking about the unseen entities relating to me in an adverse way, or that the person would demand certain ways of doing things, and as a nurse you are already very flexible, but not to the degree that you have to completely let go of your own insights. So it's not only the patient you're dealing with. You have to protect yourself, sometimes — very often, actually — in order to be able to go on living your own life in your own authentic way, and not to be of service in such a way that you would lose yourself in your job. It takes tremendous strength of your own being.

One way to articulate this experience is in terms of "the shadow", and many examples of this difficult experience were disclosed by my collaborators. Angelique said:

> Some of the challenges that I have faced — and it's a long, ongoing process — are of discovering that not all that you see and that you encounter is of a benevolent nature. And especially with diseases — and physical and mental diseases — it resonates with areas that are in the astral fields. And in the astral fields there are many different energies that can behave in ways that may be very challenging — to your own health, to your own focus, to your own wish to be aligned with something that I would call "Source", or "Christ", or anything in that direction.

Illustrated by the above from my conversation with Angelique, a significant aspect of opening to spirit, for some of the nurse healers (Angelique, James, Moira, Emma, Rose, Rachel, Ruth, and Gabrielle) was the experience of "the shadow", or spiritual darkness. In Jungian terms, "the shadow" refers to unseen aspects of everyone's psyche, or even the collective psyche, which affect one's thoughts, feelings and behaviours, typically in unwanted or unpleasant ways.[87] When opening to spirit, for some people, there comes a direct consciousness of shadow, which has a projection in spirit. This can be particularly challenging for healers, shamans, therapists and other spiritual adventurers who have a rapid and deep entry to spiritual experiencing, and may still be at the early stages of coming to terms with their own shadow.

Finding ways to work with "the shadow" presents as a vital aspect of healers' work, and is discussed in this section as well as later in this book in Chapter Eighteen 'Wounding and healing journey'.

James discussed his experience of shadow at depth, and identified areas of shadow in himself with which he had cultivated a relationship (discussed under Living as a healer). He spoke of having a number of experiences, in non ordinary reality, of spiritual darkness, some of which were very dangerous and inspired great fear.

As noted above, Angelique talked about encountering the shadow in her work as a nurse in others' homes, particularly when nursing the dying. She reported finding herself uncomfortable at times with the energy associated with the spirits drawn to the dying, having to work as a nurse in that energy.

As people sensitive to the unseen aspects of experience, my collaborators reported a number of experiences associated with darkness in spirit. For instance Rose recounted a story about being psychically attacked; and Moira spoke of being influenced by the thoughts of others, particularly men, projected at her. The manifestation of thought forms, as an aspect of spiritual darkness many healers deal with, was also discussed by Emma. This experience is also discussed below, under the theme, Living as a healer.

Emma spoke of dealing with the shadow when it presents, but not seeking it out:

> *I think when it comes up, it's important for me to explore it. I'm not going to go digging for it, just like I'm not going to go digging in past lives. If something comes up, then great — then it's time for me to learn that lesson.*

James discussed keeping balance in approaching spiritual shadow phenomena and of the importance of being alert to the complexity of the human spiritual experience. The personal shadow will likely influence how the healer engages with its more transpersonal aspects:

> *When I hear people swanning about, talking about "love and light" and stuff like that... that's not the way it is. And I don't think we can be as fully available in service, with those in need, unless we recognise the shadow in ourselves — in them, in how it works, how it is playing itself out. Because the healing process is about transforming shadow into light. And so I think if one is more aware of that, maybe that's one dimension of the experience of those, if they serve me in some way, which is to make me more aware when I am working with people, of a degree of humility. This cannot be me whacking light into somebody. There is something going on here, of which I am but a servant.*

The subject of working with shadow is fascinating to me, and would be worthy of a book in its own right. It does sit right against the edges of a healer's experience of the personal and transpersonal in journeying in alternative realities, where healers and their healees are both growing. And these are glimpses into some of the most outlandish, intractable and quite likely unknowable aspects of the many possible realities.

My own experiences of shadow have been so awkward and "out there" that I am shy to write about them here. I have felt very vulnerable around these experiences, and also ashamed at how I struggled with protecting myself from them. And these experiences made me isolate myself from other people, as I was vulnerable to the unconscious shadows connected to others. Interestingly, though, some healers report little experience with the shadow in spirit.

Related to the shadow phenomena encountered in spirit are the areas of personal shadow that is part of everybody's life journey, yet seem to have particular meaning for healers. This is touched upon in Chapter Eighteen, 'Wounding and healing journey' and explored further in Chapter Nineteen, 'Living as a healer'.

It is perhaps somewhat arbitrary to identify this Opening to spirit as a separate theme to that of living as a healer, but the sense I glean from most of my collaborator's reflections, is that the deeper and unique experience of the healer is held within this opening to the universal spiritual adventure, whilst in other aspects being quite of its own nature. Some, such as Michael and Rose, did not, in our conversation, draw a strong distinction between their deeper experiences as healers, and the spiritual realm in which it held. This accords with Dolores Krieger's account of the journey of the healer as a yoga, or spiritual path in itself,[88] as I have noted earlier. I feel this is the case with all themes — they will inevitably be arbitrary to a degree in dividing up human experience, and they all intertwine and overlap.

Chapter Seventeen

SUMMONING

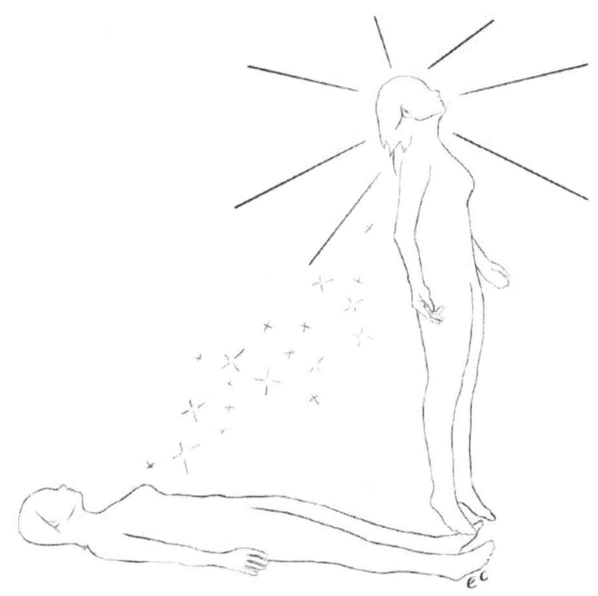

Summoning

As disclosed to me in our conversations, some of the nurse healers, particularly James, Gabrielle, Michael and Rachel — underwent dramatic personal disruption in the process of opening to and deepening into the spiritual healing experience. This is a highly distinctive pattern of experience in the deep awakening to being a healer. This was also my own experience, and from this personal upheaval I was drawn eventually to write this book.

There is a sense in James's story, and also in Gabrielle's recollections, of being challenged to overcome deep reluctance to enter into the deep domains of the spirit. In the case of James, the word summoning comes to mind, where he was commanded, against his will, by the deeper aspects of his being to change profoundly to live a life of the spirit:

> *I felt like an iron bar being bent and being made to go in a different direction. And there were long episodes of physical, emotional, mental, spiritual crisis. And I would encapsulate the whole thing as a spiritual crisis — an ongoing one lasting several years in which almost everything — my values, my ideas, my knowledge — was turned on its head. And it was terrifying.*

James described to me in detail a huge struggle where he eventually had no choice but to abandon a life focused on material success and sensory gratification, in favour of a life path centred on profound spiritual experience. And during that process his health deteriorated dramatically, he became unable to function in some of his professional activities, his relationships all changed, his values were challenged, and he began to undergo therapy. He described the process as becoming possessed by a part of himself that was unwilling to permit him to live as he'd conducted his life until then. And then followed an intense spiritual awakening.

Gabrielle also reported being deeply disturbed, initially, by an inner call to awakening. She said:

> *I had an experience which was the most terrifying of my life. I don't know how to describe it, except I had a sense of being called by the divine. The sense was a female sense, and the word that comes to mind is 'siren', of the soul, and the call was piercingly sweet, and utterly frightening. And all I could say at the time was, "Fuck off, God!"*

Rachel also disclosed a difficult process in coming to balance her spiritual experiencing with living in the ordinary world. She spoke to me of an extended period of dysfunction on the physical level of existence following her abrupt awakening to the spiritual world of visitors and other phenomena. Understanding it in terms of "dropping her baggage", of letting go of emotions and beliefs which restricted her from coming to a deeper self-knowledge and personal authenticity, Rachel reflected on that struggle:

> *So as I was unloading baggage, my health was deteriorating; the spiritual experiences were coming; my emotional being was in crisis, because the relationship that I had had broken down. It was like a total stripping me back to my bones.*

For Rachel, the spiritual experience became her main focus in a time when other aspects of her life were extraordinarily chaotic and confusing. One of the difficult aspects was the way that her sensitivity to unseen aspects of health, for instance, intruded on her ability to maintain equilibrium.

An example she gave was of difficulty she encountered in her employment as a nurse, when she was becoming:

> *… more vulnerable, being impacted more, or being aware more from an energetic point of view; realising that the chest pain I had might not be physical chest pain — that it might be an emotional pain [from another person] that I was registering in my heart…*

Rachel recounted to me how it took an extended time before she gained mastery over her spiritual impressions. As she was going through an intense period of counselling and personal reflection and re-evaluation, she was at the same time thrown powerfully into the spiritual realms. For Rachel, the world of spirit became her refuge, but this in itself created problems. She reflected how it was addictive in its beauty and security, and she came to lose interest in tending to the business of living:

> *I was slipping so far down into the spiritual realms that I could have easily taken my own life and gone to spirit. Because it was such a fine line between staying in a physical existence — because spirit seemed so much better. It was such a heightened experience — it made me feel good about who I was; it was friendly; it was all of those things. There were days, I remember, thinking, "If I could just kill myself, if I could just end it, I could be spirit and life would be fantastic, wouldn't it?" Because it was like they never seemed to have a problem — it was just this physical world that kept holding me.*

Similar in some ways to the experience of James and Rachel, Michael found that as he deepened his spiritual experiencing through the practice of healing, he entered into a period where he was forced to change radically. He spoke movingly about this period:

> *I felt as if I had no choice in engaging in that process. And the stronger that the healing energy came up in me, the more*

sacrifice I had to make. For a period of time. I did lose everything in my life — I lost my family, I lost all the wealth that I had accumulated. I'd lost, if you like, the relationship prior to that. So I felt a period of total loss, and detachment, really, from the physical things, aspects of life. I had to know that really wasn't enough. And that was huge, and very traumatic. But I had a great sense of calm inside, and obedience — I felt like I was peeled open and a strong search light was put on me, and all I could do was have humility and obedience to that. To really go with it. I couldn't struggle against that. So it was quite profound, and quite prolonged, and quite strong. And I felt quite broken in that time, as a human being, but quite intact in a certain way as well.

Michael voiced an understanding that what occurred was to make him more authentically himself:

It was actually blow-torching off the unnecessary, in a way. The essential me was more me. The essential knowledge that I had was stronger. Not new, really, it was like remembering. Rediscovering, not actually discovering. So I'd have to say probably more deconstruction. You know, and in that deconstruction, the scaffolding of life, social life and family life and material life that I had built and was taken away, allowed me to expand rapidly.

This above account by Michael seems emblematic of the process of deep transformation of the (nurse) healer, and illustrates powerfully how what occurs in the lives of these individuals — although extremely disruptive and painful — enables, in the end, a more deeply integrated and authentic living.

I have often wondered about this, in terms of my own journey, how what to many may seem to be a craziness or bizarreness is, at the bottom of things, how I am most real and true and honest. And how somehow, the pain and dysfunction and awfulness of the time presaging the awakening to healing must have been somehow right and needed, perhaps like the difficult passage through the birth canal that babies go through.

Writings on nurse healers also contain some reports of dramatic life disturbance in awakening to healing, for instance contributors to Lynn Keegan and Barbara Dossey's book told of their deeply personal experiences of transformation as healers. Susan Morales, for example, shared how her life was scoured in that process, as she traversed the darkness in her soul:[89]

With a twenty-four-hour period, I lost both my job and my husband. I was in a city with no support networks... I was alone. I lay on my living room floor staring out the windows for hours.

Summoning

The only thing I could do each day was to jog. Running along the ocean seemed to be a metaphor for my life. I was running for my life...

I journeyed into the depths of my being where shadows swallow any sound. There was never any choice about the descent; the only choice was to go kicking and screaming or to walk it and stay as alert as possible. I never fought it; somewhere in my being I knew it was the natural cycle of life and death. And something was definitely dying. Even in that dark place there is a glimmer of blessing, of Light. From that glimmer I was able to see that I was dying. Who I had thought I was as defined by relationships, job, locale had all been stripped away. I stood alone on my path. Or so I thought.

*That time in my life was the most awful and the most awesome. I naively named it my "dark night of the soul", assuming we only ever needed to go through **one** of them.*

Looking back, it was my first such experience and therefore the impact was great. It was an "initiation" of which I had only read about in relation to "healers". In my quest for discovering more about healers and healing, I had unconsciously given permission to the universe, God, whomever, to teach me in a way that guaranteed I would apply what I learned. What better way than to alter the vessel so that the contents will be congruent?

As the vessel of me shattered I discovered that I was not alone. There was the One who was lovingly shattering the vessel so as to free the contents which could no longer be contained in that form, much like helping a snake shed its old skin. I experienced a miracle every day for the first week following the change. At first I thought they were coincidences but then realised they were telegrams from God saying, "You okay? I'm here". It was the beginning of a healing for me and a deepening of faith that will always sustain me.

Another of the nurse healers who spoke with Keegan and Dossey was Irene Belcher, who also disclosed about the deep psychic and emotional disruption in her healer's transition, which required great courage and presence of being to negotiate:[90]

My personal time of healing was also an intense time of learning, about spirituality, faith, trust, surrender, letting go, flowing with the process. I had to be frequently reminded to "trust the process". Forced to live in the moment, my journey became truly transformational.

Alongside the research I conducted in 1998, mentioned in the introduction to this book, some nursing researchers have also written about the healer's abrupt experiences of awakening and transformation. For example, Victoria Slater and colleagues wrote about a liminal phase in some nurses' "journey to holism"[91], and Norma Geddes' inquiry into the experiences of Healing Touch practitioners, also found that these nurse healers often underwent powerful and disruptive transformations.[92]

Also, Robbie Davis-Floyd and Gloria St John, in their study into the transformation of doctors into healers, also reported on these kinds of experiences. One of the doctors they spoke with, Michael Greenberg, reported a seminal, life-changing experience of guidance:[93]

> *I was sitting in my office, ready to quit medicine. Everybody was gone for the day. I was sitting there alone because I thought I was having a psychotic break … I was looking in the Yellow Pages for a practice broker to sell my practice when I heard a voice say, "Close the book; you're not leaving". These voice things are not literally translatable, but the message was, "Of course you hate what you're doing. You've become more of a businessman that a doctor. Not just you, not just the profession, the whole consciousness. You can stay here and listen … (I knew I had a choice) or choose to run away".The voice said, "If you do this, you're never going to be rich or famous, but you'll always have enough". My life kind of turned on a dime then.*

Some of the nurse healers who underwent this process of summoning experienced significant health issues at the time. For example, James spoke of debilitating headaches and collapsing at inopportune times, Rachel spoke of worrying she was insane and having severe allergies. Possibly these experiences could be included in the next theme, Wounding and healing journey, but there is something different about these kinds of illness which attend the summoning experience. This type of experience is common for shamans. Below I include some examples of reports of this by anthropologists.

Ake Hultkrantz noted that some shamans experienced convulsions and other hysterical symptoms, sometimes associated with a well-known disorder known as "Arctic hysteria" which was prevalent in the arctic regions of Eurasia. Hultkrantz was not convinced that shamans suffered any lasting and pervasive psychopathology, stating:[94]

> *Still, the shaman does not succumb to these attacks, he conquers them by adapting them to the role he assumes, the role of the shaman. It has often been said that the shaman heals himself from his hysterical disease during the vocation process, and this seems to be true to a certain extent.*

Summoning

Like Hultkrantz, Joan Halifax[95] (quoted in Chapter Two), wrote how shamans powerfully transcend the traumas attending their coming to the role.

Much as was experienced by some of the nurse healers I spoke with, shamans typically undergo powerful and disruptive transitions at the start of their careers. In the anthropological discourse, terms like "recruitment" and "initiation" [96] or "making" [97] or "calling" [98] signify the transformational pathways followed by individuals coming to the role of shamans/healers in traditional societies.

Studies have documented how this process typically entails a dramatic transformation, often involving severe social disruption, life-threatening illness or temporary insanity for the potential shaman. Some neophyte shamans, notably among the Chuckchee tribes of Siberia, underwent androgyny, and many go off into the wilderness for a time.[99]

Other experiences of the shaman-elect reported in the literature included supernatural and quasi-supernormal events like being struck by lightning or bitten by a spider; frightening encounters with supernatural beings; and dreams and visions involving sacred, supernatural or symbolically significant entities, such as serpents or spirits; or spiritual journeys through metaphysical realms which might involve death, dismemberment and reconstitution.[100-109]

Mircea Eliade, a seminal contributor to this field, whose interest was the history of religions, pointed out that the dramatic and traumatic experiences described amongst neophyte shamans are found amongst initiates throughout the world's religious traditions. Such an experience, Eliade claimed, was a typical psychological response to a person's contact with the divine. In response to the commonly held assertion that the shaman's experiences were invariably manifestations of psychopathology, Eliade wrote:[110]

> *Like any other religious vocation, the shamanic vocation is manifested by a crisis, a temporary derangement of the future shaman's spiritual equilibrium. All the observations and analyses that have been made on this point are particularly valuable. They show us, in actual process as it were, the repercussions, within the psyche, of what we have called the "dialectic of hierophanies" — the radical separation between profane and sacred and the resultant splitting of the world.*

The experience of being called to shamanise against their will is frequently part of this experience of disruption experienced by neophyte shamans. For instance, Laurel Kendall wrote of *miansin* — women shamans in Korea:[111]

> *No woman claims to have wilfully embarked upon this career. Rather, the gods torment destined shaman with visions, voices, mysterious illnesses, and general ill luck. A "god-descended" woman and her family may deny the signs, but only for so long; those who resist the calling die the deaths of crazy women whose thwarted destinies yield ominous ghosts. But once a woman is initiated as a miansin [shaman], the spirits that tormented her become allies who send her divination visions and the power to cure.*

This overwhelming summoning was also the case for the *yuta* (shamans) of Okinawa, reported by Koichi Naka and colleagues:[112]

> *One does not become a yuta of her own will, but rather, she is forced to become a yuta by the notification of, or by the will of the god. In many cases, however, one would try to ignore or reject becoming a yuta to perform her pre-destined duties. It is known that unless she seeks her own guardian spirit, serves him, and seriously endeavours to do her ritual duties, she can never be freed from her sufferings, and what is worse still, she may sometimes become insane, or as good as the living dead, or various misfortunes may fall on to her children and even down to her posterity.*

I resist the temptation to include here a number of examples of these descriptions of the summoning of shamans, they are such thrilling and confounding stories, particularly when the words of the shamans themselves are used. Below I do include two vivid examples, one of the Australian Aboriginal people of my homeland, and one of the Inuit, which is simply wondrous.

A P Elkin wrote about the Aboriginal "men of high degree", including their transformational experiences. In the following account from the Yaralde people, he recorded the "psychic terrors" undergone by some recruits in their coming to terms with their relations with the spirit world:[113]

> *When you lie down to see the prescribed visions, and you do see them, do not be frightened, because they will be horrible. They are hard to describe, though they are in my mind and my miwi [psychic force], and though I could project the experience into you after you had been well trained.*
>
> *However, some of them are evil spirits, some like snakes, some are like horses with men's heads, and some are spirits of evil men*

which resemble burning fires. You see your camp burning and the flood waters rising, and thunder, lightning and rain, the earth rocking, the hills moving, the waters whirling, and trees which still stand, swaying about. Do not be frightened. If you get up, you will not see these scenes, but when you lie down again, you will see them, unless you get too frightened.

If you do, you will break the web [or thread] on which the scenes are hung. You may see dead persons walking towards you, and you will hear their bones rattle. If you hear and see these things without fear, you will never be frightened of anything. These dead people will not show themselves to you again, because your miwi is now strong. You are now powerful because you have seen these dead people.

To conclude this section on summoning, the following is from the arctic explorer and ethnographer Knud Rasmussen who recorded this account of an Eskimo shaman's introduction to the spirit world. The neophyte had sought inspiration in the wilderness, and recalled:[114]

I soon became melancholy. I would sometimes fall to weeping and feel unhappy without knowing why. And for no reason I suddenly changed, and I felt a great, inexplicable joy, a joy so powerful that I could not restrain it, but had to break into song, a mighty song, with room only for one word: joy, joy! And I had to use the full strength of my voice. And then in the midst of such a fit of mysterious and overwhelming delight I became a shaman, not knowing myself how it came about.

But I was a shaman. I could see and hear in a totally different way. I had gained my enlightenment, the shaman's light of brain and body, and this in such a manner that it was not only I who could see through the darkness of life, but the same bright light also shone out from me, imperceptible to human beings but visible to all spirits of earth and sky and sea, and these now came to me to become my helping spirits.

Chapter Eighteen

WOUNDING & HEALING JOURNEY

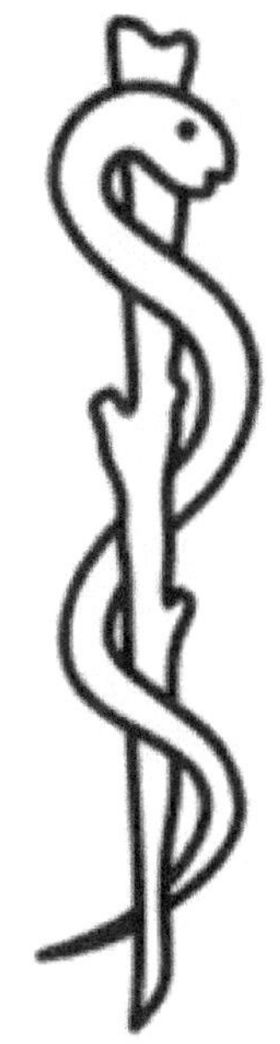

Your joy is your sorrow unmasked.

And the selfsame well from which your laughter rises was oftentimes filled with your tears.

And how else can it be?

The deeper that sorrow carves into your being, the more joy you can contain.

Is not the cup that holds your wine the very cup that was burned in the potter's oven?

And is not the lute that soothes your spirit the very wood that was hollowed with knives?

When you are joyous, look deep into your heart, and you shall find that it is only that which has given you sorrow that is giving you joy.

When you are sorrowful, look again in your heart, and you shall see that in truth you are weeping for that which has been your delight.

Kahil Gibran – The Prophet[115]

I was constantly overwhelmed, during these deep disclosing conversations with my collaborators, and transcribing the tape recordings of them, by the shocking emotional woundings that a number of them disclosed to me. For instance, of the eleven nurse healers I spoke with, Angelique, Chris, Emma, Heloise, Gabrielle and Rachel did not disclose to me that they'd experienced sexual abuse — the others all spoke of that experience, the pain it caused them, and, in most cases, the healing of the wounds.

Above, in 'Belonging and connecting', I mentioned how a majority of the co-creators of this work had reported a deeply painful sense of isolation and loneliness in early life. Other difficult life experiences reported by the nurse healers included physical abuse by parents or partners (James, Rose, Ruth), murdered (attempt) by a parent (Ruth), death of a child (Moira), death of a partner and/or close family member (Emma, Gabrielle, Moira, Ruth), pent up grief of working with trauma victims (Michael), abuse from other nurses (Gabrielle, Michael), taking on the pain of a parent (Gabrielle), drug abuse (James, Rose), dysfunctional relationships with partners or families of origin (James, Emma, Michael, Rose, Ruth, Moira), traumatic or chronic physical injury or illness (Chris, James, Moira, Rachel, Ruth), and, for most collaborators in this study, deep spiritual and emotional distress.

I mention this not to catalogue the traumas of the nurse healers, but rather to convey a sense of the difficult life experiences of the nurse healers. The only nurse healer I spoke with who did not disclose a significant personal journey around wounding was Heloise.

Among the others, Moira and Rose certainly experienced the devastating traumas of their lives, and the healing of them, as the absolute core of their journeys as healers. Chris, Gabrielle, James, Michael, Rachel, Emma and Angelique also saw the healing of their wounds as critical to their understanding of themselves as evolving humans in the experience of spiritual healing.

How the nurse healers responded to their wounding was highly significant for their life paths as healers. Angelique, for instance, spoke of being sent away from her family as a small child, and how she responded to the lack of a mother figure by mothering herself:

> *The way people are doing now — the other way around, you know — that you've grown up, and you're letting your inner child talk to you. I have done that the other way around.*

Wounding and healing journey

Later, she reflected how that resilience and self-nurturance she developed at that time enabled her to act as a healer to others:

> I know that my patients really like to have me around — I know I'm a very good nurse. And it comes from this background story that I just told, of being alone, being lonely, and having to delve very deep inside myself — to keep my balance, and to grow in a harmonious way. And I feel that that is part of what I can share with other people who are sick, also. To turn it into healing qualities.

The literature on wounded healers at end of this chapter corroborates the sense in the nurse healers' accounts of the woundedness and its healing, funding the ability to contribute to the healing of others.

Moira voiced a recognition of a progression in her evolution as a healer, concurrent with her own healing journey. She said:

> I think the healing work that I do becomes stronger, as I work through my own stuff.

Still further, Rose, who had disclosed to me a life of multiple traumas with intense personal suffering and deep emotional disruption over decades, spoke of the blessing of her woundings:

> I don't regret any of [those experiences of wounding]. ...I don't even think, "Oh wouldn't it be nice if that hadn't happened". I feel really grateful, and I feel in a sense that I'm quite privileged to have been through those things, because they just served to make me a better person, or a greater person, or more capable of serving other people.

Similarly, James reflected on his healing journey:

> ... part of the forgiving process is, when looking back, upon terrible things that happened in one's life, and looking back on them now with appreciation — one loses the anger. Part of forgiveness is that you don't see them as terrible things through which you hold anger, or victimisation, or anything like that. You just let them go.
>
> Because it's the alchemical process — one turns lead into gold. You look back at them and say, "Oh, wow". If that hadn't happened then I wouldn't be here talking to you now. I wouldn't have.

This was recognised by a number of the nurse healers I spoke with, who, like Rose, came eventually to be healed of the deep hurts they had carried within. Another insight on the wounding experience and its healing, came from Emma, who spoke of the woundings being the "coming home" experiences:

> *Some of the experiences of being wounded, eventually are the "coming home" experiences... So the strongest presence of angels was there, around the most painful times.*

Ruth also spoke of the spiritual support which came to her when her need was greatest. She recollected this example:

> *There were many times where [Baba] actually protected me in the physical from getting very very badly hurt. When my husband would see a wall of light around me, and he'd say to me, "If I could get through that, I'd kill you!" But wouldn't dare to come close.*

The actual healing journeys of the nurse healers were deeply significant, and they described numerous kinds of healing. Examples of approaches which helped were psychotherapy (James, Rachel, Michael, Moira), EMDR therapy (Rose), Healing Touch, Therapeutic Tough, Reiki and other energy healing approaches (Emma, Rachel, Gabrielle), rebirthing (Michael, Heloise), contact with spiritual teachers (James, Michael), and contact with beings and masters on spiritual planes (Rachel, Moira, Ruth, Gabrielle). Chris spoke of the existential meaning of others bringing healing to her (and her to others) at times of life threat, putting their shoulder to her life:

> *I had always worked in intensivist situations, with people who were in that kind of fight for their life. In that situation I absolutely had an awareness that you used your life, you put your shoulder to their life to fight, because without you doing that, they would die. I wouldn't have survived without other people doing that for me. And I mean people had clearly done that when I was born.*

With the healing of their own emotional wounds, most of the nurse healers I spoke with reported experiencing increased capacity to heal others and the deepening of spiritual consciousness. Rose spoke of her own experience of this:

> *Having dealt with the emotional traumas and blockages — that means I'm freer in the spiritual sense and in the healing sense. Like there's a sort of an opening now. It's like seeing the light, but being in the light as well. And, yes, I do feel on the brink of something great, of greatness. I don't mean that in any egocentric way at all. It's just more a spiritual knowledge, I suppose.*

Wounding and healing journey

And furthermore, most of the nurse healers I spoke with expressed the experience of the healing impact on their lives of learning healing modalities, and reaching out to heal others. So that was quite a reflexive process, where their ability to channel healing for others increased with their own healing, and the healing of their own wounds was moved ahead by reaching out as healers to others. This phenomenon is fascinatingly articulated by the English academic David Brandon. Drawing on the work of writers on shamanism such as Joan Halifax and Michael Harner, Brandon saw the separation between the wounded healer and the wounded healee bridged by the wounds themselves. He wrote:[116]

> *In the shamanic tradition, the "client" and the "healer" exist in the same person; wounds are the conduit to healing. As Kalweit[117] puts it, "In tribal society, the healer experiences the illnesses of his patients and then heals himself. It is of the essence of the primal healer that, through the deepening of his inner consciousness, he is linked with his body and the illness, with himself and the patient".*

Discussions on the transformative experiences of healers often include reference to the notion of the "wounded healer", as an archetype, and a model for understanding the healer's path of transformation. One example comes from Dolores Krieger's book Living the Therapeutic Touch,[118] where she identified the "wounded healer" as a transitional stage in the evolution of a healer.

Krieger saw two expressions of the wounded healer archetype. One is where an individual has suffered, and finds her own healing through helping others; the second is where the healer, who has herself suffered, reaches out compassionately to others so that they themselves need not undergo the same hurts experienced by the healer.

The Australian nurse scholar Jane Hall brought a wide-ranging mythological, historical and transcultural exploration of the phenomenon of the wounded healer to a discussion of nurses as wounded healers. She elaborated a pattern of the wounded healer, which involves:[119]

a call to healing

- wounding
- self-awareness — becoming aware of wound
- exploring wounds

journey towards healing

- seeking healing, involves whole of self — body, mind, soul and spirit
- letting go of cherished view of self (disintegration)
- the process of growth (reintegration)

healing

- wounds are healed
- transformation of self
- ongoing process repeated over time

healer

- personal qualities
- healing relationship
- healing knowledge and skills

Hall maintained that a healer is usually a healer throughout the stages of the model, and therefore faces the considerable challenge of working to deal with her own wounds whilst also caring for others. In this, the healer is not an end point or finished product, but is constantly evolving and expanding in understanding of, and insight into, self.[120,121]

In many cultures, Hall pointed out, a shamanic experience of woundedness is a natural and necessary precursor to the shaman's ability to serve as a healer and mediator with the spirit world. Furthermore, drawing upon the experience of modern-day therapists, Hall asserted that for any healer to ignore their woundedness is to invite serious imbalance in the healing relationship.[120,121]

Such an imbalance has the potential to cause significant harm, such as the unconscious enactment by the healer of power-over behavioural patterns, like the "vengeful earth mother or the aloof and frozen ice maiden".[122] Hall also cautioned how holistic nurses who ignore their own wounds could foster unhelpful dependence in their patients. Further, ignoring her own wounds could "lead to the activation of the darker or shadow side of the healer who then may actually wound others".[123]

Chapter Nineteen

LIVING AS A HEALER

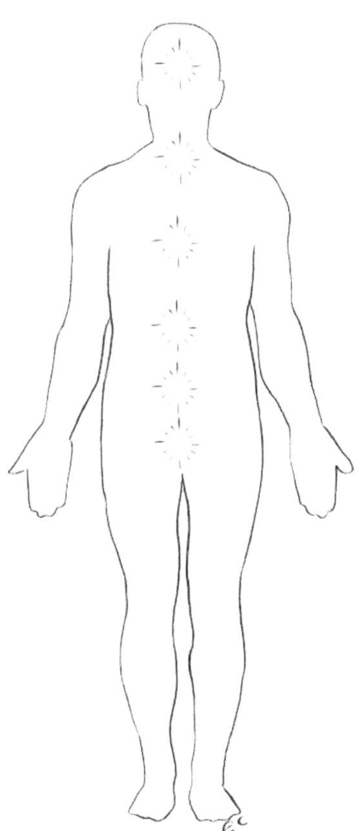

All the nurse healers who co-created this research with me spoke of the everyday lived reality of being a healer. This occurred on multiple dimensions, from how they integrated the identity of a healer, to how they managed the inner and outer transformations, to what the world tends to throw at someone who faithfully walks the path of the healer

Dolores Krieger, the founder of Therapeutic Touch, in an interview published in a holistic journal, spoke to this matter of the practice of healing bringing about transformational changes in the practitioner's life when she said, seemingly reflecting on her own experience:[124]

> It seems that what happens is that, if you become accustomed to being in center [a key aspect of the practice of TT], it can change your worldview. And if that happens, you begin to find that your lifestyle must also change. And if your worldview and lifestyle change, you are edging into a nice definition of transformation of personality. This is what can happen to people who use Therapeutic Touch. It's a dual process.
>
> One aspect involves helping and healing the person who is ill, the other concerns what happens within the therapist.

As I outline below, the changes nurse healers experience in their lives can be both remarkable and challenging.

Am I a healer?

Almost paradoxically, some of my collaborators, notably James and Chris, were adamant about not being called "healer". This was for slightly different reasons. James spoke of the fundamental nature of healing, and the complete mystery of what occurs in healing exchanges, when he asserted that nobody is really a healer:

> First of all, I don't think I'm a nurse healer. I don't think I'm a healer. I don't think anybody is. I think we can participate in healing, and we have certain skills, intention, consciousness, that we bring to a healing context. … We perceive ourselves to be channelling, or we perceive, "I'm somehow doing healing". But in practice, in reality, I think something deeper might be taking place.

Chris had a slightly different take on not wanting to be called a healer, related to not wanting to place her work in a frame which might bind up its meaning, and related to her not liking to be herself labelled. She said:

Living as a healer

I don't talk about myself as being a healer. I tried out lots of labels for myself. And I actually thought to myself at some point, none of them actually express me, or who I am. And every time I used the label, people approached me in a certain way. And I'd think, "Oh no, I'm not like that!". So I decided, probably about twenty years ago now, not to use any titles. I would just use my name. For that reason. Yet you and I know that we have this absolute passion about healing.

Whilst it may seem contradictory, it is meaningful, I believe, to call these nurses I spoke with "healers", even though all would at some level agree that the healing exchange is far deeper and more complex than suggested by the notion of "a healer healing a healee". Perhaps the words of Michael can add texture to this mysteriousness of healing as we understand it, as he reflected on his own experience of using words to heal another:

… while it comes through my mouth, sounds like my voice, and it doesn't feel like anybody else — the knowing is greater than me.

I'm not instructed — I'm not given words that I just spit out. They are inherent at the time. I know it, and I speak it and it comes with great love and clarity.

Moira reflected:

Healing power is not from me. Even though people will say, "Oh, gee, you really fixed that", I'll say, "No I didn't — I'm the vessel. Universe is doing everything else". Or God, whoever you to say is helping. It's not me — we're just the means of application. I think it's important people know that, too. Because otherwise it becomes a very egotistical thing, for some people to say, "I'm a healer", "I'm this", "I'm that". Really, we are just the vessels, and the means.

Rose also tried to describe what was occurring when she was aware of playing a part in healing of others:

I have a very intense feeling. It's not sympathy, and it's not emotional. It's definitely not deeply emotional; I feel a bit detached, but I do feel something moving through though it's not coming from me in total. Some of it's coming from me, but a lot of it's coming from — I would like to think — external, divine realms and moving through.

Unlike James, for Rose, there was a time in her life when she found it to be important to acknowledge herself as a healer. This was central to her self-concept and she felt the requirement to honour herself as playing a part in being able to function as a healer.

Inside the healing

The experience of participating in healing exchanges was seen as a great blessing for both herself and the other, Heloise reflected, and she spoke of her personal joy when that occurred. She also spoke beautifully of the spiritual nature of these healing connections which happened in her working days:

> *I don't have a conscious belief of, you know, that I work for God, but I sometimes feel like God comes in, somehow. And sometimes I feel like whoever I'm with, or the combination of both of us, is bigger — that there's some otherpresence there. So it's not like I'm working for God, but... it's like He does the connections.*

Regarding the essential nature of the healer and her role in healing, Rachel expressed the belief that people have an ontological recognition of the healer — they "read your bones", Rachel said. She saw the path of the healer as one of coming to know her own bones, so that they are clear to be read by others. The deep self-knowledge of being Rachel referred to automatically puts the nurse into a healing relationship with the other which is both authentic and grounded. She said:

> *Before, I could say, "Yes, you've got an energy block in your heart," or "around your liver," — whatever. Now being — sitting next to that person — can help balance all that out. I don't have to do anything. It's more than presence ... it's actively being there... this is an active thing. An actual valuing of what my bones can show you, communicate with you. There is an exchange of something. That exchange then brings me to ask things of a spiritual nature, or of a more holistic nature, as a nurse healer.*

All the nurse healers I spoke with had lovely accounts of healing occurrences. The experience of being a healer, as described by the nurse healers participating in this study, had a number of dimensions, beyond the actual experience of participating in the healing exchange.

This reached into the lives of these people in a myriad of ways. Some discussed being connected to a spiritual heritage, or lineage, of healers (Angelique, Chris, Gabrielle). As Gabrielle's words illustrate, this was significant to their self understanding as healers:

> *... it was my deep inheritance. That somehow — and of course, I can feel the tears coming because I always know the energies around it — what I am to do now, and have been doing, is*

accessing something that's deep within me and beyond me and part of what I have inherited.

Evolving in the healer role

My collaborators spoke of growing into the healer role, or evolving. Aspects of this have been discussed earlier under 'Wounding and healing journey' (Chapter Eighteen), but there were a number of reflections from the nurse healers regarding what was involved personally in moving deeper into that experience. For instance, Michael revealed how he went through a period where his obvious impact on other people frightened him. He did not know all that was occurring, and feared for a time that he was being used in some way by an unseen force. Moving past that anxiety was a significant step for Michael. He recalled:

> *When I sit on buses and trains and boats and planes, people would cathart next to me, quite regularly. I got upset about that for a long time, but realised it was just spiritual energy.*

Grounding

Growing into the healer role for the nurse healers I spoke with was often associated with being grounded. There was an understanding that being unbalanced by not having a strong grip on material living was an impediment to functioning as a healer. Rachel spoke in great detail about her struggles around being ungrounded for a time. Emma reflected on the grounded nature of what she offered in her work:

> *The more experiences of spirit I have, the more important it is I remain grounded. Because what I wish to offer people who come to me for healing, or students, or people in my life, needs to be grounded.*

Chris made the clear distinction that being grounded absolutely did not mean being un- connected to spiritual realities, but means being balanced in relation to earthly life. She reflected:

> *I was a child who was quite fey, there would be some people who'd say "not very grounded". But I was very grounded, and very practical. Very much in the gumboots. But I just had a big map in my head. ... So my learning was how not to let other people reframe my reality, and turn it into a negative or pathologised space.*

Living as a healer

Protection

For a number of the co-creators of this study, the issue of protection played an important role in their being healers, as they discussed that with me. This hearkens to the issue of the shadow, discussed in Chapter Sixteen, 'Opening to spirit', and is a significant aspect of the esoteric lived reality of the spiritual healer. Heloise spoke of how the issue might come up for her, and how she would respond to it:

> *If I was working in a violent, or aggressive or really confronting situation, part of my intuition might tell me to contract Sometimes I flatten my chakras — I get a hint to shut down psychically, so that I don't take in all this stuff.*

The sense of being very open, for healers, can lead to a sense of being vulnerable to being adversely affected by the energy, or thought forms or entities associated with a person, or a situation. This is particularly in times of unbalance, as Rachel's account of being physically vulnerable to the suffering of others bears out. Some of the healers, such as Moira and Rose, reflected on becoming less vulnerable to the energy and projections of others as they moved ahead in their own healing journeys.

Nonetheless, as Moira reflected, being open and sensitive to the suffering of others is a native attribute of a healer:

> *I think we're very sensitive, because I don't think we would be healers if we weren't sensitive. And especially, if you can put your hands on somebody and feel where their body is not well, or to feel something that isn't quite right within them — whether it's in their aura, or in the shell of their body. I think we have to be sensitive to that, to recognise it.*

As with Moira and Rose, I found my own healing journey, in my case through psychotherapy, was helpful in moving me past vulnerability to others' energy. Prior to therapy, I was much more focused on needing to be protected from the unseen energies associated with the distress of other people. One of the reasons for this, I feel, is that therapy has helped me to able to create healthy boundaries.

Boundaries

> *If I am yearning for freedom, I will*
> *find it by way of boundaries.*
> *— Liz Scarfe[125]*

Another issue discussed by some of my collaborators was that of personal boundaries, which highlights a key feature of the healer's experience. For instance, Michael spoke about his struggle to create healthy boundaries between himself and others:

> *I've been crashed all my life in emotional ways, without knowing it. So I had no boundaries, and I didn't know how to declare boundaries, until my mid-to-late thirties.*

However, he made the important reflection that the healer experience by its nature involves the dropping of one's boundaries, and the healer at some point learns to create healthy boundaries:

> *I think that declaring boundaries is an inherent part of healing. I think you've got to experience "boundary-lessness" in order to allow incoming energy. I think you learn to control it later — Most of the wounded healers have boundary issues as well....*

> *I think "boundary-less-ness " is part of the kit and caboodle of healing. I think that if we had strong boundaries all our life, I don't think that you can be a very good healer. I don't think that you get incoming energy. I think it's too filtered. So, I think when I talk to the healers, especially the Indigenous model healers … most people that deal with hands on or energetic healing have a fairly similar story about having no boundaries, and having to find the boundaries later on. In the beginning when the gifts pour in, and you get overloaded, if you like, swamped, even caved in, that you've actually then got to physically — consciously start to erect them.*

Another nurse healer who gave a strong account of boundaries was Angelique. Her account revealed a high degree of mastery of boundaries, where she was in the experience of travelling in many dimensions of existence. She reflected about creating healthy boundaries in her nursing practice, involving the choice to hold back some of her spiritual perceptions:

> *I have been able to have a clear boundary in my work. In my profession as nurse, I go "this far". In my inner being, I can be limited or unlimited. Most of the time I've been able to know exactly what has been required of me, as nurse. But then, at the same time, I have a whole other level of information about my*

*patients, and about my relationship with a patient in the
moment, and what I need to learn in that situation.*

Angelique's thoughts (above) point to a key element in the healers' capacity
to sojourn in multiple realities. There are boundaries between the worlds,
which are both personal and transpersonal, and it is the healer's mastery of
boundaries which enables them to safely traverse the worlds.

Being able to drop one's personal boundaries around the experience of
Consensus Reality enables one to channel healing, and also to enter into
non-ordinary realms to know oneself more completely and to serve others.
Bringing forth one's boundaries again enables one to safely and comfortably
live in the everyday.

The mastery of boundaries enables a creative and textured experience of
Self, and as Liz Scarfe (above) suggests, is a key to personal freedom.

Shadow dancing (growing edges)

As I mentioned earlier, there is a personal dimension to the "shadow", which
as a Process Worker I might call "growing edges". Healers, Process Workers,
shamans and therapists of most persuasions are confronted by these in their
work, and their challenge is to come to terms with them, or process them. In
that way, for example, a healer has some hope of knowing whether what
they are experiencing in a healing encounter relates to their own process or
psychology, or that of their healee, or something else entirely. Thereby they
may have some hope to be a clear channel for healing.

The nurse healers spoke of pitfalls on the path, some of which I have written
about in earlier chapters. For instance, Rachel spoke of being addicted to
spiritual experience, and how in order to live a balanced life she had to grow
through that experience:

> *It was very addictive. The energy work was gorgeous — I had
> sensations through my body that just were such a high, it was so
> lovely, it was so nice! And then, to come back to earth was such a
> bummer! And all this was being juggled with trying to work as a
> nurse.*

James emphasised the crucial importance of coming to terms with shadow,
and also discussed some aspects of the shadow side of the spiritual path. He
said:

> *One of the shadow sides of this spiritual awakening is it's like an
> addiction. Wanting more experiences.*

He spoke of how he maintained an intimate and vigilant relationship with his personal shadow, characterising this relationship as a key spiritual practice:

> *And so that, while one has terrible experiences — frightening, dangerous — there is meaning and purpose in them. They are offered to us as teachings. I've talked with many wise people about this, all people I trust and they don't dismiss these as illusions. Ram Dass said that to me. "The more you unfold, the more you are challenged — so, where the light is strongest, there the darkness grows strongest too. That's your work, and your spiritual practice is how you work with it".*

Emma similarly spoke of a quite difficult process in balancing the different aspects of her life as she came to accommodation with living in two worlds. For her also, there were issues in functioning materially:

> *… the illusion that being in a spiritual realm — or being in this place — seems to negate having to look after the other section. As if it's all taken care of. Now, I know on one level it is all taken care of. But on another level I am required to actively participate in this human life.*

Others have reported healers' disclosures on their relationship with the personal shadow. For instance, in Keegan and Dossey's book on nurse healers, Dorothea Hover-Kramer spoke of the shadow side of her work:[126]

> *My biggest obstacles have been my own lack of trust, lack of hope, and lack of resourcefulness in getting help for myself. While I can look at external obstacles, such as loss of loved ones, pain, and divorce with some candor, there is always a personal shadow part that remains hidden, outside of my awareness. Like the proverbial blind spot when one is driving a car, I have learned to assume that there is an area I cannot see, a part I might be missing.*

The well known author on shamanism, Joan Halifax, wrote of experiencing serious illness as a child and, as an adult, exploring non-ordinary states of consciousness which led her to look deeply at herself and seek explanations for her experiences in the anthropological literature.

Later, she met shaman healers who brought their teachings of "earth wisdom" to her, and she also learned the "sky wisdom" of Buddhist teachings. She offered insights into some pitfalls concerning the path of the healer:[127]

> *There is a trap in the extraordinary. One begins to feel special and self-important, along with an absence of compassion. Maybe it is disappointing, this talk of simplicity in favour of the more dramatic aspects of being shaman. What we all want at our core*

is to be free from suffering; we want to be in a situation of simplicity. We don't want to be driven by desire, or hate; nor do we wish to be caught in confusion. Moving past these three positions means that we discover simplicity, harmony, relaxation, compassion, and wisdom. From this awakening arises the impulse to help others.

If I am to be honest, I should disclose that I too, as reported above by Joan Halifax, was caught up for a time in feeling special around the shamanic healing experiences, and was lacking in compassion. This remains something I need to be conscious of.

Healing in the workplace

A publisher friend who reviewed some of the accounts of my collaborators marvelled at how these nurse healers managed to work in the midst of their spiritual crises. This makes me think about how I was unable to keep working in an acute mental health inpatient ward when visited by my own initiatory crisis. Each nurse healer experienced being a healer in the workplace in their unique way, but there are a couple of general themes to this aspect of living as a healer.

The collaborators all, at some point, had been employed within health care services, typically public-run under the medical model of treatment. As I noted in Chapter Two, there has often been hostility and ridicule expressed towards those who openly operated as healers in these settings. In addition to that, some nurse healers have found it very challenging, at some parts of their evolution, to function in those environments.

Some nurse healers described being covert, even subversive, healers in their workplaces. Heloise recalled:

> *If you have, as I do, a concept of spirituality and energy healing and psychic phenomena, or other things and live outside the limitation of a lot of medical people's ideas — and a lot of nurses' as well. I went and did Reiki because I wanted to be able to give more than what I was giving, without inviting the criticism or the judgment of people around me.*
>
> *And that meant I could be talking to someone, and put my hand on their shoulder or I could, you know, say, "Gee, you've got a headache. Let me just hold your head, and just see if I can find any tension there". But I could do Reiki, and nobody would know. So I guess I did it to become a secret healer — to save myself*

*from some of the, not so much criticism, as being made fun of.
You know, "Oh gee, you've got wacky ideas".
You know, "Heloise's crystal ball gazing".*

Heloise also reported how she brought healing approaches to patients experiencing spiritual emergencies, strongly contradicting the pathologising medical model approach of the psychiatric system she worked in.

The reality for all the participants was that the nursing profession within their workplaces was not supportive of healing by nurses. The nurse healers in large part learned healing and even practised it outside of the health care systems.

Angelique spoke of how nursing and healing work were very much separated for her in her evolution as a healer. Nonetheless, Angelique described challenges in keeping her healing work and her everyday nursing work separate. She felt pressure from her patients and their families, and the spirits around them, to go beyond her established role as a mental health nurse in their homes.

Rachel disclosed how the simple reality of being a healer at a certain point in her evolution — having overwhelming experiences in her workplace such as picking up the symptoms of her very ill patients — posited intense challenges to her ability to nurse professionally.

James reported being similarly unable to conduct his professional activities at a point in his spiritual evolution.

However, some nurse healers I spoke with found some support within nursing. Rachel described the excitement of her colleagues at the creative way she approached her work. Michael also acknowledged how his development as a healer had its roots in how he learned and went on to practice nursing:

> *I was lucky to be in a very good training school. … I learned from one of our tutors, a beautiful Maori woman, about the spiritual aspect of nursing. She spoke — openly and eloquently about caring, and about the importance of touch, and healing.*
>
> *So from day one that was just a given in the curriculum; not necessarily an established curriculum, her curriculum. I had a clear understanding of the spiritual aspect of nursing from the start.*

The non-ordinary in the everyday

Michael reflected on what living as a healer looked like in his everyday life:

I talked about the process of coming to be a healer. Living as a healer. I do identify myself as a healer now — I wouldn't have, once. It's quite a strange, chaotic life at times. If I had anyone staying with me for period of time, they'd see the different people that come and go, spontaneously, from this house and they'd laugh. There is a lot of mystical, and the metaphysical joke is alive in lots of ways. It's like a series of one-act plays. And that's not me being displaced from it, it's just what is attracted to my door. Sort of spontaneously.

Blessing of being a healer

My collaborators spoke of the blessings that come from being a healer, how that experience has graced their lives. Heloise disclosed to me the wonder of expanded consciousness she would experience following a healing encounter:

I don't know if it's God, I don't know what it is, it's like energy it's like I'm walking down the street, and right down the other end of the street, walking towards me, is some energy that's really light. And that's like an aspect of God, or something. And I get renewed by being out there, rather than losing energy going out there.

A number of the nurse healers disclosed how being a healer had come to mean living their lives in radically different ways. Michael reflected on how his life patterns had changed, how he was more conscious in his connections with others; how he was learning to live without labels, and more in harmony and accord with nature; to live more lovingly. Rachel spoke of being more grounded and authentic in her living and working.

Gabrielle spoke of being true to her journey, and learning to trust and deepen her connection to spirituality. James indicated improved

relationships and could point to a life lived in a way entirely transformed from the hedonistic life he lived prior to his awakening. He spoke of learning to live with uncertainty, of coming to terms with his shadow side, his flaws and faults, and of living in two worlds. Rose spoke of finding new levels of self-worth, balance, and living with integrity.

Doing the personal work

James, in his characteristically sober way, cautioned that healers must continue to work on themselves emotionally as well as spiritually to keep balance in their journeys through non- ordinary reality to participate in the healing for others:

> *I don't think you can get it unless you've done the work. There ain't no short cuts, there are no bypasses, no quick leaps. While I think it is important to have the techniques and the approaches — like I've learned Energy Healing — without the personal work, in psychological terms it's working on the ego or the emotional work, or spiritual terms it's deepening one's connection with the Divine or "All That Is". I think all of them are needed to develop discernment. Everything in a holistic universe is all enmeshed, it's all connected. Holism is about absolutely everything connected with everything else. Everything, everything is connected. There is no separation — of anything. And I don't think one can truly grasp that unless you've trodden non- ordinary reality*

The rivers ran

All the co-creators of this work spoke of coming to live in more authentic and integrated ways through their sacred journeys as healers. Michael's poetic words exemplify and sum up this deep journey of transformation as a healer:

> *I think, through loss, pain, and personal suffering I got to blend. The rivers ran, you know, all the rivers ran. It all became one, rather than lots of different parts of me. … So healing was part of that process too. You know, it's part of that expansion.*
>
> *Because all creation expands. And so I'm expanding with it, and I see that, very much. That's a good thing.*

Chapter Twenty

WALKING TWO WORLDS

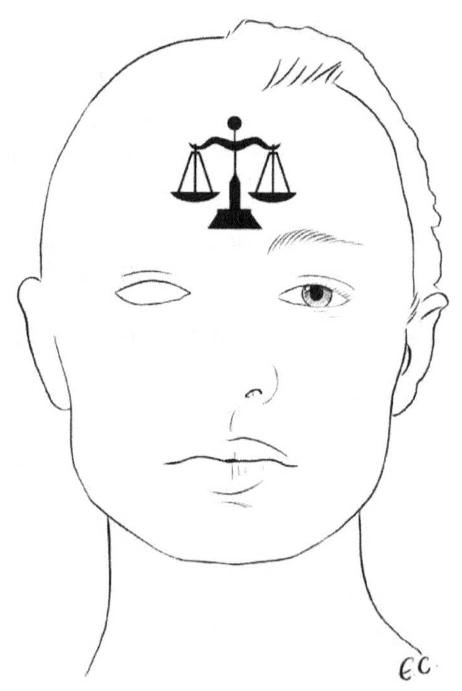

Walking two worlds

If there were one phrase to voice the quintessence of the stories of the nurse healers I spoke with, it might well be 'Walking Two Worlds'. This is the supertext and the subtext to the other themes, being the primary experience of the nurse healers I spoke with in their deeper, transformative life path as healers. For most, this is where they arrive to, in that journey, if they weren't already there, and it is also the journey itself.

Walking two worlds is the title of the work from which this book is drawn, and I thought initially to so name this book. It is also a theme running through the accounts of the co- creators of this work, and below I explore how it plays out in these stories.

I guess the first thing to say is that there are, as voiced by some of the healers I spoke with, as well as by healers and shamans and spiritual adventurers throughout the world, more than two worlds that healers have access to. Angelique, for instance, spoke a lot of spiritually travelling and working in a number of dimensions of existence. She spoke of the other dimensions, suggesting also how experience of other worlds is not a passive thing but one requiring intelligence and vigilance to negotiate:

> *I travel many different dimensions. I achieve balance by using my intelligence to seek out what I know that I need.*

When we spoke together, James told me how his constant experience was of living in two worlds:

> *Somebody once sent me a card a few years ago. A birthday card, when I hit fifty. ... A picture of a man, a long grey-haired bearded man, halfway between a wall; he was walking through the wall. There were two distinct worlds on one side. She said the card was for a man who truly walked in two worlds. ... In my existence now, my life is one of being in two worlds simultaneously — ordinary reality, and non-ordinary reality. I walk between both; I've a foot in both camps. Sometimes I'm more in one than t'other, and sometimes more in t'other. But most times, it's just moving backwards and forwards.*

Michael also disclosed his experience of non-ordinary or esoteric reality alongside the everyday world:

> *I guess it's like the temporal world and the esoteric. Really, it's walking two worlds. So, I started to walk two worlds as a nurse, and do healing. You know, there was this temporal, socially constructed, organised thing called "nursing". And the other deeper spiritual stuff, and it was about aligning the two. The Indigenous at home taught me to walk two worlds.*

Ruth spoke very movingly of the love and support she experienced in her being in spiritual reality:

> *It was like I had two lives, in a way... like being in two places. There is always this other one, always. So I might be in one world, talking, but there's always this other spirit world, where I can be me. Where I don't have to play a part and there's nothing to do; there is total acceptance, no such thing as good and bad. There is just acceptance. Where our souls meet.*

Angelique spoke about the transpersonal boundaries that delineate the inner realms that healers as spiritual adventurers must learn to traverse:

> *It is all part of exploring who we are — who I am, and what I am — because I am much more than the body, and the life that I'm having in this moment in time. That is connected to my identity — who I am. The "I ", or the "id-entity" that I am, deep inside myself.*

Judging by the accounts of the nurse healers I spoke with, living in more than one reality is a very varied and multifaceted experience. Chris, when I spoke with her, did not use that phrase — "walking two worlds" — but clearly this was her experience. Being born into a heritage of healers and wise women, receiving detailed messages from spiritual realms an early age led to her being very surprised by aspects of the ordinary reality lived by most of humanity.

As the following quote attests, on occasion this could be affirming about her inner experiences:

> *As a sixteen-year-old I stayed with a Jewish family for a time and they had the sacred Jewish texts. I remember finding in these books and thinking, "Oh my God, it's written down! These things are written down. How amazing!". When you have a big map of things where you see things, and you see it actually written down in a text, or you see something that the words are not dissimilar (they belong to the Jewish tradition), yet I had complete comprehension of what was there in the text.*

Much of what I have written about in this book concerns the journey of finding balance in living between the worlds, be it about balance, the shadow, boundaries, or their personal journey of healing, etcetera. The world of spiritual experience is universally described as being populated by beings and sensations of great wonder and beauty, and it could be hard for those I spoke with to move back and forth from that to a world more mundane and troubled by human concerns. Emma spoke about this aspect of the journey:

Walking two worlds

And part of mine is the balance between living in the human everyday world, and living in the spirit world. … One friend said she could actually see me moving right into that spiritual space, and that I really needed to make a choice about whether I wanted other people to look after me or not. Because that's what I could do — and they would, because of my contribution to their welfare on a spiritual level. But, of course, the human side of Emma took over there. "No way, Jose! No way! I want to do it myself, my way!". And my friend said, "Well, you'd better make some choices then, hadn't you?"

Earlier in her journey as a healer, Rachel had experienced living in the spiritual world to the detriment of her everyday ordinary living. At the time we spoke, the balance of this had turned around, and, while missing the constant experience of spirit, she saw that as positive. She reflected that balance in living between the two worlds is at the heart of the healer's journey:

My life circumstances now ground me in the physical — and I wish I was more in the spiritual. It's forever going to be, I believe, that balance — that to be a nurse healer, you need to have the balance. So many evolving healers, and people that I thought were so endearing and loving, and so spiritual — and they were so good, you know — they were the people, like me, who were having these experiences, talking to the angels, and seeing stuff — they were tantalising. I could have sat with them, and talked with them for ever. And now, what I know is that that is an addictive quality, to escape while you're here.

I still don't like it! I don't like having to be so focused on the physical. Yet the work, the spiritual healer's work, gets done on the physical body, energetically. Like that's the problem that we all have. No matter whether we bring in issues from past lives, from dual realities — it impacts us in the physical.

So, a healer needs to understand the physical reality in order to get their life organised. I guess that my journey as a nurse healer has been about that swing. And today you find me focused on a physical reality, because I have two young children now, and dependent people keep you focused on the physical. And I'm incorporating a spiritual life into that.

So it's almost like it's swung. Now when I think about the nurse healers I admire — they're the ones who are grappling with that spiritual experience in the physical. Not the physical experience in the spiritual world. It's like, it's that movement and that, I think, makes a mature healer.

For myself, there is a fierce tension in my experience of multiple realities. Nowadays I think of this as my life myth; a collection of experiences that seem to run through my life and give it structure in some ways. There is a battle between the worlds of ordinary and non- ordinary me, which has preoccupied me over the years. Exploring it in therapy has helped me lessen the uncomfortableness of this tension, and I notice, over time, a beginning friendliness between these elements.

Still, I am yet to comfortably acknowledge to the world my shamanic nature, and still my shaman is not always understanding of my ordinary living.

Angelique also spoke of aspects of finding balance living in multiple worlds, such as living in the ordinary world whilst in the experience of impinging aspects of the non-ordinary. She reflected:

> *There is a balancing act between one world and the other — between one dimension and the other, because I need time that I can spend. I need time for myself, to be able to do that. And I must say that I've become really good at integrating — I've integrated a lot inside myself. Even when I do this private nursing... Like, four days in a row I'm in someone else's house, I sleep in someone else's bed, someone else's room, someone else's completely psychic field. And every time, over and over again, I need to create my own "space bubble". I need to energetically clear the energy from the bed, from the room. I need to clear the space for myself.*

This concludes the thematic analysis of the stories gifted me by the eleven nurse healers I spoke with at the beginning of this millennium, about their sacred journeys, the extraordinary and transformational experiences they underwent around coming to be healers.

The themes I found in these stories — Belonging and connecting, Opening to spirit, Summoning, Wounding and healing journey, Living as a healer, and Walking two worlds, all attest to the awesome but very human and fallible undertaking of the healer's sojourn. I am very grateful for the openness and generosity of my collaborators in this exploration.

In the following chapter, I look back at this investigation and its findings and personal implications. With that, I can dream forward into how it might affect the world of nurses, Process Workers and others interested in these phenomena.

Chapter Twenty-One

HARVEST

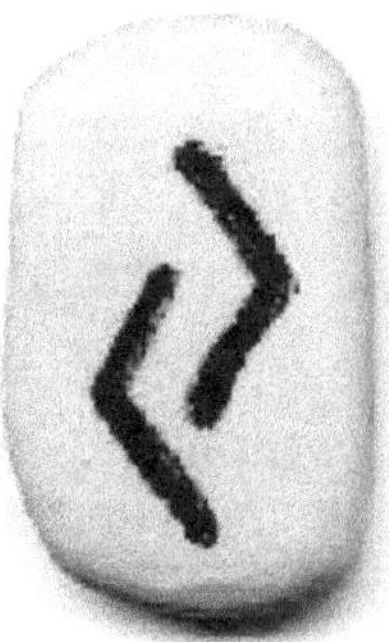

JERA — Harvest

A rune of beneficial outcomes, Jera applies to any endeavour to which you are committed. Receiving this rune encourages you to keep your spirits up. Be aware, however, that no quick results can be expected. You have prepared the ground and.planted the seed. Now you must cultivate with care. To those whose labour has a long season, a long coming to term, Jera offers encouragement of success.[128]

Gazing back and dreaming forward

The American novelist and cultural critic Michael Ventura, who inspired the title of this book, may not have been referring precisely to the worlds depicted in these pages when he wrote of the "unknown terrain that psychotherapy must either explore or become meaningless".[129] He was writing about recent historical movements in the human psyche, the implications of how our dreams have become manifest through cultural and technological change.

In this, he appealed to the force of Yeats' resonant declamation: "In dreams begin responsibility". Ventura's words do, nonetheless, resonate powerfully with the phenomena under exploration in this book.

Like all Process Workers, influenced by Jung, I, too have a deep interest in dreams. I marvel at how unfolding them enriches our lives and expands our self understanding. The founder of Process Work, Arny Mindell speaks of the Dreaming background to experience, and how important it is to live it, at least in part:[130]

> *After many years working as a therapist with people from all over the world, it seems to me that ignoring the Dreaming is an undiagnosed global epidemic. People everywhere suffer from a chronic form of mild depression because they are taught to focus on everyday reality and forget about the Dreaming background.*

There is something dream-like, aligned to Dreaming reality in the accounts in this book, and in the skeptical Consensus Reality of this culture they might be easy to dismiss, disregard, minimise, even forget. But as with ordinary dreams and Dreaming reality, they are also mysterious, creative, generative, sacred. They point to solutions for intractable problems and struggles of living in a world which can be so unsupportive of our need to live close to our always-deeply-dreaming natures.

In these concluding pages I invite you to join with me in gazing back on the ideas and experiences of these nurse healers' sacred journeys, and dreaming forward to how these can make a difference to nurses and to Process Workers, and to deep dreamers everywhere.

Gazing back

It has been an immense privilege to receive the disclosures of the co-creators of this work. These are of the deep and tender and sacred parts of their life journeys, their encounters with the divine and the improbable. I feel responsibility to do my utmost to be faithful to these stories entrusted so generously to me, and to honour their meaning and exposure to the world.

The essences I distilled from the accounts gifted me by my collaborators are the answers to the research questions I raise at the start of this book. These essences are: Belonging and connecting, Opening to spirit, Summoning, Wounding and healing journey, Living as a healer and Walking two worlds.

Belonging and connecting, is about the journey experienced by a number of the nurse healers of a disrupted sense of connection with other people leading, ultimately, to a very deep connecting, and a satisfying sense of belonging.

The second, Opening to spirit, investigates the deep spiritual connection and awakening experienced by my collaborators, encompassing the various kinds of esoteric experiences and challenges they reported, such as visionary experience, spiritual entities, and experience of the shadow side of spirit.

Summoning, concerns the radical transformative process experienced by some of the nurse healers, where they underwent deep personal disruption and confusion in the process of becoming transformed to live more authentic lives as healers.

Wounding and healing journey is about the trauma and pain suffered by nearly all of the co- creators of this work, and their healing journey. This theme also explores their deep understanding of this experience, where some see their wounds as blessings that enables them to have deeper insight and a greater capacity to help others.

Living as a healer explores the aspects of the deeper journeys of the nurse healers which relate to their identifying, practising and living as healers.

In the final essence or theme, Walking two worlds, I looked at how the nurse healers were living and functioning in two (or more) realities, and explored some of the implications of that on their lives.

Gazing back and dreaming forward

That these essences amount to a depiction of a process of deep transformation is axiomatic (and indeed is assumed in the research questions). There are a lot of writings on the esoteric path of life, but not so many which delve so specifically into its implications for living, the balancing act of serving as a healer or a shaman and being an ordinary human trying to steer a course on an extraordinary and poorly charted voyage.

The advantage of exploring in this way is that first-hand personal accounts — compelling and illuminating — have a resonance missing in more theorised or quantified reports. Of course, presenting a number of different accounts is valuable in corroborating these experiences and providing a multifaceted picture of this domain of experience. I sense that such a way to explore these matters provides opportunities for you, the reader, to see yourself in the stories, and ultimately your own transformation, if that is your process, might be more possible.

The process of transformation for some of the nurse healers — coming to live in more than one reality — was chaotic and confusing at times. This makes sense when you consider the change in self-concept with these transformations demanded of the psyche which has developed in the cultures of the modern West. Eliade[131] believed that this disruption to self concept, which he named the "dialectic of hierophanies", is universal as individuals confront the sacred. How new and challenging, in the coming to be a healer or shaman, to find oneself needing to drop one's personal history and trust the gifted empowerment that booms and resonates down the inner chambers and corridors of one's inner being. To accept the imperative to not only serve and treat with the powers and the gods, but enter the various worlds and command the ghosts and dream figures, spirit creatures, entities, diseases, thought forms and even demons who come forward to teach, challenge, bedevil, protect, and to serve healers and shamans. All this is needed, in many cases, to participate in the healing process as healer, therapist or shaman.

The accounts of the eleven nurse healers reveal how intentionality of healing is a significant path to spiritual evolvement. It opens the heart and mind in ways that are intrinsically selfless, invoking for others the loving powers of the transcendent realities. To participate in that is, of necessity, transformative.

This is a book about the experiences of healers, not so much about their power to heal or channel healing, but about how entering into the

Gazing back and dreaming forward

mysterious and wondrous field of healing has thrown them into places they may never have dreamed existed. How in offering the healing to others, most have become exposed to their own wounds and flaws, and as they attended to the healing of these, their capacity to be channels for the healing of others has increased and also taken them further into the other, non-ordinary realities.

While each sacred journey is unique, the journeys do have certain commonalities. I should acknowledge that not all the nurse healers held the same views on the precise nature of their experiences of coming to be and live as healers. Some did not refer to shamanism directly and would discuss their experiences in other frames, such as certain healing or mystic traditions. I truly hope what I have written in these pages honours all of their journeys; it has been my goal throughout to achieve this.

The nature of the book

I have wondered about the nature of what I am presenting here, this book about the sacred journeys of nurse healers. For me, it has its genesis in an immense, awful and passionate inner shift, and burning desire to bring to the world what was birthed in that time. It comes from an explosion in my life that revealed to me my love of healing, from the awesomeness and brokenness of this journey. It comes from my love of truth and my bewilderment that such experiences can be real. It also comes from my long intense search for empowerment and agency in all the worlds I am thrown into. I speak here about not only the detonation which impelled me on this path, but also the ten-year journey as a student of Process Work, of which this book is in some ways the culmination.

It is a presentation of an investigation, research report, which is its primary identity. The practical origins of this book lie in a highly structured, rationalised, rigorous research project. Permission was sought from approval bodies at the university, participants were formally approached, interviewed, consulted and re-consulted. The interviews were transcribed and analysed acording to specific protocols. It was closely monitored by my supervisor, sent out to markers in different parts of the world, finally graded and also disseminated in research papers, producing knowledge which is highly circumscribed in its nature and applicability in the world. This process was duplicated as it morphed into my Process Work Diploma thesis.

Gazing back and dreaming forward

But I do wonder if it has more to offer, or perhaps something a little different, along the leylines of what has propelled me to write this? And this also harkens to certain understandings of the nature of knowledge. The philosopher Hans-Greorg Gadamer wrote about the emancipatory, ontlolgical nature of knowledge, talking about "fused horizons" where to assimilate knowledge one is somehow changed in the process.[132]

I have wondered if this is somehow a self-help book? I have not set out to instruct on how to do things, how to live life differently, how can your life be improved by this? I have not provided any exercises for the reader to follow. I have not embarked to do this, and yet it might be important to acknowledge that you could possibly be changed in reading these stories. If you are having certain experiences in your connections with other people, or in your inner life and dreams, that are out of the ordinary, maybe this information could encourage you to feel safer, less marginalised, not so alone, more confident that this can be survived and supported to unfold.

Still more powerfully, you might experience on reading this, the initiatory nature of such accounts, and find yourself gradually, or even suddenly having for the first time the kinds of experiences reported in these pages. If you are excited by these stories of nurse healers, this could be something that helps to open you to your nature as a healer or a shaman. This cannot be ruled out, although it has not been my goal. It may well be one of the secondary processes of this work, perhaps more interesting, frightening and generative than its conscious intent. I don't know for sure.

It is not a book about how to be a healer, although there are descriptions of healings in the preceding pages. I wonder whether in reading this book you may in some ways come to better know the healer you are, for, as I have said, there is an initiatory power in certain stories. If that does happen to you, I hope you find the wise and loving support you need to live this life. You, the reader, are an essential part of that.

This is worldwork

Similarly, reading this (and maybe you identify with some of what I have reported) will change the field of your own experiences. It may awaken something in you, the reader, or it may even awaken the clarity that such experiences are not for you. Arny Mindell said, "Every Process Work session, even opening up to something new or wild or ecstatic in yourself, is worldwork".[133] Hence, exploring, experiencing and working with such deep experiences and movements in consciousness and transformations, will inevitably be working on the field of the world. Thus, it is Worldwork, and in some ways must change the world.

Dreaming forward

Don't turn your head. Keep looking
At the bandaged place. That's where
The light enters you.
And don't believe for a moment
That you're healing yourself.

— *Rumi*[134]

The stories have been told and I have made what sense I may of them, through discussing the essences or themes I found therein. It remains to reflect about how this knowledge might shine out on the world, on Process Work, and on nursing. On healers and others interested in what is not ordinarily experienced but which is, nonetheless, of vital importance.

Process Work

Process Workers in their everyday supporting of the processes of those they work with may be familiar with much of what has reported in these pages. This is because Process Work is one modality which will not pathologise these experiences as they unfurl from the wounds and other disturbances people bring forward to work on. For many, the healing gift does uncoil from deep pain and confusion, such as someone might bring to therapy to investigate and seek solace and integration. The nurse healers' accounts in these pages attest to this.

Nonetheless, despite the potential familiarity of these processes for experienced Process Workers, I feel this investigation and expression of the sacred journeys of nurse healers can have important messages for Process Work. When I reflect upon how devoted the healers I spoke with are to their journeys, to the dreamland and sentient work of healing, I am reminded that

CR reality is only one aspect by which "this amazing world" (as Don Juan would say) can be experienced.

Like other Process Workers, I can be very much in the thrall of the CR, which has remorselessly hypnotised us all from birth.

However, writing this book has pointed me back home to the wilder, unpredictable, terrifying, creative tracts of experience. I hope this can also inspire other Process Workers so. To live on the edge of things, in big states and in weird and unknown lands takes courage and strength. And it craves and thirsts for the support and the stories of others on this path.

I have mentioned the dream-like nature of personal zeitgeist of nurse healers, how their experiences often don't fit in with the consensus picture of how things work. Arny Mindell suggests that dreams are needed for us to "live in a way that feels balanced yet exciting, peaceful yet fun, satisfying yet terrifying".[135] We need to follow our night-time dreams.

Mindell suggests that following these connects us to our shamanic natures. Attending to these "dream-like" stories, the sacred journeys of nurse healers, might thus entice us back closer to our own dreaming, and not only help us to live more fully, but be better Process Work therapists and facilitators.

While Process Work already has a rich theoretical and practical association with shamanism,[136] there is still opportunity to deepen and enrich PW's engagement with alternate paths of awareness. There is particular value in putting forth accounts of these kinds of life path from the inside, in the words of those who have undergone these life journeys. Process workers and others have the opportunity thus to see close-hand how healing and shamanising play out in people's lives. These accounts paint a picture, or fashion a model over the edge of ordinary experiencing. Therapists and supervisors and facilitators and educators can thus see how it is the experiencing which is so very important, and also how that plays out in people's lives in all the myriad multifaceted ways. Thus, they can be better informed to facilitate such journeys in themselves and others.

Perhaps these accounts can add texture to the deeper sentient experience Process Workers and other therapists enter into — the wild and wide possibilities, and the challenges and pitfalls presenting on the paths. Having familiarity and trust and soberness around the entering into these worlds can only be helpful, and I hope this book can contribute to those.

Gazing back and dreaming forward

I do reflect, also, how Process Work could have helped me and the other nurse healers co- creating this work, in their crucial transitions. I believe seeing a process oriented therapist would have been immensely helpful for me as I went through that dark night of the soul. And when I think on all the savage and deep wounding, bewildering experiences and lack of understanding the nurse healers I talked to went through, how helpful might it have been to be supported by someone with the knowledge, understanding, skills and meta-skills to support the unfolding of these immense and awesome processes. Perhaps the advent of this work might make such help for emerging shamans and healers more accessible.

Nursing

As I touched on in Chapter Two, nursing as a profession has shown itself to be profoundly ambivalent about spiritual healing. Striving to assert its professionalism and independence from medicine, nursing has sought status from academic theory and knowledge based upon rigorous research projects. Nonetheless, many prominent nurses have pointed out that nursing has tended to distance itself from its spiritual and healing roots in its unequivocal affiliation with and reliance upon knowledge founded in conventional scientific paradigm.

The stories and analysis of the nurse healers presented herein present a facet of nursing which seems to be fading from the zeitgeist of the profession. However, as theorists such as Jean Watson[137] have pointed out, healing is intrinsic to the fundamental nature of nursing practice. As such, the information in this book is important nursing knowledge. It is important to bear in mind, also, that practical nursing expertise, as has been pointed out by nurse researchers, is healing, as it supports the experience of wholeness in the recipients of care.[138,139]

Clear in the stories of the nurse healers, is not being supported in their difficult, painful and confusing experiences, particularly by the profession. I reflected, when first presenting the research issuing from the nurse healers' stories,[140] that by setting out a rigorous and theoretically informed study, there may be opportunities for nurses in clinical, educational, administrative and research roles to have information before them which may assist them to support nurses going through such experiences.

Gazing back and dreaming forward

As I have suggested above, this knowledge harkens to the archetypal roots of nursing. The act of making visible that, which by its subtle and tender nature, has been held secret is itself significant. Perhaps, by this research, disseminated in this form, the deeper experience of nurse healers might be supported to resonate and reverberate in the overt consciousness of the profession.

There may be thousands of nurses throughout the world who self-identify as healers, and it is appropriate that the profession begins to be more appreciative of the blessing and blossoming occurring within it of those who are giving so deeply of their beings to bring healing to their patients. In serving to illuminate and flesh out the lived terrain of the healer, and the immense challenges faced by those whose primary tool of practice is their open and sensitive and honest self, research such as this could support the profession to acknowledge the great expertise such nurses bring to their work. For administrators and educators, having some knowledge of the nature of the healers' deeper experiences can inform their supporting the practitioners on the ground who may need practical assistance, understanding, validation and information in order to prosper.

There is a need for knowledge in nursing to support its affiliation with holism, often espoused as a theoretical basis for practice. With that in mind, nurse healers, as providers of fundamental holistic knowledge, are precious indeed for the nursing profession, and ought to be treasured and embraced wholeheartedly. Perhaps this book, based on research, can make an important contribution by setting out some of that fundamental holistic knowledge provided by the eleven nurse healers participating in this study.

In Process Work terms, perhaps, this book may be seen as representing one side of a polarity existing in nursing. Bringing it forth so forcibly offers the opportunity for it to dialogue with other aspects, such as the more materialistic point of view, to support the emergence of more harmony and respect regarding the different ways nurses approach their practice.

Process work and nursing

This is a book about nurse healers, and it is directed to Process Work. I believe there is much for both nurses and Process Workers in these pages, but I have a dream of speaking to both simultaneously. I imagine nurse healers would make good Process Workers, for the act of healing involves

Gazing back and dreaming forward

following the flow of a powerful process, into the unknown. And this a good description of a Process Worker phenomenologically following a process.

I have dreamed about positing a role in nursing of something like "Nurse Process Worker". Process Work has a lot to offer nurses, and nurses practising in a process-oriented way would bring much to their patient care, or to whatever other role the play as nurses. The process-oriented approach follows and unfolds what nature is already working towards, so it interrupts the authoritarian and controlling ways of providing patient care which have rightly engendered so much criticism of health care settings.

In important ways, Process Work is a program about empowerment. It proffers a potent body of skills, metaskills and theory in promoting mutual empowerment with enhanced awareness as means to resolve conflict. Empowerment is a huge issue for nurses, whose agency is so very subservient to medicine's.

Further, there is a considerable literature about the misuse of power amongst nurses, pointing to horizontal violence as well as the authoritarian nature of nurses' relationships within structures in health and educational organisations. Nearly all nurses have been painfully subject to misuse of power, from other nurses, doctors, administrators. Difficult conflict with doctors and other nurses, even from patients and visitors, and members of other professions such as Emergency Services and the legal profession can all affect nurses in our professional lives.

I believe that If we nurses learned to be Process Workers we could be so much better equipped to practice effectively in such challenging work settings; in the process, too, we could be more effective healers to our patients and clients.

Final reflections: Waking and dreaming — Life myth, deep democracy and a shamanic path

Orienting this work to Process Work has highlighted how I am deeply one-sided in favour of the sacred and non-ordinary. This is a very biased work, and has been so from the beginning of this project. Mindful of the marginalisation of healers by the dominant cultural voices, I have been combative in standing for the non-ordinary experiences of others and myself.

Throughout my earlier life my interest in spirituality has led me to be nonmaterialist in outlook, and I had embraced the tenet that material existence is illusory and true reality is to be found in unitary consciousness. I recall feeling horrified when I first read the words of Arny Mindell criticising a spiritual guru for being too much aligned with spiritual experience, Arny reflecting that he was, "a phantom, a real person with the potential to grow to completion without identifying as such".[141]

There have been good reasons for being so one-sided in this work. Its original target audience had been the highly critical world of academe, and the nursing profession which largely holds to the rigidly materialist world view of scientific research. In that context it was important to hold very strongly to the world view in which healing makes sense. In this I have also stood up against my own inner critics imbued in the consensus view of normality.

Notwithstanding the clear value of standing so strongly for experience so marginalised in this culture, as a Process Worker I am informed by Deep Democracy, which invites all points of view to have their say. I have outlined Deep Democracy earlier, in Chapter Two, as a guiding tenet in PW. Liz Scarfe[142] puts its value and importance clearly:

> *The concept of deep democracy represents a profound valuing of diversity. All roles and voices within a context/issue, etc. are not just welcome or tolerated, but seen as necessary to resolve or transform conflicts and dynamics of oppression.*

I have striven to marginalise the voice of the dominant paradigm of this culture, both regarding the reports of the nurse healers and, possibly more significantly, within myself. In the understanding of Process Work, that which I marginalise in my interactions with the world, I holographically marginalise in myself. Therefore, a valuable part of reflecting on the sacred journeys of nurse healers, my own included, must be the acknowledging of dissenting voices in the field, particularly those which stand against this reality. Another take is to say that my own journey with this work is incomplete without seeking to process the figures which come against this.

And as I write this I feel somehow relieved, for there are within my being, within the worlds I inhabit, tracts which are oppressed and marginalised by taking such a one-sided approach. It helps to have that out, and to see the value in other perspectives, even those opposed to my own predominant attitude to life. In previous sections of this book I wrote of my life myth, and of my struggles in reconciling the parts of my being which dwell in different worlds.

The part of me which lives an ordinary life has been so often horrified by the shamanic part, even though I feel empty when not living it. And the shamanic part has been so often unreasonable and uncompromising in its relating to the ordinary world. In the face of this I have feared insanity, a dream figure which strides the edges of my experience of multiple worlds. Deep Democracy, as a powerful precept in resolving conflicts, prompts me to value dialogue amongst these points of view and figures, in my personal processes and in the field of healing and shamans in the world.

Holographic theory suggests that the boundary between my own and the wider world field of this conflict is mutable, or that these experiences are linked. This proffers other ways to look at and process this. In particular, it offers some relief of the loneliness of my inner conflict between the views that healing and other worlds are "real", versus being "ridiculous" or "crazy". This conflict belongs holographically to the world as much as to me; it not solely a feature of my psychology, but is just as much an aspect of the wider world field.

An implication is that processing my own conflict helps relieve the conflict in the field of the world. Similarly, supporting the world field to process its conflict will help me and others affected by this conflict. I sense that, even simply metacommunicating about this, as I have been doing in these paragraphs, is somewhat relieving to the wider field and it is also helpful for me.

While this discussion could be the subject of another complete book, I think it is worth fleshing out the conflicting roles a little, heeding these dissenting voices. Honouring the point of view which stands against the strange, seemingly reality-denying perspective of the healer, invites more ease and comfort to an area of human discourse which is vexed and irritated.

Thus, for instance, I must acknowledge the clear and reasoning voices of the Enlightenment, which once freed the mediaeval West from superstition, ignorance and (to an extent) oppression. In a way, these voices created an environment in this culture where I am unlikely to be exiled, imprisoned, or burned at the stake for what I have written in these pages.

Gazing back and dreaming forward

I do imagine these voices now contemptuously dismissing the world view of the healer; yet I feel quite safe presenting what is, in many ways, "heretical" and dismissive of some of the grounds of reason which is the Enlightenment's legacy. This plays out within my own psychology, the Enlightenment part of myself takes umbrage, and is ashamed, at the outrageous sounds and movements and powers of the shamanic me. Yet, it is helpful to all of me for this to be vocalised.

Still, it seems a fitting way to end this book by bringing these disparate viewpoints into the open, and ratifying the necessity of each for the full exposition of my topic — the sacred journeys of nurse healers. Those who walk the ways of many worlds know that they must be open to questioning, if only from themselves. To have a rich and fulsome conversation about these pathways of human experience, I think it is not enough to simply honour and recount them faithfully.

There is also immeasurable value in supporting these wondrous voices of healers and shamans to engage with those of the consensus. This is because the everyday experience of life is impoverished and incomplete without embracing at least a little of the magic humming beneath its surface. And the human experience of other worlds within is incomplete and ephemeral without the worldly yoke. Thus, utterly preposterous and completely necessary, these almost incommensurate parts of human existence should move us separately and in union through the astonishing dance of being.

Gazing back and dreaming forward

Glossary of Terms

Altered and extreme states

In Process Work, **altered states**:

> *refer to a state of consciousness which is different from the state connected to collective primary process. For example, if ordinary waking consciousness is our primary state, altered states include nocturnal dreaming, hypnotic conditions, drunken and drugged states, states centred around strong emotions like rage, panic, depression, elation, or states induced by meditation.[143]*

— **Extreme states**:

> *are normally antagonistic or unusual in a given community, for example, a psychotic episode or altered state of consciousness.[144]*

Mindell has differentiated Extreme States as those occurring when there is a missing metacommunicator role in the individual or community; the state is experienced without awareness of itself. Other examples of extreme states are coma and other near-death experiences, and war and racial hatred.

Archetype

Archetypes are "Primordial, structural elements of the human psyche".[145] The Fontana Dictionary of Modern Thought *defined the archetype as follows:[146]*

> *A Jungian term for any of a number of prototypic phenomena (e.g. the wise old man, the great mother) which form the content of the collective unconscious (and therefore of any given individual's unconscious), and which are assumed to reflect universal human thoughts found in all cultures.*

Arnold Mindell, founder of Process Work, defined archetypes in process-oriented terms:[147]

> *The implicit structure and organisation of processes which may appear in dreams, body problems, relationships, synchronicities and hallucinations.*

Awakening

In spiritual traditions, awakening refers to a change in consciousness and life orientation due to a realisation of the fundamental unity of the individual with the divine.

Being

The fundamental concept of ontology, being refers to the existence of an entity.

Boundaries

In the psychological or energetic sense appearing in this book, "boundary" refers to the propensity of an individual to experience the self as separate and distinct from others. Psychological theorists such as John Bradshaw[148] have emphasised the role of the effective development of boundaries in healthy personal growth. Further, they associate an undeveloped or distorted sense of boundaries between self and others with disrupted and traumatic childhood experiences, leading to difficulties in forming healthy relationships, and other psychological problems through adult life, such as chemical dependence or workaholism.

Healers and mystics have associated the dropping of all personal boundaries with experience of the numinous and the channelling of healing energies. It may be the case that healers enter the healing experience with poor personal boundaries, which enables the channelling of healing for others, but can bring problems such as uncontrolled experiencing of the pain and illness of others. This then challenges the healers to address their own childhood issues so they maintain healthy boundaries in ordinary living, but may choose to drop at times of healing practice. This can, ideally, lead to a mastery of boundaries characteristic of highly evolved healers, mystics and therapists.

CR (Consensus Reality)

Consensus Reality. In Process Work, CR is one of three co-existent levels of reality. In CR we identify with the culture we live in, the shared meanings, and agreed reality of the everyday.

Brahman

The Absolute, God (Hinduism).

Chakras

Chakras are the seven circular or conical energetic structures, visible to some people, situated on the body. They are part of the energy fields of people, and are associated with the energising and balancing of our psychic, spiritual, physical and emotional functioning.[149]

Channel (Spiritual healing)

Healers channel by allowing spiritual energy to flow through them from Divine source to another to facilitate healing.

Channel (Sensory grounded signals)

Process Workers conduct therapy phenomenologically, focusing on sensory grounded signals apparent in the moment. From NLP, these signals are said to occur in channels — visual, auditory, movement, proprioceptive (feeling and sensation). As well as those channels, Process Workers utilise composite channels — relationship channel and world channel.

Cosmic /Universal / Divine consciousness

The state of being aware of one's unity with all that is.

Don Juan

In Carlos Castaneda's famous books, Don Juan is the Yaqui Indian "Man of Knowledge" to whom Castaneda is apprenticed. The teachings on spiritual power and evolvement in Castaneda's books come from Don Juan. Below are some concepts from Don Juan, used by Process Workers in their work.

— Second attention

A term originating in the writings of Castaneda, second attention is important to Process Workers in perceiving their and their clients' dreaming processes. As Salome Schwarz reported:[150]

> Process work training advances the ability to track experiences which a person doesn't pay attention to, including seemingly nonsensical experiences. This ability is called "second attention". Second attention can be used in a focused and sharp or diffuse and relaxed way.

— Shifting the assemblage point

An important concept pointing to a profound transformation of perspective, also originating in Castaneda's writings.

— Sensing the atmosphere

Taking note of the underlying feeling in a room, group etc.

Dreamland

One of the three levels of reality in which Process Workers operate. Arnold Mindell defined it as: "A general level of awareness including dreams, dreaming while awake, and non-consensual experiences (relative to a given community)".[151]

Dreaming

In terms of Process Work, dreaming is, "The metaphysical or spiritual experience and meaning behind behaviour, signals, symptoms, and disturbances".[152] The influence of the shamanism of the Australian Aboriginal peoples is evident in Arny Mindell's adoption of this term.

Edge (The edge)

An edge is the experience of the boundary of the person's known identity. "An edge is the limit of what we can perceive, think, communicate, or believe we can do. Structurally speaking, an edge separates the primary from the secondary process".[153]

— Growing edge

An edge on which a person is challenged over time. For example, it may be manifesting an unproductive personality trait or addiction or persistent relationship issue or body symptom.

Ego (Self)

In common parlance, we find ego as a synonym for self-worth, or an excess or imbalance in self-worth. Also, it can signify self-centredness, selfishness or arrogance.

Technically, ego is often an ambiguous term, used somewhat differently in the various world traditions of psychology (particularly analytical psychology of Freud and Jung), as well as Buddhist and other Eastern mystical traditions. Whereas the Buddhist devotee might see the destruction of the ego as the ultimate goal of their spiritual journey, to the Western psychologist, this is anathema, and a nonsense signifying insanity. To the psychologist, the ego is the means by which the individual balances the various psychic forces of id and superego whilst negotiating with the social world; whereas the mystic views the ego as illusory, maintaining that the assumption of a true separation or individuation is a misperception of the nature of reality.

Perhaps this disagreement is caused in part by the conflation of two slightly separate concepts into the same term, ego. For example, it seems that a healthy ego is a prerequisite for successful mystical exploration. Commentators on mystical transformation contend that it is only a well integrated ego (i.e. a person with a strong sense of self-worth) which can be transcended in a mystical sense, and those with unbalanced or immature self-perceptions risk psychosis by intensively applying themselves to mystical practices.[154]

EMDR: Eye Movement Desensitisation and Reprocessing

An innovative method of psychotherapy. The focus of EMDR treatment is the resolution of emotional distress arising from difficult childhood experiences, or the recovery from the effects of critical incidents, such as automobile accidents, assault, natural disasters, and combat trauma. Other problems treated with EMDR are phobias, panic attacks, distress in children, and substance abuse.[155]

Energetics

In energetic experience, consciousness is expanded beyond a self contained in a body. Here, healers often report a sense that they are linked with others in a shared field of energy.

Further, energetics, as discussed in this book, points to the direct experience of a sense of truth of being, which both guides and funds the unfolding of one's healing journey. In this journeying with energetics, the fundamental joinedness of all in consciousness becomes increasingly evident, as the healer is brought to a hearkening of the astounding Source of all healing.

Energy field

In esoteric spirituality and spiritual or "energetic" healing, there is the perception that the human is not simply a physical body, but a number of bodies, most of which are not

ordinarily visible, which interpenetrate. The non-visible bodies, or human energy field, are said to extend beyond the physical body, and interact directly with the energy fields of other humans and other entities, and with the "universal energy field". The human energy field equates approximately to the human "aura", which is visible to some individuals at all times, and to most individuals under certain circumstances.[156,157]

Essence

In Husserl's phenomenology, essence denoted that which for a phenomenon makes it uniquely itself, and this is what phenomenological reduction strives to elucidate. This has been adopted by Max van Manen[158] in his approach to phenomenological research, where the researcher seeks the essential nature of experience as it manifests linguistically as themes in the data.

Expanded consciousness

Often interpreted as spiritual or religious experience, expansion of consciousness occurs when there is a direct experience of the individual being greater than the boundaries of ordinarily perceived existence. Sometimes this is perceived to be an instance of sensing closeness to God. It may occur at any time, but perhaps is most often associated with certain spiritual practices such as prayer or meditation, or during intimate inter-human connection or at times of extreme stress and emotion or in the perception of great aesthetic beauty such as a lovely sunset.

Healing

What is of deepest interest to me is that wholeness, when traced to its essence, must mean the utter indivisibility of everything — that nothing is apart. This is the underlying reality of healing, and a key implication is that healing is not something that anybody really enacts, or even happens — it is more something that becomes obvious, something that is realised, something that is remembered. The apparent activity of a healer reminds the participants in the healing exchange that in reality, in truth, they have never ever been separate or apart, never been alone.

This realisation of oneness, completely beautiful, utterly right, is the true meaning of healing, which may also entail improvement in physical or psychological wellbeing.

Higher self

In a number of spiritual traditions, the higher self is said to be the part of the individual which is in direct communication with the Source, or God, and may act as an intermediary between the individual and God. There is an understanding that one's higher self provides necessary guidance. The higher self is said to be available for channelling, or speaking through the mouth of the individual, who is in an expanded state of consciousness at the time.

Holism

The philosophical position that humans are indivisible wholes who cannot be correctly understood in terms of their constituent parts.

Kundalini

The Encyclopaedia Britannica Online stated:[159]

> In some Tantric (esoteric) forms of Yoga, the cosmic energy that is believed to lie within everyone, pictured as a coiled serpent lying at the base of the spine. In the practice of Laya Yoga ("Union of Mergence"), the adept is instructed to awaken the kundalini, also identified with the deity Shakti.

Associated with powerful spiritual transformation, the rising of the kundalini can also bring on considerable psychological disruption, even severe psychosis, if the individual is not prepared for the dramatic personal changes attending this spiritual opening.[160]

Life myth

Drawing on Jungian concepts, for Process Workers, life myth refers to long-term processes and edges which pattern and structure life experiences. They are the underlying stories running through our lives.

Metaskill

Identified by Amy Mindell,[161] Metaskills are the overarching qualities or feelings guiding therapeutic skills. According to Mindell, whose therapeutic practice Amy Mindell studied to arrive at this concept:

The way you say something or do something is a metaskill that can be harsh, helpful, compassionate, playful, scientific, etc.[162]

Ontological

This pertains to ontology, the philosophical study of being, the existence of entities. Ontology is one of the two core concerns of philosophy, the other being epistemology, the study of meaning.

Ontology

Refers to exploring the nature of reality or a general orientation to life and, for me, this means asking the question: "What does it mean to be a person?".

Phenomenology

Phenomenology is the study of phenomena. As such, it can be philosophy, methodology or approach. The phenomenological method, as conceived originally by Husserl, involved attending faithfully to phenomena as they present themselves to consciousness, outside of the preconceptions or theoretical concerns of the investigator. Although there are great philosophical differences amongst those who espouse phenomenology, it remains a vehicle for thinkers who are deeply committed to keeping philosophy and method in touch with the deeper human concerns.

Power animal

In Indigenous spiritual traditions, often shamanistic, the individual will commonly be associated with an animal whose attributes reflect the individual's character, and also bring strength and wisdom to that person when that animal is invoked through meditation or visualisation. The shaman or spiritual practitioner may undertake a spiritual journey out of their body to discover someone's power animal and connect that animal, spiritually, to the individual for healing.

Practice

Amongst some groups of people engaged in a deliberately worked at spiritual life, practice is often the word used to denote the techniques and habits, even rituals employed.

Process

As defined by Arnold Mindell, the founder of Process Oriented Psychology, process is:[163]

> *The flow of signals and of information as defined by those who perceive it. Process is differentiated into primary and secondary information which is closer to or further from the sender's awareness.*

— Primary process

The body gestures, behaviour and thoughts with which one identifies oneself or which it can be assumed one would identify with if asked.

— Secondary process

All the verbal and nonverbal signals in an individual's or community's expressions with which the individual or community does not identify. The information from secondary processes is usually projected, denied, and found in the body or outside the sender.

Protection

In esoteric spiritual traditions, and in a number of healing practices, the adept adopts certain attitudes or practices to protect them while in open and vulnerable states, especially during healing sessions.

Protection may be from the negative emotions or other energies associated with illness and distress, or from other unseen spiritual entities which may become attached to the unwary or unguarded practitioner. Protection may also be from the deliberate non-local acts of other people.

Reiki healing

A common healing modality involving the laying of hands and specific meditative techniques.

Sentient reality

In Process Work, sentient reality (also called 'Essence') is the holistic consciousness where there are no polarities. Along with consensus reality and dreamland it forms the multiple realities in which Process Workers are trained to function.

The shadow

In Jungian psychology, the shadow refers to unconscious — often repressed — aspects of the self which may be unwelcomed or denied by the individual when eventually revealed to consciousness. This may include unproductive personality traits, or past painful experiences which have been discounted or unexamined and which are yet influential on a person's behaviour, relationships and self-concept.[164]

In this book, the shadow also refers to spiritual darkness — unseen entities and thought forms of a less-than-helpful nature. This may in some cases be the same as the abovementioned Jungian conception of shadow, where the unconscious processes, through projection, manifest in spiritual experience. It must be noted that in recent times Process Workers are enjoined to avoid use of this term as it can be experienced as disparaging by people of colour.

Shaman

Healer and/or mediator between the material and spiritual worlds, practising in Indigenous societies throughout the world. Originally specifically associated with certain Siberian tribes.

Shamanism

The practices of shamans in certain Indigenous societies, having some of the features of a religion.

Soul birth

Spiritual transformation.

Soul loss

Condition of spiritual dis-ease recognised in some Indigenous societies, usually diagnosed and treated by shamans.

Synchronicity

The *Fontana Dictionary of Modern Thought* defined synchronicity as: "Jungian term for an acausal principle that would give meaning to a series of coincidences ... not explicable through notions of simple causality".[165]

Thought forms

In esoteric spirituality, thought forms are described as energetic structures which are constructed by human thoughts and emotions. Barbara Brennan described them as visible as blobs in the human aura which can act powerfully to affect an individual's wellbeing.[166]

Transformation

Personal change at a fundamental level, often involving change of attitudes, emotional responses, and self-concept. The individuals may come to experience themselves and their relations with others and the spiritual in completely new ways.

TT: Therapeutic Touch

Healing modality involving the laying-on of hands, developed by Dolores Krieger and Dora Kunz in the 1970s and now practiced by tens of thousands of nurses throughout the world.[167]

Yoga

Spiritual pathway, particularly the practices employed by the aspirant, distinguished from the philosophical teaching or doctrine.

Bibliography

Abelson RP & Schank RC. 1995. *Knowledge and Memory: The Real Story.* In *Knowledge and Memory: The Real Story. Advances in Social Cognition*, edited by RS Wyer Jr et al. Hillsdale, NJ: Lawrence Erlbaum Associates.

Andrews L. 1985. *Jaguar Woman.* New York: Harper & Row.

Andrews L. 1983. *Medicine Woman.* New York: Harper & Row.

Bailey A. 1978. *Esoteric Healing.* St Paul, MN: Lucis Publishing.

Benner P. 1984. *From Novice to Expert: Excellence and Power in Clinical Nursing Practice.* Menlo Park, California: Addison-Wesley.

Blum R. 1982. *The Book of Runes.* London: Angus & Robertson.

Bradshaw J. 1990. *Homecoming: Reclaiming and Championing Your Inner Child.* New York: Bantam.

Brandon D. 1999. *'Wounded Healers'.* Nursing Standard 13 (28): 99279723.

Brennan BA. 2017. *Core Light Healing.* Sydney: Hay House.

Brennan BA. 1993. *Light Emerging: The Journey of Personal Healing.* New York: Bantam.

Brennan BA. 1988. *Hands of Light: A Guide to Healing Through the Human Energy Field.* London: Bantam.

Bruyere, R. 1994. *Wheels of Light: Chakras, Auras, and the Healing Energy of the Body.* New York: Fireside.

Bullock A & Stallybrass O (eds). 1977. *The Fontana Dictionary of Modern Thought.* Sixth Impression ed. London: Fontana.

Carlson R & Shield B. 1989. *Healers on Healing.* New York: Tarcher/Putnam.

Castaneda, C. 1972. *Journey to Ixtlan: The Lessons of Don Juan.* New York: Simon & Schuster.

Castaneda C. 1968. *The Teachings of Don Juan: A Yaqui Way of Knowledge.* Berkley: University of California Press.

Courcey K. 2001. *'Further Notes on Therapeutic Touch'* [Web Page]. "Quackwatch", http://www.quackwatch.org/01QuackeryRelatedTopics/tt2.html, 2001 [viewed 6 May 2003].

Davis-Floyd R & St John G. 1998. *From Doctor to Healer: The Transformative Journey.* New Brunswick, NJ: Rutgers University Press.

Diamond J & Spark Jones L. 2005. *A Path Made by Walking.* Portland: Lao Tse Press.

Dossey BM Keegan L Guzzetta CE & Kolkmeier LG. 1988. *Holistic Nursing: A Handbook for Practice.* Rockville, MD.: Aspen publishers.

Dubin-Vaughn S. 1991. *'Elizabeth Cogburn: A Contemporary Shaman'.* In *Shamans of the 20th Century,* edited by R-I Heinze. New York: Irvington Publishers Inc.

Eliade M. 1964. *Shamanism: Archaic Techniques of Ecstasy.* Translated by W. Trask. Princeton, NJ: Princeton University Press.

Eliade M. 1959. *The Sacred and the Profane: The Nature of Religion.* Translated by WR Trask. San Diego, New York & London: Harcourt Brace.

Elkin AP. 1977. *Aboriginal Men of High Degree.* 2nd Edition. (1st edition 1945). Brisbane: University of Queensland Press.

EMDR International Association. Accessed on 19/8/2019 at: https://www.emdria.org/page/what_is_emdr_therapy.

Encyclopedia Britannica Online, The. Accessed online on 7/12/2003 at: http://www.britannica.com/eb/article?eu=47504&tocid=0&query=kundalini&ct=.

Gadamer H-G. 1975. *Truth and Method.* Translated by Joel Weinsheimer & Donald G Marshall. Second, Revised ed. London: Sheed & Ward.

Geddes NJ. 1999. *The Experience of Personal Transformation in Healing Touch (HT) Practitioners: a Heuristic Inquiry (Unitary Paradigm).* PH.D, Virginia Commonwealth University.

Gibran K. 1980 (1926). *The Prophet.* London: Heinemann.

Glazer S. 2001. *'Therapeutic Touch and Postmodernism in Nursing'.* Nursing Philosophy 2 (3):196–212.

Griffiths B. 1989. *A New Vision of Reality.* London: Fount.

Grof S & Grof C. 1989. *Spiritual Emergency: When Personal Transformation Becomes a Crisis.* New York: Putnam.

Grof S & Bennett HZ. 1992. *The Holotropic Mind: The Three Levels of Human Consciousness and How They Shape Our Lives.* New York: HarperCollins.

Halifax J. 1982. *Shaman. The Wounded Healer. London: Thames & Hudson.*

Halifax J. 1979. *Shamanic Voices: A Survey of Visionary Narratives.* New York: EP Dutton.

Hall J. 1997. *'Nurses as Wounded Healers: The Journey to Healing the Person and Profession'.* Australian Journal of Holistic Nursing 4 (1):11–16.

Hall J. 1996. *'Challenges to Caring: Nurses as Wounded Healers'.* Australian Journal of Holistic Nursing 3 (2):12–18.

Harvey A. 1998. *The Essential Mystics: The Soul's Journey into Truth.* Edison, New Jersey: Castle Books.

Heinze R-I (ed). 1991. *Shamans of the 20th Century.* New York: Irvington Publishers Inc.

Hemsley M. 2003. *Walking Two Worlds: Transformational Journals of Nurse Healers: A Hermeneutic Phenomenological Investigation.* PhD thesis, Southern Cross University: Lismore, NSW.

Hemsley M. 1998. *Exploring the Fused Horizons of Healing and Nursing: An Hermeneutic Phenomenological Study.* Unpublished Honours Thesis, School of Nursing and Health Care Practices, Southern Cross University: Lismore, NSW.

Hemsley M. & Glass N. 2006. *'Sacred Journeys of Nurse Healers'.* Journal of Holistic Nursing. 24(4):256-268.

Hemsley M., Glass N. & Watson J. 2006. *'Taking the Eagle's View: Using Watson's Conceptual Model to Investigate the Extraordinary and Transformative Experiences of Nurse Healers'.* Holistic Nursing Practice. 20(2):85–94.

Hillman J. 1975. *Re-Visioning Psychology.* New York: Harper & Row.

Hillman. J. & Ventura M. 1993. *We've Had a Hundred Years of Psychotherapy & the World's Getting Worse.* HarperOne.

Horrigan B. 1998. *'Conversations: Dolores Krieger, RN, PhD; Healing with Therapeutic Touch'.* Alternative Therapies in Health and Medicine 4 (1):86–92.

Horrigan B. 1996. *'Janet Quinn, RN, PhD: Therapeutic Touch and a Healing Way'.* Alternative Therapies in Health and Medicine 2 (4):69–75.

Hover-Kramer D & Shames KH. 1997. *Energetic Approaches to Emotional Healing.* Albany, New York: Delmar.

Huber BR. 1990. *'The Recruitment of Nahua Curers: Role Conflict and Gender'.* Ethnology 29:159–176.

Hultkrantz A. 1978. *'Ecological and Phenomenological Aspects of Shamanism'.* In Shamanism in Siberia, edited by B Dioszegi & M Hoppal. Budapest, Hungary: Akademiai Kiado.

IAPOP: International Association of Process Oriented Psychology. Glossary. Accessed on 28/11/2018 at: http://www.iapop.com/glossary/

Ingerman S. 1991. *Soul Retrieval. Mending the Fragmented Self.* New York: HarperCollins

Jamal M. 1987. *Shape Shifters: Shaman Women in Contemporary Society.* New York: Arkana.

Jobe K. 1994. *'An Interview with Arny Mindell on Extreme States'.* The Journal of Process Oriented Psychology Volume 6 (1) pp 7–10.

Johnson M. 1999. *'Observations on Positivism and Pseudoscience in Qualitative Nursing Research'.* Journal of Advanced Nursing 30 (1):67–73.

Joy B. 1979. *Joy's Way.* Los Angeles: JP Tarcher.

Jung.CG. 1965. *Memories, Dreams, Reflections.* New York: Vintage Books.

Keegan L & Dossey B. 1998. *Profiles of Nurse Healers.* Series editor, L. Keegan, Nurse as Healer. Albany, New York: Delmar.

Kleinman A. 1980. *Patients and Healers in the Context of Culture.* Berkley: University of California Press.

Krippner S. 1991. *Foreword.* In *Shamans of the 20th Century, edited by R-I Heinze.* New York: Irvington Publishers Inc.

Krieger D. 1975. *'Therapeutic Touch: The Imprimatur of Nursing'.* American Journal of Nursing 75 (5):784–787.

Krieger D. 1987. *Living the Therapeutic Touch: Healing as a Lifestyle.* New York: Dodd Mead.

Krieger D. 1993. *Accepting Your Power to Heal: The Personal Practice of Therapeutic Touch.* Santa Fe, New Mexico: Bear & Co.

Kunz, D. 1995. *Spiritual Healing.* Wheaton, IL : Quest Books

Lewis IM. 1989 (1971). *Ecstatic Religion: An Anthropological Study of Spirit Possession and Shamanism.* 2nd ed. Baltimore: Penguin Books.

Martin M. 1997. *'Aotearoa, New Zealand and the Centre for Human Care'.* Advanced Practice Nursing Quarterly 3 (1):85–7.

Merel P. 2003. *Tao Te Ching: An English-Language Interpolation 1995* [cited 10 July 2003 2003]. Available from http://www.clas.ufl.edu/users/gthursby/ taoism/ ttcmerel. htm.

Miller J. 1965. *'Living Systems. Basic Concepts'.* Behavioural Science 10 (3):213.

Mindell, Amy. 1995. *Metaskills: The Spiritual Art of Therapy.* Tempe, AZ: New Falcon Press.

Mindell, Arnold. 1985. *River's Way: The Process Science of The Dreambody.* London. Routledge and Kegan Ltd.

Mindell, Arnold. 1988. *City Shadows: Psychological Interventions in Psychiatry.* New York: Routledge.

Mindell, Arnold. 1990. *Working on Yourself Alone: Inner Dreambody Work.* London. Penguin Group.

Mindell, Arnold. 1992. *The Leader as Martial Artist: An Introduction to Deep Democracy Techniques and Strategies for Resolving Conflict and Creating Community.* San Francisco. HarperCollins.

Mindell, Arnold. 1993. T*he Shaman's Body: A New Shamanism For Transforming Health, Relationships and The Community.* New York. HarperCollins Publishers.

Mindell, Arnold. 2000. *Dreaming While Awake: Techniques for 24-Hour Lucid Dreaming.* Charlottesville, VA. Hampton Roads Publishing Company, Inc.

Mindell, Arnold. 2000. *Dreaming While Awake: Techniques for 24-Hour Lucid Dreaming* (Kindle Edition).

Mindell, Arnold. 2000a. *Quantum Mind: The Edge Between Physics & Psychology.* Portland, Oregon. Lao Tse Press.

Mindell, Arnold. 2002. *Working with The Dreaming Body.* Portland, Oregon. Lao Tse Press

Mindell, Arnold. 2004. *The Quantum Mind and Healing: How to Listen and Respond To Your Body Symptoms.* Charlottesville, VA. Hampton Roads Publishing Company, Inc.

Mindell, Arnold. 2007. *Earth-Based Psychology: Path Awareness from the Teachings of Don Juan, Richard Feynman and Lao Tse.* Portland, Oregon. Lao Tse Press.

Mindell, Arnold. 2010. *Coma: The Dreambody Near Death.* Portland, Oregon: Lao Tse Press (Kindle Edition). (First published in 1989 by Shambala Publications, Inc.)

Mindell, Arnold. 2010a. *Process Mind: A User's Guide to Connecting with the Mind of God.* Wheaton, Ill.: Quest Books.

Myss C. 1996. *Anatomy of the Spirit: The Seven Stages of Power and Healing.* New York: Harmony.

Ngaanyatjarra Pitjantjatjara Yankunytjatjara Women's Council Aboriginal Corporation. 2013. *Traditional Healers of Central Australia: Ngangkari.* Broome, W.A. Magabala Books.

O'Mathuna DP, Pryjmachuk S Spencer, W Stanwick M & Matthiesen S. 2002. *'A Critical Evaluation of the Theory and Practice of Therapeutic Touch'.* Nursing Philosophy 3 (2):163– 176.

Osborne A. 1970. *Ramana Maharshi and the Path of Self-Knowledge.* York Beach, Maine: Samuel Weiser.

Plotinus. 1952. *The Six Enneads.* Translated by S MacKenna & BS Page, *Great Books of the Western World.* Chicago: Encyclopedia Britannica.

Quinn JF. 1979. *'One Nurse's Evolution as a Healer'.* American Journal of Nursing 79:662– 664.

Rama S., Ballentine R., and Ayjaya S. 1981. *Yoga and Psychotherapy.* Honesdale PA: Himalayan International Institute.

Reid J. 1983. *Sorcerers and Healing Spirits.* Canberra: Australian National University Press.

Rogers ME. 1970. *An Introduction to the Theoretical Basis of Nursing.* Philadelphia: F.A. Davis.

Romanian Association for Psychoanalysis Promotion, The. Dictionary of Jungian Terms. Accessed on 27/11/2018 at https://www.carl-jung.net/glossary.html

Rosa L Rosa E Sarner L & Barrett S. et al. 1998. *'A Close Look at Therapeutic Touch'.* Journal of the American Medical Association 279 (13):1005–1010.

Rumi Childhood Friends h ttp://andylal.blogspot.com/2011/04/childhood-friends-by-rumi.html (Accessed 6 January 2019)

Sayre-Adams J & Wright SG. 1995. *Therapeutic Touch.* Edinburgh: Churchill Livingstone.

Scarfe L. 2015. *Pointing at the Moon Exploring the Question: What is Psychological Freedom?* A thesis submitted in partial fulfilment of the requirements for the Diploma in Process Work. ANZPOP.

Schwarz S. 2006. *Shifting the Assemblage Point: Transformation in Therapy and Everyday Life.* PhD Thesis. The Union Institute: Cincinnati, Ohio.

Sharp D. 1991. *Jung Lexicon: A Primer of Terms & Concepts.* Accessed on 17/11/2018 from https://www.psychceu.com/jung/sharplexicon.html

Singer M & Garcia R. 1989. *'Becoming a Puerto Rican Espiritista'. In* Women as Healers, edited by CS McClain. New Brunswick: Rutgers University Press.

Slater VE Maloney JP Krau SD & Eckert CA. 1999. *'Journey to Holism'.* Journal of Holistic Nursing 17 (4):365–383.

Struthers R. 2000. *'The Lived Experience of Ojibwa and Cree Women Healers'.* Journal of Holistic Nursing 18 (3):261–279.

Tansley DV. 1985. *Subtle Body.* New York: Thames and Hudson.

Taylor BJ. 1994. *Being Human: Ordinariness in Nursing.* Melbourne: Churchill Livingstone.

Van Gennep A. 1960. *The Rites of Passage.* Chicago: The University of Chicago Press.

van Manen M. 1990. *Researching Lived Experience: Human Science for An Action Sensitive Pedagogy.* New York: State University of New York Press.

Vitebsky P. 2000. 'Shamanism'. *In Indigenous Religions, edited by G Harvey.* London: Cassell.

von Bertalanffy L. 1950. *'The Theory of Open Systems on Physics and Biology'.* Science 111:23–25.

Watson J. 2002. *'Intentionality and Caring-Healing Consciousness: A Theory of Transpersonal Nursing'.* Holistic Nursing Practice 16 (4):12–19.

Watson J. 2000. *'Postmodern Era/Paradigm III, and Beyond'* (Unpublished conference presentation). In *Embracing the Spirit of Wholeness in Healing*: 4th International Conference of the Australian College of Holistic Nurses Inc.

Wilber K. 1996. *The Atman Project: A Transpersonal View of Human Development.* Quest Books Theosophical Publishing House

Wright SG. 2001. *'Beyond "Being With"'* (editorial). Sacred Space Journal 2 (4):1–7.

Yogananda P. 1972 (1946). *Autobiography of a Yogi.* First Paperback Edition. Los Angeles: Self-Realization Fellowship.

Yutang L. 1949. *The Wisdom of India.* 2nd ed. London: Michael Joseph.

Zweig C & Abrams J (Eds). 1991. *Meeting the Shadow: The Hidden Power of the Dark Side of Human Nature*: Tarcher Books: Los Angeles.

Notes

1. Quote from James Hillman & Michael Ventura (1993). *We've Had a Hundred Years of Psychotherapy & the World's Getting Worse*. HarperOne, p 123–124.
2. The author's PhD dissertation: Martin (Sananda) Hemsley (2003) *Walking Two Worlds: Transformational Journeys of Nurse Healers, a Hermeneutic Phenomenological Investigation*. PhD thesis, Southern Cross University: Lismore, NSW. [Online at: https://epubs.scu.edu.au/cgi/viewcontent.cgi?referer= https://www.google.com. au/&httpsredir=1&article=1024&context=theses].
3. Martin Hemsley & Nel Glass (2006). 'Sacred Journeys of Nurse Healers'. Journal of Holistic Nursing. 24(4):256–268.
4. Martin Hemsley, Nel Glass &. Jean Watson (2006). 'Taking the Eagle's View: Using Watson's Conceptual Model to Investigate the Extraordinary and Transformative Experiences of Nurse Healers'. Holistic Nursing Practice. 20(2):85–94.
5. See notation on Life Myth in the Glossary of Terms
6. Mindell, Arnold. (1993). *The Shaman's Body: A New Shamanism for Transforming Health*, Relationships and The Community. New York. HarperCollins Publishers.
7. See Chapter Four, 'Chris'
8. Quote about Viking Rune — Kano — appears multiple times on the internet. Unable to locate original attribution.
9. Quoted in Piers Vitebsky (2000), 'Shamanism'. In Indigenous Religions, edited by G Harvey. London: Cassell, p 60–61.
10. The author's Honours thesis: Martin Hemsley (1998). *Exploring the Fused Horizons of Healing and Nursing: An Hermeneutic Phenomenological Study*. Unpublished Honours Thesis, School of Nursing and Health Care Practices, Southern Cross University: Lismore, NSW.
11. Op cit. Hemsley (1998), p 65–66.
12. Op cit. Hemsley (1998), p 65.
13. Op cit. Hemsley (2003)
14. Quote from Margi Martin (1997). 'Aotearoa, New Zealand and the Centre for Human Care'. Advanced Practice Nursing Quarterly 3 (1):85–7, p 86.
15. Robert Abelson & Roger Schank (1995). 'Knowledge and Memory: The Real Story'. In *Knowledge and memory: The real story. Advances in social cognition*, edited by RS Wyer Jr et al. Hillsdale, NJ: Lawrence Erlbaum Associates.
16. See Chapter Four, 'Chris'
17. Quote from Max Van Manen (1984). 'Practicing Phenomenological Writing. Phenomenology and Pedagogy 2 (1):36–69. p 59
18. Viking Rune — Perth. Quote from Blum (1982). *The Book of Runes*. London: Angus & Robertson, p 67.
19. Bonnie Horrigan (1996). 'Janet Quinn, RN, PhD: Therapeutic Touch and a Healing Way'. Alternative Therapies in Health and Medicine 2 (4):69–75.
20. Dolores Krieger (1987) Living the Therapeutic Touch: Healing as a Lifestyle. New York: Dodd Mead.

21. For example, Dolores Krieger, in (1975) 'Therapeutic Touch: The Imprimatur of Nursing'. American Journal of Nursing 75 (5):784–787, wrote about her research measuring certain changes in immune factors following TT sessions.
22. Op cit. Krieger (1987).
23. Janet Quinn (1979). 'One Nurse's Evolution as a Healer'. American Journal of Nursing 79:662–664.
24. Martha Rogers (1970). *An Introduction to the Theoretical Basis of Nursing.* Philadelphia:
F.A. Davis
25. eg Ludwig von Bertalanffy (1950) The Theory of Open Systems on Physics and Biology. Science 111:23–25.
26. eg James Miller (1965) Living Systems. Basic Concepts. Behavioural Science 10 (3):213.
27. Op cit. In Bonnie Horrigan (1996).
28. There are numerous published articles aiming to discredit TT by asserting that it is a "pseudoscience" with little or no verifiable evidence of efficacy. Examples are by D. Ónal P.O'mathÚna, Steven Pryjmachuk, Wayne Spencer, Michael Stanwick & Stephen Matthiesen (2002); Kevin Courcey (2001); Donal O'Mathuna (2000); Martin Johnson (1999); Sarah Glazer (2001); and the remarkable "school project" research report by Linda Rosa, her daughter Emily Rosa, Larry Sarner et al (1998).
29. Quoted in Kevin Courcey (2001) Further Notes on Therapeutic Touch [on the. "Quackwatch" website].
30. Quoted from Peter Merel's (2003) interpolation of the Tao T Ching by Lao Tse.
31. ee Wikipedia: https://en.wikipedia.org/wiki/Advaita_Vedanta.
32. See, for example, Osborne (1970). *Ramana Maharshi and the Path of Self-Knowledge.* York Beach, Maine: Samuel Weiser.
33. Bede Griffiths (1989). A New Vision of Reality. London: Fount, p 176.
34. Op cit. Osborne (1970).
35. Quoted in Lin Yutang (1949). *The Wisdom of India.* 2nd ed. London: Michael Joseph, p 32.
36. Op cit. Griffiths (1989).
37. From Isaac Shapiro (1997), on his website: http://www.isaacshapiro.de/.
38. Op cit. Griffiths (1989), p 181.
39. Quoted in Harvey (1998). The Essential Mystics: The Soul's Journey into Truth. Edison, New Jersey: Castle Books, p 8.
40. Op cit. Griffiths (1989), p 184.
41. These following three citations do not exhaust Arny Mindell's writings on Quantum Theory's relevance to understanding unitary consciousness: Arny Mindell (2007). *Earth- Based Psychology: Path Awareness from the Teachings of Don Juan, Richard Feynman and Lao Tse. Portland, Oregon. Lao Tse Press*
42. Arny Mindell (2004). *The Quantum Mind and Healing: How to Listen and Respond To Your Body Symptoms.* Charlottesville, VA. Hampton Roads Publishing Company, Inc.
43. (2000a). Quantum Mind: The Edge Between Physics & Psychology. Portland, Oregon. Lao Tse Press.
44. See, for example, Arny Mindell's (2000). Dreaming While Awake: Techniques for 24-Hour Lucid Dreaming (Kindle Locations 75–77). Kindle Edition.

Notes

45. Arny Mindell (1992). The Leader as Martial Artist: An Introduction to Deep Democracy Techniques and Strategies for Resolving Conflict and Creating Community. San Francisco. HarperCollins.

46. Quote from James Hillman (1975). *Re-Visioning Psychology*. New York: Harper & Row.

47. Quoted in Richard Carlson & Benjamin Shield (1989). *Healers on Healing*. New York: Tarcher/Putnam, p 124.

48. See, for example, the clear detailing of the theory and practice of Process Work in Julie Diamond & Lee Spark Jones (2005). *A Path Made by Walking.* Portland: Lao Tse Press.

49. Barbara Brennan (2017). *Core Light Healing.* Sydney: Hay House.

50. (1993). *Light Emerging: The Journey of Personal Healing.* New York: Bantam.

51. (1988). Hands of Light: A Guide to Healing Through the Human Energy Field. London: Bantam.

52. See for example books by Dorothea Hover-Kramer & Karilee Halo Shames, (1997); Caroline Myss (1996); Dora Kunz (1995); Rosalyn Bruyere (1994); Alice Bailey (1978); David Tansley (1985); Swami Rama, Rudolphy Ballentine and Swami Ayjaya (1981) and
W. Brugh Joy (1979).

53. Op cit. Brennan (1988).

54. Op cit. Brennan (1993).

55. Op cit. Brennan (1988), p 51.

56. Op cit. Brennan (1988), p 45.

57. Op cit. Griffiths (1989), p 198–199.

58. Ken Wilber (1996) *The Atman Project: A Transpersonal View of Human Development.* Quest Books Theosophical Publishing House

59. Stanislav Grof and Hal Zina Bennett (1992) *The Holotropic Mind: The Three Levels of Human Consciousness and How They Shape Our Lives*. New York: HarperCollins.

60. Carl Jung (1965) *Memories, Dreams, Reflections*. New York: Vintage Books, p 86.

61. This is expressed in very many places. One example is in Barbara Dossey, Lynne Keegan, Cathie Guzzetta and Lesl Kolkmeier (1988). *Holistic Nursing: a Handbook for Practice*. Rockville, MD.: Aspen publishers.

62. This is famously articulated in the work of Stanislav and Christina Grof, particularly through their (1989) book: *Spiritual Emergency: When Personal Transformation Becomes a Crisis*. New York: Putnam.

63. Quote from Robbie Davis-Floyd and Gloria St John (1998) *From Doctor to Healer: The Transformative Journey*. New Brunswick, NJ: Rutgers University Press, p 159.

64. See for example in writings by Piers Vitebsky (2000), Stanley Krippner (1991), Brad Huber (1990), Ioan Lewis (1989), Joan Halifax (1982, 1979), Janice Reid (1983), Arthur Kleinman (1980), A.P. Elkin (1977), and Mircea Eliade (1964). Mircea Eliade, in particular, investigated the psychological disruption attendant upon those who embrace the sacred, across religions worldwide.

65. Joan Halifax (1982) Shaman. The Wounded Healer. London: Thames & Hudson, p 16.

66. Op cit. Griffiths (1989), p 232.

67. Plotinus (1952) *The Six Enneads*. Translated by S MacKenna & BS Page, Great Books of the Western World. Chicago: Encyclopedia Britannica.

68. Ibid.

Notes

69. Op cit. Halifax (1982).

70. See Amy Mindell (1995) *Metaskills: The Spiritual Art of Therapy Tempe,* AZ: New Falcon Press.

71. These ideas are present in most of Carlos Castaneda's books. Mindell most commonly cited his (1968). The Teachings of Don Juan: A Yaqui Way of Knowledge. Berkley: University of California Press; and (1972). Journey to Ixtlan: The Lessons of Don Juan. New York: Simon & Schuster.

72. See also the dissertation by the Process Worker Salome Schwarz (2006), *Shifting the Assemblage Point: Transformation in Therapy and Everyday Life.* PhD Thesis. The Union Institute: Cincinnati, Ohio.

73. Arny Mindell (2010). Coma: The Dreambody Near Death. Portland, Oregon: Lao Tse Press (Kindle Edition), Location 1016–1023.

74. Op cit. Krieger (1987).

75. Op cit. Brennan (2017, 1993, 1988).

76. Op cit. Griffiths (1989).

77. Op cit. Griffiths (1989), Plotinus (1952).

78. Eg op cit. Halifax (1982).

79. 'Dreamed by Dragons' previously unpublished poem by the author.

80. Jean Watson and Margaret Newman are prominent nurse theorists who each posit holistic frameworks for nursing practice and research.

81. See, for example, Jean Watson (2000). Postmodern Era/Paradigm III, and Beyond. (Unpublished conference presentation). In 'Embracing the Spirit of Wholeness in Healing': 4th International Conference of the Australian College of Holistic Nurses Inc. The concept has come from the idea of 'Era II Medicine' which was articulated by holistic doctor, Larry Dossey.

82. Patricia Benner (1984). F*rom Novice to Expert: Excellence and Power in Clinical Nursing Practice.* Menlo Park, California: Addison-Wesley.

83. Op cit. Blum, p 100.

84. Quote from: Sarah Dubin-Vaughn (1991). Elizabeth Cogburn: A Contemporary Shaman. In *Shamans of the 20th Century*, edited by R-I Heinze, p. 70–71. New York: Irvington Publishers Inc.

85. Stephen Wright (2001). 'Beyond "Being With"' (editorial). Sacred Space Journal 2 (4):1–7, p 1–2.

86. Op cit. Krieger (1987) p 38.

87. See, for example, Connie Zweig & Jeremiah Abrams (Eds). (1991). Meeting the Shadow: The Hidden Power of the Dark Side of Human Nature: Tarcher: Los Angeles.

88. Op cit. Krieger (1987).

89. Lynn Keegan & Barbara Dossey (1998). Profiles of Nurse Healers, p 75–76. Albany, New York: Delmar.

90. Ibid, p 55.

91. Victoria Slater, Joseph Maloney, Stephen Krau & Carol Eckert (1999). Journey to Holism. Journal of Holistic Nursing 17 (4):365–383.

92. Norma Geddes (1999). *The Experience of Personal Transformation in Healing Touch (HT) Practitioners: a Heuristic Inquiry (Unitary Paradigm).* Ph.D, Virginia Commonwealth University.

Notes

93. Robbie Davis-Floyd & Gloria St John (1998). *From Doctor to Healer: The Transformative Journey*, p. 158-159. New Brunswick, NJ: Rutgers University Press.
94. Ake Hultkrantz (1978). 'Ecological and Phenomenological Aspects of Shamanism. In Shamanism in Siberia, edited by B Dioszegi & M Hoppal, p. 50. Budapest, Hungary: Akademiai Kiado.
95. Op cit. Halifax (1982), p 16.
96. Mircea Eliade (1964). Shamanism: Archaic Techniques of Ecstasy. Translated by W. Trask. Princeton, NJ: Princeton University Press.
97. A P Elkin (he preferred to be called 'AP.') (1977). *Aboriginal Men of High Degree*. 2nd Edition. (1st edition 1945). Brisbane: University of Queensland Press.
98. Ruth-Inge Heinze (ed). (1991). *Shamans of the 20th Century.* New York: Irvington Publishers Inc.
99. Joan Halifax (1979). *Shamanic Voices: A Survey of Visionary Narratives.* New York: EP Dutton.
100. Piers Vitebsky (2000). *Shamanism. In Indigenous Religions*, edited by G Harvey. London: Cassell.
101. Stanley Krippner (1991). Foreword. In *Shamans of the 20th Century,* edited by R-I Heinze. New York: Irvington Publishers Inc.
102. Brad Huber (1990). 'The Recruitment of Nahua Curers: Role Conflict and Gender'. Ethnology 29:159–176.
103. Ioan Lewis (1989) (1971). *Ecstatic Religion: An Anthropological Study of Spirit Possession and Shamanism.* 2nd ed. Baltimore: Penguin Books.
104. Op cit. Halifax (1982).
105. .Op cit. Halifax (1979).
106. Janice Reid (1983). Sorcerers and Healing Spirits. Canberra: Australian National University Press.
107. Arthur Kleinman (1980). Patients and Healers in the Context of Culture. Berkley: University of California Press.
108. Op cit. Elkin.
109. Op cit. Eliade (1964).
110. Ibid, p xii.
111. Laurel Kendall (1989). Old Ghosts and Ungrateful Children: A Korean Shaman's Story. In Women as Healers, edited by CS McClain, P.139. New Brunswick: Rutgers University Press.
112. Koichi Naka, Seijun Toguchi, Toshihiro Takaishi, Hiroshi Ishizu & Yuji Sasaki (1985). Yuta (shaman) and community mental health on Okinawa. International Journal of Social Psychiatry 31 (4):267-74, p 267–268.
113. Op cit. Elkin, p 58–59.
114. Op cit. (Lewis 1989, p 37).
115. Kahil Gibran (1980) (1926). The Prophet, p 36. London: Heinemann.
116. David Brandon (1999). Wounded healers. Nursing Standard 13(28):17; quiz 18, p 199.
117. Brandon, quoting Holger Kalweit (1992). *Shamans, Healers and Medicine Men*. Boston: Shambala.
118. Op cit. Krieger (1987).
119. Jane Hall (1996). 'Challenges to Caring: Nurses as Wounded Healers'. Australian Journal of Holistic Nursing 3 (2):12–18, p 14–15.

120. Op cit. Hall (1996).

121. Jane Hall (1997). 'Nurses as Wounded Healers: The Journey to Healing the Person and Profession'. *Australian Journal of Holistic Nursing* 4 (1):11–16.

122. Op cit. Hall (1997), p 15.

123. Ibid.

124. Bonnie Horrigan (1998). 'Conversations: Dolores Krieger, RN, PhD; Healing with Therapeutic Touch'. *Alternative Therapies in Health and Medicine* 4 (1):86–92, p 88.

125. Liz Scarfe (2015). *Pointing at the Moon Exploring the Question: What is Psychological Freedom?* A thesis submitted in partial fulfilment of the requirements for the Diploma in Process Work. ANZPOP, p 112.

126. Op cit. Keegan & Dossey (1998), p 65.

127. Joan Halifax, quoted in Michelle Jamal (1987). *Shape Shifters: Shaman Women in Contemporary Society*. New York: Arkana, p 18.

128. Viking Rune — Jera. Op cit. Blum, p 81.

129. Op cit. James Hillman & Michael Ventura, p 123–124.

130. Arny Mindell (2000). *Dreaming While Awake: Techniques for 24-Hour Lucid Dreaming*. Kindle Edition (Kindle Locations 75–77).

131. Op cit. Eliade (1964).

132. Hans-Georg Gadamer (1975). Truth and Method. Translated by Joel Weinsheimer & Donald G Marshall. Second, Revised ed. London: Sheed & Ward.

133. Arny Mindell, quoted in Kate Jobe (1994) An Interview with Arny Mindell on Extreme States. The Journal of Process Oriented Psychology. 6 (1) pp 7–10, p 9.

134. Rumi, excerpt from Childhood Friends http://andylal.blogspot. com/2011/04/childhood-friends-by-rumi.html (Accessed 6 January 2019).

135. Arny Mindell (1993). *The Shaman's Body: A New Shamanism for Transforming Health, Relationships and The Community*. New York. HarperCollins Publishers, p 19.

136. See, for example, op cit. Mindell (1993) and Salome Schwartz (2006) Shifting the Assemblage Point: Transformation in Therapy and Everyday Life. PhD Thesis. The Union Institute: Cincinnati, Ohio.

137. Jean Watson (2002). 'Intentionality and Caring-Healing Consciousness: A Theory of Transpersonal Nursing'. Holistic Nursing Practice 16 (4):12–19

138. Op cit. Benner.

139. Beverley Taylor (1994). *Being Human: Ordinariness in Nursing*. Melbourne: Churchill Livingstone.

140. Op cit. Hemsley (2003).

141. Op cit. Mindell (1993), p 186.

142. Op cit. Scarfe, p 108.

143. Arnold Mindell (1988). *City Shadows: Psychological Interventions in Psychiatry*. New York: Routledge, p 173.

144. Ibid, p 176.

145. Daryl Sharp (1991). Jung Lexicon: A Primer of Terms & Concepts. Accessed on 17/11/2018 from https://www.psychceu.com/jung/sharplexicon.html.

146. Alan Bullock & Oliver Stallybrass (eds). (1977). *The Fontana Dictionary of Modern Thought*. Sixth Impression ed. London: Fontana, p 54.

147. Op cit. Mindell (1988), p 174.

148. John Bradshaw (1990). *Homecoming: Reclaiming and Championing Your Inner Child*.

New York: Bantam.

149. Op cit. Brennan (1988).

150. Op cit. Schwarz, p 29.

151. Arny Mindell (2010a). *Process Mind: A User's Guide to Connecting with the Mind of God*. Wheaton, Ill.: Quest Books.

152. IAPOP: International Association of Process Oriented Psychology. (2018). Glossary. Accessed on 28/11/2018 at: http://wwwiapop. com/glossary/.

153. Ibid.

154. For example, see Op cit. Bradshaw; Stanislav and Christina Grof (1989). *Spiritual Emergency: When Personal Transformation Becomes a Crisis.* New York: Putnam.

155. EMDR International Association. Accessed on 19/8/2019 at: https:// www.emdria.org/page/what_is_emdr_therapy.

156. Op cit. Brennan (1988).

157. Op cit. Rogers.

158. Op cit. van Manen.

159. The Encyclopedia Britannica Online. Accessed online on7/12/2003 at: http://www. britannica.com/eb/article?eu=47504&tocid=0&query=kundalini&ct=.

160. Op cit. Grof & Grof.

161. Op cit. Amy Mindell (1995).

162. Op cit. Mindell (2010a), p 274.

163. Op cit. Mindell (1988), p 178.

164. Op cit. Zweig & Abrams.

165. Op cit. Bullock & Stallybrass, p 618.

166. Op cit. Brennan (1988).

167. Dolores Krieger (1993). *Accepting Your Power to Heal: The Personal Practice of Therapeutic Touch*. Santa Fe, New Mexico: Bear & Co